MEDICAL
MEANINGS

MEDICAL MEANINGS

A Glossary of Word Origins

William S. Haubrich, MD, FACP

American College of Physicians
Philadelphia, Pennsylvania

A|C|P

Manager, Books Program: David Myers
Acquisitions Editor: Mary K. Ruff
Production Supervisor: Allan S. Kleinberg
Production Editor: Amy L. Cannon
Interior and Cover Designer: Larry DiDona

Printed in the United States of America.

Composition by Techsetters, Inc., Cherry Hill, New Jersey
Printing/binding by R. R. Donnelly, Glasgow, Kentucky

Library of Congress Cataloging-in-Publication Data

Haubrich, William S.
   Medical meanings : a glossary of word origins / William S.
Haubrich. — Rev. & expanded ed.
     p.   cm.
   ISBN 0-943126-56-8 (alk. paper)
    1. Medicine—Terminology.   2. English language—Etymology—Dictionaries.   I. Title.
   [DNLM: 1. Dictionaries, Medical.   2. Nomenclature.   W 15 H368m 1997]
   R123.H29   1997
   610'. 1'4—dc21   96-29494
   DNLM/DLC   CIP
   for Library of Congress

Also Available from the American College of Physicians

On Being a Doctor
This Is Our Work
Who Has Seen a Blood Sugar? Reflections on Medical Education

Publications from the BMJ Publishing Group are available to members through the American College of Physicians.

Our *Resources for Internists* catalog and ordering information for the American College of Physicians and BMJ Publishing Group are available from

Customer Service Center
American College of Physicians
Independence Mall West
Sixth Street at Race
Philadelphia, PA 19106-1572
215-351-2600
800-523-1546, ext. 2600

5 4 3 2 1

*Dedicated to
the curiosity of all students
of medicine,
young and old*

ACKNOWLEDGMENTS

Frequently in this work I note my debt to Professor Henry Alan Skinner (1899–1967) and his seminal book *The Origin of Medical Terms*, published by Williams & Wilkins in 1949 and followed by a second edition in 1961. Professor Skinner's book, preeminent among former glossaries of medical etymology, unfortunately is no longer in print. With *Medical Meanings*, first published by Harcourt Brace Jovanovich in 1984, I hope to fill this gap in medical source material, covering somewhat different ground in a currently relevant way. In this new edition I update meanings of terms, describe new words, and freely explore origins tangential to those more commonly associated with the terms. However, I do owe much to the scholarship of my worthy predecessor.

Anyone seeking to learn about biomedical words must have access to various sources. A shelfful of dictionaries, in English and other languages, comes in handy. *The Oxford English Dictionary* will be the most frequently thumbed. *Dorland's Illustrated Medical Dictionary*, now in its 28th Edition, is in my opinion the most authoritative source of precise definitions. For background information, Skeat's *Etymological Dictionary of the English Language*, *Brewer's Dictionary of Phrase and Fable*, *Bulfinch's Mythology*, Partridge's *A Short Etymological Dictionary of Modern English*, and the *Oxford Dictionary of English Etymology* are indispensable.

A fascination with words, how they came to be and how they are used, is not a genetically determined trait; it must be instilled. I am mindful that my early interest was prompted by exacting schoolteachers and by my preceptors at Franklin and Marshall College, particularly Dr. James M. Darlington in biology and Dr. W. Nelson Francis in English. My professor of pathology at Western Reserve University, the late Howard T. Karsner, was a demanding, erudite, and inspiring taskmaster when it came to precise description of disease.

I must mention, too, the help given by my medical and professional colleagues, at home and abroad, who advised me on words peculiar to their special fields. Howard Sandrum of New York, a perceptive editor, initially urged me to systematize my notes collected over a number of years, then shepherded production of the original edition of this book. Opportunity to bring out the currently revised and expanded edition has been generously afforded by Mary K. Ruff, acquisitions editor in the publishing division of the American College of Physicians.

Finally, I am mindful of my gratitude to my wife Eila for her encouragement and forbearance.

William S. Haubrich, MD, FACP

INTRODUCTION

When that prodigious 18th century savant Samuel Johnson compiled his monumental *Dictionary of the English Language,* he archly defined a lexicographer as "a harmless drudge." Whether one who compiles a medical etymology merits flattery as a lexicographer is arguable, but I can honestly say I have meant no harm in putting together this book, and at no time have I thought of the task as drudgery. Rather, the work has been fun and illuminating. I hope the reader, too, will be entertained as well as enlightened by the work.

A Word of Caution

Although the title of this book is *Medical Meanings,* and comment is offered on the past and present usage of biomedical terms, I emphasize the provenance or origin of these terms rather than their precise definitions. Accepted definitions can be found in standard medical dictionaries. Moreover, the etymology of a word should never be confused with its current definition. Indeed, it comes as a surprise, in some instances, that the ancient origin of a word and its current usage closely coincide, considering the centuries that have elapsed since the word was coined.

An example is the Greek *amnēsia,* which to the ancients meant "forgetfulness." Now, the English word "amnesia," borrowed directly from the classical Greek, means a lapse of memory. Moreover, both the Greek *amnēstia,* "oblivion," and its English derivative "amnesty" can convey a sense of "forgive and forget."

In contrast, "artery" is known to us as a term for a vessel serving to transport blood away from the heart. But its Greek predecessor was derived from a combination of *aēr-,* "air," + *tērēo,* "I carry," and to the Greeks *arteria* was "windpipe" or "trachea." The explanation for the misapplication of "artery" to a particular type of blood vessel is that early anatomists conducting postmortem dissections usually found thick-walled vessels empty and, lacking knowledge of the circulation of blood, mistakenly assumed they were conduits of air. It goes without saying that no one would contend that artery really means an air duct simply because of its origin.

Also, there is such as thing as folk etymology. This is a mistaken attribution, seemingly logical but false nonetheless. "Tip," a word commonly used for a gratuity given to one who performs a personal service, is sometimes said to have been derived as an acronym for the phrase "to insure promptness." Sound reasonable? Well, not really. A tip customarily follows, it does not precede, the service rendered. It is more a reward than a stimulus. The truth is that the real origin of "tip" is not known, which is often the case when folk etymology has been contrived. The *Oxford English Dictionary* suggests that "tip" may have survived from rogues' cant, or it may have come from the use of the word in the sense of touching lightly. But "to insure promptness" it is not (and does not).

How to Use This Book

This volume is not intended to be read from cover-to-cover, front-to-back, although a few brave souls may try. It is intended for reference, to help answer the question, "Now where did *that* word come from?"

Individual words as well as important combining forms appear alphabetically as main entries. Many explanations include additional terms that relate directly, indirectly, or incidentally to the main entry.

Additional and incidental words also are listed alphabetically; the suggestion (*see ...*) occasionally is offered as a guide to the principal entry or to an entry that further explains the word. Some categories of words, such as colors, numbers, and phobias, are grouped together, according to their particular category.

How Words Appear

Within the explanation of some entries, derivations and words for which an explanation are given are printed in **boldface** type. Words from languages other than current English, particularly classic or foreign words from which English words are derived, are printed in *italic* type.

Greek words, which figure prominently in etymology, are composed of letters originating in the Greek alphabet: alpha, beta, gamma, delta, and so on, for a total of 24. ("Alphabet" is a slightly contracted combination of the first two letters, as if we referred to our set of letters as "ABs.") To be quite proper, Greek words should be printed in Greek letters: α, β, γ, Δ, and so on. Purists would insist. But for most of us, Greek letters are difficult to recognize at a glance, and most lend themselves to a fairly easy transliteration. So, Greek words in this book are printed in letters corresponding to the more familiar Roman alphabet:

A, α	alpha	= a
B, β	beta	= b
Γ, γ	gamma	= g
Δ, δ	delta	= d
E, ε	epsilon	= e
Z, ζ	zeta	= z
H, η	eta	= ē
Θ, θ	theta	= th

I, ι	iota	= i
K, κ	kappa	= k
Λ, λ	lambda	= l
M, μ	mu	= m
N, ν	nu	= n
Ξ, ξ	xi	= x or z (both pronounced as "z")
O, o	omicron	= o
Π, π	pi	= p
P, ρ	rho	= r or rh
Σ, σ ς	sigma	= s
T, τ	tau	= t
Y, υ	upsilon	= y or u
Φ, φ	phi	= ph (pronounced as "f")
X, χ	chi	= kh (pronounced as "k")
Ψ, ψ	psi	= ps
Ω, ω	omega	= ō

Note that there are two distinct Greek letters equivalent to the Roman "e" and two distinct Greek letters equivalent to the Roman "o." These have been distinguished in the text by using a macron (a horizontal line over the letter) for the second of the two vowels in each instance. Thus, the Greek "ε" (epsilon) is presented as "e," and the Greek "η" (eta) is represented as "ē," the Greek "o" (omicron) is represented as "o," and the Greek "ω" (omega) is represented as "ō." The Greek "γ" (gamma) becomes an "n" when it precedes another gamma, a kappa, a xi, or a chi. When this is necessary to understanding a connection between the Greek word and the derived word, the substituted "n" has been inserted as [n].

How to Improve This Book

Although the publisher has provided highly expert and much appreciated editorial help in readying my typescript for the press, there may still be pockets of controversy here and there. The publishers and editorial consultants have joined me in trying to ensure accuracy, but where errors remain, the responsibility is ultimately mine. My response to whomever might call such an error to my attention likely will be the same as that of Samuel Johnson when a knowledgeable reader discovered an error in his *Dictionary* and remonstrated, "Tell me, Dr. Johnson, how could you have made such a mistake?" His reply: "Ignorance, madam, pure ignorance."

Readers who wish to dispute points that are made in this book or who can suggest additions or amendments (or perhaps deletions) are invited to write to me forthwith. Your advice will be welcomed and most kindly considered.

William S. Haubrich, MD, FACP
The Scripps Clinic and Research Foundation
10666 North Torrey Pines Road
La Jolla, CA 92037

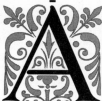**ā** is an abbreviation used in writing pre-scriptions and means "of each." These letters instruct the pharmacist to use equal parts of the several ingredients listed. The use of "āā" is more of a disguise than a time-saver. It stands for the Greek *ana*, a preposition meaning "up, again, or throughout." This is not the same *-ana* that is derived from the Latin suffixes *-anus, -ana, -anum* meaning "of or belonging to" and used to indicate a collection of items or observations as in, for example, "Americana."

A-1 (*see* **under the weather**)

abdomen is the Latin word for "belly" and is related to the Latin verb *abdodere*, "to hide," the implication being that whatever is ingested is hidden or tucked away in the abdomen. The Latin *abdomen* also was used figuratively to mean gluttony. Although for us "abdomen" encompasses all structures between the diaphragm and the pelvis, the ancients probably used the term in a more restrictive sense to refer to the ventral or belly wall. **Belly**, incidentally, comes from the Anglo-Saxon word meaning "bag or sack." This is yet another instance in which the Anglo-Saxon term has become somewhat vulgar whereas the Latin is considered more delicate. The patient says, "I got kicked in the belly!" whereas the doctor says, "This man sustained a nonpenetrating injury to the abdomen." Both describe the same event, but the patient's account is more vivid.

abduct comes from the Latin *abducere* (*ab-*, "from" + *ducere*, "to draw or to lead"), hence "to draw away from." An abductor muscle is one that draws a part away from the body. The **abducens**, or sixth, cranial nerve is so called because it supplies the lateral rectus muscle that "draws away" the eyeball toward the side of the head.

abhor is not really a medical term, yet it has a physiologic significance. It comes from the Latin *abhorrere*, "to shrink back, as with aversion." This, in turn, is a combination of *ab-*, "away from," + *horrere*, which as an intransitive verb means "to stand on end, to get gooseflesh." When one is confronted with horror, one may experience a sympathetic nervous response; one's hair may stand on end. Although originally "abhor" meant a reaction to horror, it now signifies a lesser repugnance.

ablation is from the Latin *ablatum*, the past participle of *aufere*, "to carry away," and represents a combination of *ab-*, "from, away," + *latum*, the past participle of *ferre*, "to carry or bear." The French *ablation* means "a removal or excision." In surgery, to ablate is to remove, especially by cutting away.

ablatio placentae refers to a detachment, or "carrying away," of the placenta. When this occurs because of a precipitous tear, it is an **abruptio placentae** (from the Latin *abrumpere*, "to sever").

abnormal (*see* **normal**)

abortus is the Latin word for miscarriage. The Latin verb *aboriri* means "to miscarry or fail," particularly in the sense of not completing a full course. This, in turn, is a combination of *ab-*, "away, from," + *oriri*, "to descend from or to be born."

abrasion comes from the Latin *abradere, abrasum*, "to scrape off, to shave." The Indo-European root is postulated to have been *rēd, rōd*, "to scratch." This is presumably related to the Latin verb *radere*, "to scrape," of which the past participle is *rasum*. From this come such familiar words as "rash" and "razor." The advertisement that warns of "razor rash" unwittingly combines two words of common origin. A rasher of bacon is a thin slice. Medically, an abrasion is an area of skin or other surface where the covering membrane has been scraped off.

abruptio placentae (*see* **ablatio placentae**)

abscess might be thought to come from the Latin *abscedere*, "to depart or go away." Not really. Rather, it began with the Greek *apostēma*, "a throwing off or drawing off," as of "bad humors." The Greek *apostēma* was then rendered as the Latin *abscessus*, both terms referring to a suppurative collection anywhere in the body.

absorb comes from the Latin *absorbere*, "to devour." This, in turn, is a combination of *ab-*, "away or from," + *sorbere*, "to suck, swallow, or gulp." This keeps with the sense of a process whereby, for example, the intestinal epithelial cells take nutritive fluids into their own substance. "Absorb" and its congeners have a puzzling resemblance, perhaps accidental, to the Arabic *sharaba*, "to drink," from which our word "sherbet" is derived. **Adsorb**, on the other hand, means to attract and retain other material on the surface without altering the nature of the recipient. An example would be mopping with a sponge that can be then wrung out. The difference is a fine one, but the distinction is there.

a.c. are the initials representing *ante cibum*, Latin for "before a meal." When written in a prescription, this is a convenient shorthand way of directing that a medication is to be taken before eating. The initials **p.c.** represent the Latin *post cibum*, "after a meal."

academe as the term for the scholarly environment of a college or university comes from the name of a Greek farmer. In Greek mythology the story is told that Helen of Sparta was kidnapped by Theseus, hero of Attica. Helen's twin brothers, Castor and Pollux, searched in vain until they learned from a farmer, Akademus (whose name means "on the side of the people"), where they might find their sister. As a reward, the gods gave a special blessing to the grove tended by Akademus. The grove, bearing the farmer's name, became a park situated north of ancient Athens. It was to this park that Plato retired with his students. Hence, an academy is now an association of scholars, young or old, who share a similar cultural or professional pursuit.

acanthosis comes from the Greek *akantha*, "thorn," and refers to any thorny, spiny, or prickly surface. **Acanthosis nigricans** is a black roughening of the skin, usually in the axilla or other skin folds, which, in some cases, may be a harbinger of visceral cancer.

acapnia is derived from the Greek *a-*, "without,"

+ *kapnos*, "smoke." The word was devised not to mean "smokeless" but as a reference to diminished carbon dioxide in the blood. Insofar as carbon dioxide is a major component of the common smoke produced by combustion of carbon-containing fuels, and recognizing the lack of a classical term for carbon dioxide, the contrivance makes sense. **Hypercapnia** is an excess of carbon dioxode in the blood.

accessory as the name for the 11th cranial nerve was given because it receives an additional or accessory root from the upper part of the spinal cord. "Accessory" comes from the Latin *accessio*, "an approach."

accident comes from the Latin *accidere*, "to happen, occur, or befall." The root verb is *cadere*, "to fall." This implies, in a remote sense, that unlikely happenings result from a "falling out" of the heavenly bodies. Ancient writers used the term *accidentia* to mean symptoms, the implication being that such were unexpected and extraordinary departures from a state of health.

accommodation comes from the Latin *accommodare*, "to adjust or adapt," and fits nicely with the ophthalmic reference to adjustment of the eyes, particularly of the lenses by constriction of the ciliary fibers to varying visual distances.

accoucheur is the French word for a male obstetrician and was first used in the 17th century. An *accoucheuse* could be either a female obstetrician or a midwife. The word literally means "one who attends at a couch or bed," the couch, of course, being the bed of confinement for labor. The word would be of only passing interest to English-speaking physicians were it not for the term "accoucheur hand," used to describe the posture of the hand in tetany wherein the metacarpophalangeal joints are flexed and the fingers extended. Presumably, the allusion is to the manner in which an obstetrician holds his hand when delivering a baby.

acetabulum is the name of the cup-shaped cavity on the lateral surface of the hip bone in which the rounded head of the femur articulates. "Acetabulum" is a direct borrowing of the Latin word for a vinegar cup or cruet and is related to the term **acetate**.

acetate is derived from the Latin *acetum*, "sour

wine." In French this is *vin aigre* (*aigre* being the French word for "sour or bitter"). By only a slight change in spelling and pronunciation, this becomes our word "vinegar." The acid in vinegar, called acetic acid, was the earliest known and, until the late 18th century, was thought to be the only organic acid. An acetate is any salt of acetic acid. **Acetone** was concocted from the Latin root *acet-* and the Greek ending *-ōne*, denoting a female descendent or a weaker derivative. One might conclude that acetone was first thought to be a "weak sister" of acetic acid. (*see* **ketones**)

achalasia is a combination of the Greek *a-*, designating "absence or failure," + *chalasis*, "relaxation," and we use the word in its literal sense, "a failure of relaxation." The condition known as achalasia is most commonly found in the esophagus, where it is specifically a failure in relaxation of the lower esophageal sphincter muscle as distinguished from diffuse esophageal spasm. There is a nice distinction between achalasia and spasm, the difference being immediately clear to one who knows the derivation of "achalasia."

ache has, curiously, two origins, one for the verb and another for the noun. The verb "to ache" comes from the Anglo-Saxon *acun* and should be spelled "ake." For the derived noun, however, the "k" becomes "ch," as in "to speak" and "speech" or "to bake" and "batch." The *Oxford English Dictionary* blames Samuel Johnson for confusing the origin of the verb "ake" with the Greek noun *achos* meaning "pain or distress." The esteemed lexicographer decreed that henceforth the verb should be spelled with "ch." All of this is an etymologic tempest in an epistemologic teapot. Aching is miserable no matter how it is spelled. The exclamation "Ouch!" or the German "*Ach!*" may be distantly related to the Greek *achos*.

Achilles tendon is the common and fanciful name given to the structure more properly designated as the tendo calcaneus, that tough sinew at the back of the heel by which the triceps surae muscle is attached to the tuberosity of the calcaneus or heel bone. The common name refers to the Greek legend that tells of the babe Achilles being dipped in the River Styx by his mother Thetis. The immersion was intended to make the boy invulnerable. The mother naturally had to keep a grasp on the dangling infant, so she held fast to his heels. Alas, this small, unimmersed, hence vulnerable, area was, years later, the target for Paris' well aimed arrow. Thus was felled the hero Achilles. Ever since, any small and unobtrusive point at which an otherwise stalwart person might be subject to attack has been known as his or her "Achilles heel."

achondroplasia is a cause of dwarfism wherein long bones fail to grow as a consequence of an epiphyseal defect. The word is derived from the Greek *a-*, "absence," + *chondros*, "cartilage," + *plassein*, "to form."

achromatic applied to an optical lens means it is free of the disturbing aura of colors that tends to distort microscopic or telescopic images. The construction of such lenses was achieved as early as the 18th century by combining elements of flint and crown glass. The word combines the Greek *a-*, "absence of," + *chroma*, "color."

acid comes from the Latin adjective *acidus*, meaning "sour, tart," that doubtless was used to describe the taste of acidic substances. *Acidus*, in turn, may have come from the Greek *akidos*, meaning "pointed or sharp."

acid test can mean a test for acid, but in common parlance an acid test refers to any critical or decisive examination. The expression comes from the old method of testing for gold: nitric acid was poured on the substance in question. Iron pyrite, called "fool's gold," would promptly dissolve. True gold, being a "noble metal," would remain inert and thus would pass the "acid test."

acinus is a Latin word for a berry. A round cluster of epithelial cells known as an acinus, as in the salivary glands or pancreas, does closely resemble a knobby berry.

acne is of uncertain origin. According to Professor H. A. Skinner, Hippocrates used the Greek word *achnē* in the sense of "lint" to describe scaly lesions. Also, it has been considered a corruption of the Greek word *akmē*, meaning "the highest or critical point," the allusion presumably being to that stage in life when acne typically occurs. But this would seem a highly contrived derivation. "Acne" often is accompanied by a modifying term, the most common being **acne**

vulgaris, which is just that, the Latin *vulgaris* meaning "common or usual." **Acne hordeolaris** describes hard, knobby, skin lesions that occur in rows. *Hordeolum* is Latin for "barley-corn."

acoustic comes from the Greek *akoustikos*, "pertaining to hearing," the root verb being *akouein*, "to hear." Thus, the acoustic or eighth cranial nerve is the "hearing nerve."

acrodynia comes from the Greek *akron*, in the sense of "the end or extremity," + *odynē*, "pain," and is literally a pain in an extremity, usually the foot or hand.

acromegaly is a pituitary disorder that leads to enlargement of the nose, jaw, hands, and feet. The term was introduced in 1886 by the French clinician Pierre Marie (1853-1940), aptly chosen from the Greek *akron*, "extremity," + *megas*, "large."

acromion is the highest point of the shoulder, named from the Greek *akron*, in the sense of "peak," + *ōmos*, "shoulder." Anatomically, the acromion is the protruding lateral process of the spine of the scapula.

actinic is from the Greek *aktis*, "ray," and refers to the ultraviolet rays, as in sunlight, that can cause reaction in skin; sunburn is an actinic burn. An **actinic keratosis** (from the Greek *keras*, "horn") is a focal, scaly excrescence on the scalp, face, neck, or other exposed surface of skin resulting, at least in part, from long exposure to the ultraviolet rays of the sun. Similarly, certain types of skin cancer can be described as actinic in origin.

actinomycosis is an infection by the "ray fungus," the common name for the genus *Actinomyces*. The suffix *-myces* comes from the Greek *mykēs*, "fungus." **Actinomyces** is descriptive of organisms that grow as yellow granules made up of **mycelia** (again, *myk-* + *ēlos*, Greek for "ornamental nail"), typically in a radiate array. The "ray fungus" in German is *der Strahlenpilz*, which translates exactly the same.

acumen describes a talent for penetrating analysis and diagnosis. The same Latin word means "sharpness, shrewdness, ingenuity." It is a derivative of the Latin verb *acuere*, "to make sharp or pointed."

acupuncture combines the Latin *acus*, "needle," + *punctum*, "a prick or puncture."

The procedure of acupuncture could easily be called by the simple Anglo-Saxon "needle-stick," but as such it probably would lose much of whatever efficacy it is purported to have. Acupuncture is not new to the Western scene, having been first introduced to European practice in the late 17th century by a Dutch surgeon.

acute is from the Latin adjective *acutus*, meaning "sharp or pointed." There is an ancient precedent for the use of the term in the medical sense of "severe for a short period." To be acute, symptoms or illnesses must be both intense and brief. Also, the onset is typically abrupt. A **subacute** condition is "less than acute," meaning less abrupt, less intense, and somewhat more prolonged. It might just as well be "subchronic," but such a term is not used.

adamantinoma is from the Greek *adamas*, "untamed," + *-ōma*, "tumor." *Adamas* is used here in the sense of being unyielding or unmalleable, hence "hard." *Adamas dentis* is an old term for the enamel of teeth. An adamantinoma is a hard tumor of the jaw, more specifically an **ameloblastoma** (*amel* being an obsolete word for enamel), a neoplasm of the primordial cells that produce dental enamel. Incidentally, "diamond," the name of the hardest of gems, and "adamant," meaning stubborn, are both derived from *adamas*.

Adam's apple is the anterior protuberance of the thyroid cartilage, usually seen in men, and so called, according to *Brewer's Dictionary of Phrase and Fable*, from the superstition that a piece of forbidden fruit that Adam ate stuck in his throat and occasioned the swelling. There is no mention in the biblical account that the fruit was, in fact, an apple. Professor Alexander Gode points out (*JAMA*. 1968;206:1058) that the Latin term *pomum Adami*, "Adam's apple," is really an early mistranslation of the Hebrew *tappūach ha ādām*, "male bump." Whoever made the mistake might be excused on the grounds that a single Hebrew word means both "bump" and "apple" and that the Hebrew word for "man" came to be the proper name "Adam."

addleheaded is a quaint term for a person who is confused or muddled. "Addle" comes from the Middle English *adel*, which meant "urine." At that time it was believed that liquid excrement was the result of internal decomposition. An "adel egg" was a rotten egg. Muddled or confused thinking was thought to be a sign of something rotten in the brain, hence "addleheaded" or "addlepated."

adduct is from the Latin *ad-*, "toward," + *ducere*, "to draw or lead." Hence, an adductor muscle draws toward a point of reference, usually the axis of the body.

adeno- is a frequently used prefix and represents the Greek *adēn*, originally "an acorn" and later "a gland" in the shape of an acorn. **Adenitis**, then, is an inflammation of a gland, and **adenoid** means "like a gland," whereas **adenoma** is a benign tumor wherein the glandular elements closely resemble their normal counterparts. (*see* **gland**)

adiadochokinesia is a highly contrived word and a dandy to dissect for its origin. It is composed of the Greek *a-*, "without," + *diadochos*, "successive," + *kinēsis*, "motion." So, adiadochokinesia (or adiadochokinesis) is a neurologic sign of inability to perform rapid alternating movements, such as pronation and supination of the hands.

adipose is derived from the Latin *adeps*, "fat, particularly lard." The distinction between "adipose" and "obese" is a nice one. "Adipose" usually is used to refer to tissue laden with fat; **obese** (from the Latin *obesus*, "whatever has eaten itself fat," the root verb being *obedere*, "to eat away") is used to refer to the person or animal so burdened. **Adiposa dolorosa** (from the Latin *dolor*, "pain or grief") is a rare condition marked by painful, fatty swellings, typically in menopausal women.

adjuvant as a noun designates any substance, particularly a vehicle, that enhances the efficacy of a primary agent. The best known is Freund adjuvant (named for Jules Freund [1890-1960], a Hungarian-born bacteriologist working in the United States), an emulsion of mineral oil used as a vehicle for injected antigens, thus increasing the stimulus to immunity. As an adjective "adjuvant" is used in medicine to describe especially chemotherapy or radiotherapy invoked as a supplement to another mode of cancer treatment, usually surgery. Adjuvant therapy can be applied before or after operation. In both cases, the word is a near borrowing of the Latin *adjuvans*, *adjuvant* (the present participle of *adjuvare*, "to help"), especially in the sense of attaining a goal.

adolescence (*see* **adulterate**)

adrenal is the name for the small endocrine glands that sit atop the kidneys, so called from the Latin *ad-*, "toward," + *renes*, "kidneys." Occasionally, they are referred to as the suprarenal glands, from the Latin *supra*, "on top." **Adrenalin** is a registered trademark held by the Parke-Davis Company for **epinephrine** (here the Greek *epi-*, "on top of," + *nephros*, "the kidney"), the potent vasopressor hormone elaborated by the adrenal medulla. The pressor effect of extracts from the adrenal gland was demonstrated by G. Oliver and E. A. Schäfer in 1895 and reported in the *London Journal of Physiology*. John J. Abel, a professor at Johns Hopkins University, and Jokichi Takamine, a consultant to Parke-Davis, independently and simultaneously isolated the active pressor principle from the medullary portion of the adrenal gland. It was Professor Abel who conferred on this substance the name "epinephrine" in 1899. The name "Adrenalin" was given by Dr. Takamine in 1901. We can also be grateful to him as the donor of the celebrated Japanese cherry trees that adorn the boulevards of Washington, D.C.

adroit is from the French phrase (*à droit*, "rightly," and has come to mean skillful or nimble. Conversely, the French word *gauche*, "left," has been taken into English to mean awkward or lacking in grace. The common adjective "gawky" might be thought to come from *gauche* (and "gawk-handed" was an old way of saying "left-handed"), but it more likely came from the Old Norse *gaukr*, "a cuckoo." To gawk is to stare stupidly. The Latin *dexter*, "right," is the origin of the English "dexterity," meaning skill or agility, whereas the Latin *sinister*, "left," has been taken directly into English to mean ominous or portending evil. The allusion, obviously, is that most people are more facile with the right hand than with the left hand. To those good and graceful folk who happen to be left-handed, this is a prime example of the tyranny of the majority. "Lefties" are consoled by knowing the right side of the brain controls the left side of the body and, therefore, only those who are left-handed are in their right minds.

adsorb (*see* **absorb**)

adulterate shares the same Latin root as "adultery." The root verb is *adulterare*, "to defile or corrupt," from *ad-*, "to," + *alter*, "other." A substance that has been adversely changed by the admixture of a "corrupting" addition is said to be adulterated. Although adultery is usually perpetrated by adults, the two words "adult" and "adultery" are quite unrelated in origin. "Adult" is from the Latin *adultus*, "one who has grown up," the past participle of *adolescere*, "to grow up." This is also the source of our word for the period of growing up, **adolescence**.

adventitia is derived from the Latin adjective *adventicius*, meaning "foreign, strange, or extraneous." The connective tissue surrounding an artery is called the "adventitia" because it is looked upon as extraneous to the principal structure itself. At **auscultation**, adventitious sounds are those not normally heard to emanate from the healthy chest or abdomen.

aerobe is a combination of the Greek *aēr*, "air," + *bios*, "life," and describes organisms dependent on free air or oxygen to live. **Anaerobe** describes a microorganism that flourishes and, indeed, lives only in the absence of oxygen. The Greek prefix *a-* or *an-*, "without," confers a negative sense to whatever follows. The terms "aerobe" and "anaerobe" were conceived in 1863 by Louis Pasteur (1822-1895), the famed French chemist and bacteriologist. In recent times, the adjective "aerobic" has been applied to certain forms of exercise, usually strenuous, that are conceived to improve the body's utilization of oxygen.

aerophagia combines the Greek *aēr*, "air," + *phagein*, "to swallow," to aptly describe an aberrant intake of air conducive not to health but rather to belching, bloating, and flatulence.

Aesculapius is the Latin form of Asklēpios, the name of the legendary Greek god of medicine, and Aesculapians are his followers. The mythical Asklēpios was the son of Apollo and the nymph Coronis. His wife was Epiome, and celebrated issue came from this union, including Panaceia, goddess of healing; Hygieia, goddess of health; and the Homeric heroes Machaon, a surgeon of Peloponnesus, and Podaleiros, a physician of Asia Minor, both of whom are mentioned in the *Iliad*. Myths aside, there may have been an actual person known by the name Asklēpios who was celebrated for his gentle and humane remedies, such as the treatment of fevers by fasting. His disciples established temples throughout the Greek world, the most famous being at Kos, Knidos, Epidaurus, and Pergamum. The modern medical fraternity known by the Greek initials Alpha Kappa Kappa takes its name from "Aesculapians of *Kos* and *Knidos*."

afferent comes from the Latin *ad*, "toward," + *ferre*, "to carry." Afferent nerves carry impulses toward the central nervous system; an afferent limb of the gut carries its contents toward an anastomosis. **Efferent** is the opposite (*e-* or *ex-*, "away or out").

agar is a Malay word and in its native haunts is usually doubly sounded, as agar-agar. The substance was originally prepared from seaweed and was found to form a mucilaginous jelly when mixed with water, heated, then allowed to cool. It is a basic ingredient of many bacterial culture media, hence the reference to "agar plates." Agar also has been used to support emulsions and as a bulk laxative. Its use in the bacteriology laboratory is said to have been suggested by the wife of Walter Hesse, one of Robert Koch's (1843-1910) early associates. Frau Hesse had obtained samples of agar-agar from Dutch friends in Batavia.

ageusia (*see* **geusia**)

agglutination is from the Latin *ad-*, "to," + *glutinare*, "to glue." Particles that agglutinate are said to be stuck together, as if by glue. Incidentally, our word "glue" is derived from the Latin *gluten*, which means the same thing. But **gluten** for us has come to mean something else again, the sticky substance in certain cereal flours, notably wheat, that causes diarrhea in persons afflicted with coeliac disease.

agony comes from the Greek *agōn*, "a struggle or contest." The Greek *agōnia* also means anguish, and this is the nonmedical sense in which our word "agony" usually is used. The medical adjective **agonal** describes pathologic changes occurring just before or at the moment of death, implying a death struggle. When referring to muscles, an **agonist** is a prime mover, and its **antagonist** is a muscle having the opposite effect. In physiologic terms, an agonist is a stimulant to a specific action, whereas an antagonist blocks or counteracts the stimulus. Histamine, for example, is an agonist when it stimulates secretion of hydrochloric acid by parietal or oxyntic cells of the stomach; cimetidine, acting as an H_2-receptor antagonist, blocks this action. **Protagonist**, incidentally, has a quite distinct meaning, and that is "to designate the leading character in a drama or the foremost exponent of a movement or cause."

agraphia (*see* **graph**)

ague is an archaic word from Old French which, in turn, was derived from the Latin *acutus*, "sharp or pointed." A *fièvre aiguë* was an acute fever. Often this was shortened to merely "ague" and typically was used to describe an attack of malaria. Professor H. A. Skinner has pointed out that "ague" also may be connected with the Gothic word *agis*, meaning "trembling." Indeed, rigorous shivering often attends an acute fever.

AIDS is the acronym for "acquired immune deficiency syndrome." Often, when a medical condition is poorly understood, it is described rather than specifically named, and it is called a syndrome when its status as an entity is uncertain. Because descriptions often are lengthy and cumbersome, ways are sought to shorten them. Forming an acronym by taking the initial letters of a phrase is a clever means, especially useful if it seems to form a short word. Sometimes an acronym eventually becomes a word itself, though its meaning may change in the process. An example is "flak," which originated in the German *Flieger Abwehr Kanone*, "aircraft defense cannon." "Acronym," by the way, comes from the Greek *akros*, "tip or peak," + *-onym*, the combining form of *ōnoma*, "name."

ainhum is a rare disease of the digits, more often the toes and usually the fifth toe, typically seen in black African men. A narrow, circumscribed constriction of the affected

digit can lead to spontaneous amputation. The name of the disease is a Portuguese adaptation of the Yoruba (Nigerian) word *ayun*, "to saw or cut."

ala is the Latin word for "wing" and also "armpit." In anatomy, it is almost always used in the sense of "wing," and in combination with other terms, as in ala nasi, the flaring, winglike outer extension of the nostril. An old term for the mesosalpinx was ala vespertilionis or "bat's wing," the *vespertilionis* referring to a creature that flies at vesper or eventide.

albino is a derivative of the Latin *albus*, "white," but the name "albino" was first given by Portuguese traders to mottled or white Negroes encountered on the west coast of Africa. Medically, **albinism** refers to a partial or total lack of pigment in the eyes, skin, and hair. Persons so affected are sometimes called albinos.

albumen spelled with an "e" is the white of an egg; **albumin** spelled with an "i" before the final "n" refers to a protein substance, found in almost all animal and many plant tissues, that is soluble in water and is coagulable by heat. Both words obviously come from the Latin *albus*, "white." Albumen is the older word for the simple reason that eggwhite was a known substance long before biochemistry became a science. The distinctive spelling probably started as "albumine," indicating a substance derived from albumen.

alcohol traces its origin to the Arabic *al*, "the," + *kuhl*, "fine, impalpable powder." The first *al-kuhl* was a preparation of finely powdered antimony used by Arab women to tint their eyelids, much as cosmetic eyeshadow is used today. Later, the term was applied to any substance that could be pulverized to exceeding fineness. In this sense, a "perfect fineness" would be no powder residue at all, and gradually the concept of *al-kuhl* as a spirituous substance evolved. Once this idea was conceived, it didn't take long to discover that the "spirit" of wine was its alcohol content.

aldehyde is a word contrived to convey the nature of a substance that was recognized as a dehydrogenated alcohol. It was Justus Liebig (1803-1873), a pioneer German organic chemist, who coined the word in 1835. Luckily for us he did; otherwise, we might be burdened with the cumbersome term "*al cohol dehyd rogenatus.*"

alexia is from the Greek *a-*, "without," + *lexis*, "word," and means a loss of the capacity to read or understand the written word. It can be caused by a lesion that disconnects the visual cortex from certain recognition centers in the brain. **Dyslexia** (Greek *dys-*, "faulty") is a developmental disorder, sometimes familial, manifested in children (more often in boys) by impaired comprehension of written words. Although the dyslexic youngster often is mistakenly thought to be retarded, the condition is not associated with any lack of intelligence. The cause may be a lag in maturation of intricate brain circuits, and the impairment tends to be self-limited.

alexin was the name given in 1889 by Hans Buchner (1850-1902) to a bacteriolytic substance recognized in blood serum. The name was suggested by the Greek *alexein*, "to ward off," presumably in the sense of warding off infection. The substance was later renamed "complement."

alexithymia is another well appointed word that is both useful in clinical medicine and fun to dissect for its origins. The word is concocted by combining the Greek *a-*, "without," + *lexis*, "word or expression," + *thymos*, "mental state or mood." Thus, alexithymia is a condition wherein a person is unable to express emotions in words. Such a condition is prevalent among patients seeking medical help because of so-called functional disorders. Not being aware of, or unable to express, his condition as "depression," the patient complains of loss of appetite, constipation, and inability to sleep soundly.

algorithm is being used today to designate a particular sequence of procedures for solving a problem. For example, in medical instruction, a branched diagram may be used to graphically illustrate the proper array of tests needed to arrive at a correct diagnosis. The *Oxford English Dictionary* calls "algorithm" an erroneous refashioning of "algorism." Originally, algorism was simply the Arabic or decimal system of numeration, obviously a much better means of solving mathematical problems than the Greek or Roman numerations. The term "algorism" came from al-Khowarazmi, the surname of the 9th cen-

tury Arab mathematician whose translation of an early work on algebra led to the general use of Arabic numerals in Europe. Incidentally, **algebra**, as one might guess, also is of Arabic origin. It began as *al-jabr*, meaning "the reunion of broken parts" and specifically referred to the art of bone-setting. Even as late as the 17th century, "algebra" kept its original surgical meaning. Gradually, "reuniting what is broken" shifted to the sense of mathematical equations.

alienist formerly was used to designate a physician who specialized in the diagnosis and treatment of mental disorders, particularly one who advised courts of law in judgments of insanity. The insane were thought to suffer "mental alienation," the term being derived from the Latin verb *alienare*, "to make strange or set at variance." Psychiatrists probably are as glad as anyone that they are no longer referred to as alienists.

alimentary is an adjective derived from the Latin noun *alimentum*, meaning "food or nourishment." **Aliment** is an old word for any nourishing foodstuff, and **alimentation** refers to the process of feeding. Lately, **hyper-alimentation** (adding the Greek prefix *hyper*, "over and above") has come to mean the provision of nourishment over and above that which can be handled by the alimentary tract, namely that introduced through a central venous catheter. The Indo-European root has been postulated as *al*, "to grow, to nurture." This led to the Latin *alere*, "to feed or nourish." From this we have a number of words such as **alma mater** (nourishing mother), **coalesce** (to grow together), **abolish** (to do away with sustenance), **alimony** (allowance for sustenance), and **adult** (grown up, the "ul" being equivalent to "-al").

alkali suggests its Arabic origin by its beginning with *al-*. The original word was nearly the same: *al-*, "the," + *qaliy*, "ashes." Originally, a marine plant, the sea-wort, was burned to produce a basic ash. The water-soluble extract of plant ashes was, for many years, referred to as potash, presumably because the ashes were collected in pots. When the principal base metal of potash was identified, a more dignified, Latinized term was required, thus **potassium** was contrived. The ancient Romans had no such word. But in choosing a symbol for the newly discovered element, "K" was selected to stand for *kalium*, which went back again to the Arabic *qaliy* or *kali*.

alkaptonuria signifies a metabolic disorder wherein an intermediate product of the catabolism of tyrosine and phenylalanine, namely, homogentisic acid, is excreted in the urine. All of this was not known in 1861 when Karl Bödecker, a German chemist, coined the term **alkapton**. What he did know was that urine of patients with this condition turned dark brown when allowed to stand or when an alkaline solution was added. In fact, he had difficulty analyzing the substance in urine because of its avidity for oxidation in an alkaline medium. So, to name the substance, he contrived to link alk-, referring to alkali, to the Greek word *kaptein*, meaning "to gulp down or to avidly consume." In bygone days it was not unusual for a chemist to know Greek.

allantois (*see* **urachus**)

allele comes from the Greek *allelon*, "of one another," in the sense of counterparts. An allele is one of two or more contrasting genes, occupying the same locus in homologous chromosomes, that determine alternative characteristics by inheritance.

allergy is derived from the Greek *allo-*, "other or different," + *ergon*, "work." In this sense, an allergy is something that "works differently" from the normal. The word was first used in 1906 by the Austrian pediatrician Clemens von Pirquet (1874-1929) to designate what he conceived as an altered power to react. Specifically, allergy should be reserved for abnormal conditions arising from the interaction between a sensitizing substance (an **allergen**) and a peculiarly induced capacity to respond to that substance. The consequence of the interaction between an antigen and an uncommon antibody (typically an IgE immunoglobulin) represents an allergy. However, the observation that a minority of people complain of gas when they eat coleslaw does not mean that such persons are allergic to cabbage; this is not an antigen-antibody reaction. Unfortunately, "allergy" has come to be loosely used by pseudosophisticated patients for almost every idiosyncrasy, and such loose use has not always been discouraged by their doctors.

allopathy (*see* **homeopathy**)

alopecia refers to a pathologic loss of hair, as from the scalp, but distinct from the pattern of "normal" baldness in men. The word seems to be derived from the Greek *alōpēx*, "a fox." Here the story becomes murky. To the Greeks, *alōpecia* meant "fox-mange," and mangy foxes lose their hair. Or, could it be because the urine of a fox was seen to make grass disappear, thus rendering turf barren in patches?

alveolus in Latin means "a small tray or basin" and was also applied to a game board in which were engraved small depressions to hold pebbles or other markers. By extension, alveolus came to mean "any small cavity or compartment." Vesalius (1514-1564), the Flemish anatomist, is said to have first applied the word to anatomy as a term for the socket of a tooth, and we still refer to the dental alveoli of the maxilla and mandible. It was not until the 19th century that "alveolus" was used in reference to the tiny air sac that is the terminus of the finest bronchial channels in the lungs.

alyssum is the name of a modest little flowering plant to which was attributed a property it never had. The name comes from the Greek *a-*, "against," + *lyssa*, "madness." At one time there was a notion that chewing the leaves of this plant, after being bitten by a rabid dog, would prevent the rigors of rabies. Alas, there is no evidence validating this therapy, just as there is no basis for believing that wearing an amethyst is a remedy for drunkenness.

amalgam is a malleable alloy such as that used to fill dental cavities. The word was a Medieval Latin term used by alchemists to designate a combination of mercury and another metal, such as tin or silver. Amalgam is said by some to derive from the Greek *malagma*, "a soft mass, especially an emollient or poultice," the assertion being that "amalgam" was an alchemist's anagram for malagma. That sounds devious and not a little farfetched. Others have suggested an Arabic origin whereby *al-*, "the," was simply tacked on as a prefix to form almalagma, which then became "almalgam" in a manner analogous to the formation of the word "alchemy."

amaurosis is taken directly from the Greek word meaning "dark or obscure." The ancients used amaurosis to describe dullness or dimness of sight occurring without any apparent lesion in the eye. Later, the word referred to impaired vision consequent to disease in the retina, optic nerve, or brain. **Amaurotic family idiocy**, also known as Tay-Sachs disease (Warren Tay [1843-1927] was an English physician and Bernard Sachs [1858-1944] was a New York neurologist), is a neuropathy characterized by blindness, muscular atrophy, and intellectual deficiency. It results from lipid degeneration in the brain and occurs as a recessive genetic trait, usually in the offspring of Jewish parents. **Amblyopia** is another word for diminished vision, being derived from a combination of the Greek *ambly-*, "dull," + *ōps*, "eye." It is interesting to note that the currently understood meaning of amblyopia has reverted to the ancient meaning of "amaurosis," i.e., "deficient or absent vision in an intrinsically normal eye." The amblyopic eye, sometimes called a "lazy eye," does not see because the image it transmits is suppressed by the cerebral cortex. This happens in the case of marked strabismus so as to avoid diplopia or "double-vision." It happens, too, in the case of severely disparate refractory error wherein the blurred image from one eye is suppressed in favor of the clearer image transmitted by the other, good eye.

ambidextrous comes from a combination of the Latin *ambo*, "both," + *dexter*, "the right hand." An ambidextrous person can use his or her two hands as if both were right hands, referring to the **dexterity** possessed by most people in the right hand. A left-handed person who is equally facile with both hands would properly be "ambisinstrous" but that word has never caught on and probably never will.

ambulance comes from the French and began as *hôpital ambulant*, literally "a walking hospital." During Napoleon's campaigns, to bring medical aid directly to soldiers in the field, portable units were devised that contained dressings and medicines and provided for evacuation of the wounded as well. When later introduced into the British army, the name was shortened to simply "ambulance."

This was the germ of an idea that was effectively fulfilled by the U.S. Army Medical Corps in the Korean War with the establishment of the celebrated M.A.S.H. (Mobile Army Surgical Hospital) units.

ameba is a single-celled organism that, in its live trophozoite form, is observed to constantly change shape by extension and retraction of its cell wall. The name, which is classically spelled **amoeba**, comes from the Greek *amoibe*, "change." The genus is now called *Entameba*, implying that the organisms typically inhabit the intestine.

ameloblastoma (*see* **adamantinoma**)

amethyst is the name for a semiprecious gemstone that ranges in color from purple to violet and is a variety of quartz. Although the stone has no medical significance, its name has. It comes from the Greek *amethystos*, meaning "a remedy against drunkenness"; this, in turn, is derived from *a-*, "negative or against," + *methyein*, "to be drunk." Presumably, the ancient Greeks attributed to the stone a power to deter wine-bibbers, this despite the fact that in all of Greek literature there is no record of a controlled, randomized, double-blinded study to show that it ever worked.

amino acids are the organic compounds that, when linked together in various sequences, comprise proteins. **Amine** was contrived to designate a derivative of ammonia, the classical suffix "-ine" being taken from the Latin *-inus* or the Greek *-inos*, both meaning "of or pertaining to." Many of the amino acids were discovered and named individually during the early 19th century, but it was not until about 1848 that the collective term "amino acids" was introduced by Jöns Jakob Berzelius (1779-1848), a Swedish chemist. Another 30 years passed before Albrecht Kossel (1853-1927) originated the German term *Bausteine*, "building stones" for amino acids that Emil Fischer (1852-1919), another German chemist, proved to be the primary components of protein. Professor H. A. Skinner compiled explanations for the names of specific amino acids. **Cystine** was first obtained from urinary concrements by Wollaston in 1810. Braconnot in 1820 found a breakdown product of protein that had a sweet taste and called it **glycine**. In 1846

Liebig isolated a substance from casein and named it **tyrosine** (from the Greek *tyros*, "cheese"). **Leucine**, discovered by Proust in 1818, was later given its name by Braconnot because of the whiteness of its crystals. Hopkins and Cole in 1901 isolated **tryptophan**, so called because it was a product of tryptic digestion and gave a bright violet color reaction. (The Greek *phanos* means "bright.")

aminophylline (*see* **theophylline**)

ammonia in one form or another is a long-lived word and has been traced by some authorities to a temple at the ancient town of Ammon in Libya. The name of the town situated at the edge of the Libyan desert may have come from the Greek *ammos*, "sandy." Or, it may have descended from the supreme Egyptian god Amon. How the pungent odor of ammonia became associated with a temple at Ammon is not entirely clear. The ancients knew of **gum ammoniac** (the Greek *ammoniakos* means "of or from Ammon"), a plant resin used as a counterirritant and as an expectorant in the treatment of cough. Possibly it was this substance that was processed for healing purposes at the temple of Ammon. This ancient temple has another claim to fame. Ammon's horn is another name for the hippocampus, a curved structure in the medial part of the floor of both lateral ventricles in the brain. The Egyptian god Amon was often represented by a ram's head displaying large curved horns.

amnesia is loss of memory. The word is easy to remember, however, because it comes from the Greek *a-*, "without," + *mnēsis*, "memory." Because amnesia can occur in dramatic circumstances, it has been a favorite motif for storytellers. Doubtless, amnesia has been cited more often in fiction than in real life. I can't remember having known an actual case. A contrary construction is **anamnesis**, an archaic term for a patient's history. Occasionally, the word is encountered in old medical writings. It comes directly from the Greek *anamnēsis*, "a recalling."

amnion is the thin, tough membrane surrounding the fetus during gestation. Contained within the amnion is the amniotic fluid, in which the fetus is immersed. The Greek *amnion* was the bowl in which blood of sacri-

ficial sheep was collected. The derivation of this word is uncertain, but it may have come from the Greek *amnios*, "lamb." A connection, if there is one, between a lamb and the fetal membrane could well be that newborn lambs were intimately familiar to shepherding people. **Amniocentesis** is a compound of *amnio-* + the Greek *kentēsis*, "a puncture."

amorphous (*see* **morphology**)

amphetamine is a drug whose use is now more often illicit than licit. Its name is a sort of acronym for its chemical designation as *a*lpha *m*ethyl *ph*enyl *et*hyl *amine*.

amphoric describes the sound made by blowing across the mouth of a bottle. Amphoric breath sounds are low-pitched and hollow; when elicited by auscultation they may signify consolidation in the lungs. The Latin *amphora*, "a jar," comes from the Greek *amphi*, "on both sides," + *phoroi*, "handles." The common, narrow-necked jar in those days had handles at both sides.

amphoteric is borrowed from the Greek *amphoteros*, "in both ways." An amphoteric substance is one having opposite properties, for example, the capability of acting both as an acid and as a base.

ampule is known as a small, sealed, glass container used to preserve medicines in a sterile, stable condition. The word comes from the Latin *ampulla*, "flask." **Ampulla** also refers in anatomy to a dilated segment in a tubular structure. An example is the ampulla of Vater, commemorating Abraham Vater (1684-1751), a German anatomist. Interestingly, the Latin *ampulla* also means bombast or inflated discourse, as a "blowing out." Glass flasks were and are made by "blowing out" air.

amputation is borrowed from the Latin *amputatio*, "a pruning," which, in turn, is derived from *ambi-*, "around," + *putatio*, "cutting short, as in pruning." This is not to be confused with the Latin verb *putare*, "to think or reckon," from which we derive our words putative, impute, compute, and computer.

amulet is an almost direct borrowing of the Latin *amuletum*, "a talisman," usually worn as a charm around the neck to ward off evil influences. One version is that this is related to the Arabic *himāla*, "a carrier," especially as a cord bearing a small Koran or prayer book and worn about the neck. The early Christians wore amulets in the shape of a fish and bearing the Greek word *ichthus*, "fish." This was an acronym for "*Iesos Christos Theou Uios Soter*" (Jesus Christ, Son of God, Savior). In former years it was not unusual to find children wearing cords carrying little bags of asafetida around their necks. These were intended to ward off infections and may have been effective. Asafetida (from the Latin *fetidus*, "stinking") has such a foul odor it discourages mingling. Today, one occasionally finds a patient presenting himself for a reassuring physical examination and wearing a necklace bearing a saintly image as an amulet. This is known as hedging a bet.

amygdaloid usually is thought of in connection with the amygdaloid nucleus of the brain, an almond-shaped mass at the tail end of the caudate nucleus. Its shape suggested its name from the Greek *amygdale*, "almond," + *eidos*, "like."

amyl- is a combining form taken from the Greek *amylos*, "starch." This, in turn, is a combination of *a-*, "without," + *myle*, "mill," and taken to mean "not processed by milling." The explanation is that starch was originally obtained from wheat that had not been ground.

amyloid is a glycoprotein substance that when first found in certain diseased tissue was observed, when treated with iodine, to react by forming a blue color. Hence, it was thought to resemble starch and was called "amyloid" from the Greek *amylos*, "starch," + *eidos*, "like."

anabolism means "building up" in the sense of constructive metabolism, i.e., the formation of complex substances from simpler components, as in the building of tissues from nutritive elements. The term is derived from the Greek *anabole*, "that which is thrown up, a mound of earth." The Greek word combines *ana-*, "up," + *ballein*, "to hurl or throw." Anabolism is the opposite of **catabolism**, a destructive metabolic process.

anacrotic (*see* **dicrotic**)

anaerobe (*see* **aerobe**)

analgesia is an insensitivity to pain or a suppression of the sense of pain, but with the subject in a conscious state. It comes from the Greek *an-*, "without," + *algesis*, "sense of pain." An analgesic is a medication that suppresses pain without inducing a loss of consciousness.

analog (*see* **anlage**; *also* **homologue**)

analysis is a Greek word that combines *ana-*, "up," + *lysis*, "loosening." We use the word to mean breaking up a whole, either material or abstract, into its components, the usual purpose being to gain an understanding of that which is analyzed. This is what *analysis* meant to the Greeks, too, though they added the sense of dissolution, even death. It has been suggested the use of the term might have begun with the practice of loosening up earth to discover bits of gold or precious stones. In medicine, an analysis can apply either to a substance or to thoughts. **Urinalysis** (a contraction of urine analysis) is the determination of the various constituents of urine. **Psychoanalysis** (Greek *psyche*, "the mind or soul") is an exploration of psychic content, including that which may not be readily evident in the conscious mind.

anamnesis (*see* **amnesia**)

anaphylaxis is an unusual or exaggerated reaction of an organism to foreign protein or other immunoreactive substance. The word was contrived by combining the Greek *an-*, "without," + "a" + *phylaxis*, "protection." Charles Robert Richet (1850-1935), a French physiologist, first used the term in 1902 when he observed that a dog previously injected with a noxious substance would, on being given a second small injection of the same substance, react violently, often with bronchial spasm. The original concept was that the first injection had so reduced the dog's immunity to the noxious substance that the dog was left without protection against the second dose. Only later was it learned that the opposite occurred. The first dose actually heightened the animal's immune reaction to the second injection. Nevertheless, a word was born. And Richet was awarded the Nobel Prize for medicine and physiology in 1913.

anaplasia combines the Greek preposition *ana-*, here used in the sense of "backward' + the Greek *plasein*, "to mold or shape." In pathology, an anaplastic neoplasm is one that has failed to attain or has regressed from a more differentiated form. The term often connotes an exceptionally virulent or intractable type of tumor growth.

anasarca is a condition of generalized, massive edema. The term is said to have originated as the Greek *hydrops ana sarka*, literally "dropsy throughout the flesh."

anastomosis is a borrowing from the Greek word of similar spelling that referred to an opening or a junction through a mouth, as of one body of water in relation to another. The word is a compound of *ana-*, "through," + *stoma*, "a mouth." Galen is said to have used the term to describe interconnections between blood vessels in the body. Today, "anastomosis" is used to refer both to a natural opening between conduits (as in **arteriovenous anastomosis**) and to an artificially constructed connection (as in **gastrojejunal anastomosis**).

anatomy is an almost direct borrowing of the Greek *anatomē*, the Greeks being among the first to systematically dissect the human body. The Greek word is a compound of *ana-*, "up or through," + *tomē*, "a cutting." Thus, the earlier anatomy was a "cutting up," and dissection remains to this day the essential means of learning the structure of the body. The study of the human body fell into disrepute during the so-called Dark Ages. Andreas Vesalius (1514-1564), the Flemish anatomist, is generally credited with being "the father of modern anatomy," as the study was revived with his publication of *De Humani Corporis Fabrica* ("The Structure of the Human Body") in 1543, when Vesalius was only 29.

Ancylostoma (*ankylo-* + Greek *stoma*, "mouth") is a genus of nematode parasites, including the hookworms. This worm finds its way to the intestine where it hooks onto the mucosa by means of its crooked mouth.

androgen designates a sex hormone that occurs naturally in both men and women but, when present in excess from either an endogenous or exogenous source, tends to stimulate development of male characteristics. The term was contrived from the Greek *andros*, "man," + *gennaō*, "I produce." Thus, an androgen can be fancied as a "man maker." Unfortunately, there have been reports of

athletes who take this notion literally. **Androgynism** (+ Greek *gynē*, "woman") is a condition wherein both male and female traits are evident in a single person.

anemia is from the Greek *an-*, "without," + *haima*, "blood." Hence, a patient who is anemic is lacking in blood. There is a genus of plants called *Anemone*, but this is of quite a different origin. The plants were popularly known as "wind flowers," and the name presumably comes from the Greek *anemos*, "wind." Sea anemones are brightly colored polypoid creatures of the order Actiniaria and were named after the flower.

anesthesia comes directly from the Greek *an-*, "without," + *aisthēsis*, "feeling or sensation." In medicine, anesthesia (the British, more faithful to the Greek, spell it "anaesthesia") has come to have two meanings: (*a*) the symptom wherein a part of the body has lost perception of pain or touch; and (*b*) the procedure whereby a patient has been rendered incapable of sensation, either by inducing a state of total unconsciousness (general anesthesia) or by blocking the neural pathway of sensation in a part of the body (local or regional anesthesia). Both meanings were known and used in ancient times. Herodotus referred to the effect of inhaling the vapor from burning hemp, now known to be the result of liberated cannabis. A diminished but not absent perception is **hypoesthesia** (*hypo-*, "below"), whereas an enhanced perception is **hyperesthesia** (*hyper-*, "above"). To Dr. Oliver Wendell Holmes Sr. (1809-1894) goes the credit for aptly applying the Greek term to the use of ether to abolish the pain of surgery. This he did in a letter dated 21 November 1846 addressed to William T. G. Morton, the dentist who successfully demonstrated the procedure only a month before at the Massachusetts General Hospital in Boston.

aneurysm is a near borrowing of the Greek *aneurysma*, "a widening," which is derived from a combination of *ana-*, "up, through," + *eurynein*, "to widen." In pathology the term designates a localized dilatation of an artery. There are **berry aneurysms** (the allusion is obvious), **fusiform aneurysms** (shaped like spindles), **miliary aneurysms** (tiny, like millet seeds), and **racemose aneurysms** (clustered like a bunch of grapes), among other types.

angi- is a combining form derived from the Greek *a[n]geion*, "a vessel." The reference in medicine is to a conduit for any of the body fluids, notably blood, lymph, or bile. From "angi-" have come such present-day words as **angiology**, **angiogram**, **lymphangioma**, and **cholangitis**.

angina is a Latin word meaning "sore throat" and comes from the Latin verb *angere*, "to choke or throttle." In former years, submandicular infection was known as Ludwig's angina after the German surgeon Wilhelm von Ludwig (1790-1865), and "trench mouth" or necrotizing gingivitis was called Vincent's angina, after the Parisian physician Henri Vincent (1862-1950). Today, "angina" is usually associated with **angina pectoris**, the familiar crushing retrosternal (Latin *pectus*, "the chest") pain resulting from myocardial ischemia. The relation to ischemia has led "angina" far afield, and one may hear of "abdominal angina" as a reference to severe pain in the abdomen resulting from constriction of the mesenteric arteries. An etymologist might regard this as "abominable angina."

angiogenesis is a type of neovascularization (angi- + Greek *gennan*, "to produce"), particularly that which occurs in neoplasia. One means of impeding neoplasia is suppression of angiogenesis, which may also lessen the chance of metastasis.

angiorrhexis (*see* **rhexis**)

angulus is a direct borrowing of the Latin word for "angle" when referring to the bend in the stomach at the junction of its body and antrum.

animal is derived from the Latin *animus*, "breath, spirit, or soul," related to the Greek *anemos*, "wind." In this sense, an animal can be any breathing thing, but its use is restricted to those life forms distinct from plants. From the same source comes our adjective "animated," meaning spirited or full of life, but also "animosity," meaning enmity.

anion (*see* **ion**)

anisocoria (*see* **pupil**)

anisocytosis (*see* **cyto-**)

ankle comes from the Anglo-Saxon *ancleōw*, which may be distantly related to the Greek *a[n]kylos*, "bent or at an angle," referring to the relationship between the foot and the leg.

ankyl- is a combining form that means "bent," as in the form of a loop or noose, and is derived from the Greek *a[n]kylē*, "the bend in the arm" and also the looped thong by which a javelin is hurled. The Greek *a[n]kylos* means "bent or crooked." The Latin equivalent of the Greek term is *angulus*, from which we get "angle."

ankylosis refers to a fixation of joints, either by disease or design, usually in a bent position.

anlage is a German word meaning "a plan or arrangement." The noun is derived from the verb *anlegen*, literally "to lay on," particularly in the sense of "to prepare or set up." Biologically, an anlage is whatever precedes or "sets the stage" for something else. In embryology, an anlage is a forerunner or precursor of a more mature structure. This is distinct from an **analog** (or analogue), a part or an organ having the same function as another but of a different evolutionary origin. "Analog" is related to the Greek *analogos*, "proportionate, or in conformity with." (*see* **homologue**)

annulus means "a ring" but appears to be a misspelling of the Latin *anulus*, "a little ring," as that which encircles, such as a ring worn on a finger, being a diminutive of the Latin *anus*, a ring of more substantial size. Perhaps the confusion was with the Latin *annus*, "a year," thought of as a circuit. In any event, the spelling was corrected in a more recent publication of *Nomina Anatomica*, the official pronouncement of the International Congress of Anatomists. By the same token, **annular**, "shaped like a ring," should be spelled "anular," but it isn't and probably never will be.

anode (*see* **ion**)

anodyne is a word seldom heard today, but formerly it was commonly used for any painkiller. It comes from the Greek *an-*, "without," + *odynē*, "pain." Opium and its derivatives, for example, are anodynes.

anomaly refers to any deviation from the normal and comes from the Greek *an-*, "not," + *omalos*, "even or level" and, metaphorically, "average or ordinary." In biology an anomaly is usually a structure or organ that is congenitally abnormal, but the word "anomaly" can be used to refer to anything that is out of the ordinary.

Anopheles is the name of a genus of mosquitoes that is notorious for transmitting the malarial parasite, thus is directly implicated in perpetuating what is probably the commonest disease of man worldwide. The name comes from the Greek *an-*, "not," + *ophēlos*, "of advantage or use," and was bestowed on this pesky creature long before it was identified as the vector of malaria by Sir Ronald Ross (1857-1932) in 1898. Incidentally, knowing the origin of this mosquito's name also tells us the meaning of the feminine name Ophelia, "useful." **Mosquito**, by the way, is the diminutive of the Spanish *mosca*, "a fly," from the Latin *musca*.

anorexia comes from the Greek *an-*, "lack of," + *orexis*, "appetite," and it still means just that. Incidentally, Orexin is the trade name of a vitamin B supplement purveyed purportedly as a stimulant to appetite. The Greek *orexis* could also mean any other sort of yearning, and perhaps that accounts for a form of the male hormone, testosterone, being named Oreton.

anosmia comes from the Greek *an-*, "lack of," + *osmē*, "smell," and refers to the condition wherein the sense of smell is lost. The element **osmium** is said to have been so named because of the distinctive odor of its vaporous oxide (OsO_4). The Greek *osmē* is not to be confused with *osmos*, "impulse," from which is derived "osmosis."

anoxia means "a deficiency of oxygen in tissues" and is derived from the Greek *an-*, "lack of," + *oxys*, "sharp," in the sense of "acid." This sounds farfetched unless one is acquainted with the origin of "oxygen."

ansa is the Latin word for "handle" but could also mean "a loop, as used to fasten a sandal." In anatomy the word is used for various looplike structures, particularly small loops of nerves.

antagonist is used in anatomy to designate a muscle that opposes the action of another muscle, and in pharmacology to designate a substance having a blocking or opposing effect. Thus, extensor muscles are antagonists of flexor muscles, and beta-adrenergic blocking agents, such as propranolol, are antagonists of certain actions of epine-

phrine and other sympathomimetic amines. The Greek *antagōnixomai* means "to struggle against," and *antagōnistes* means "an adversary or rival." These words, in turn, come from *anti-*, "against," + *agōn*, "struggle." (*see* **agony**)

antecubital (Latin *ante*, "before or in front," + *cubitum*, "the elbow") locates the fossa or hollow in front of the elbow. A related term is "cubit," an archaic unit of measure, being the distance from the elbow to the fingertips.

anthracosis is a lung disease caused by inhaling coal dust and thereby often afflicts coal miners. The condition also is called "black lung disease." The name was taken from the Greek *anthrax*, "coal," which by direct borrowing had, much earlier, been used as the name for a quite different disease.

anthrax is an infectious disease of wild and domesticated animals that can be transmitted to man. Its principal feature is a carbuncle that can become necrotic and ulcerated. Such a lesion can have a hard, black center surrounded by red inflammation, thus resembling a burning coal and accounting for its name, taken directly from the Greek *anthrax*, "coal." The causative organism, *Bacillus anthracis*, can lurk in the hides or wool from infected animals, and human anthrax has been known as "woolsorters' disease," among other names. The development of a vaccine effective against anthrax in sheep went far to advance the career of Louis Pasteur (1822-1895), the celebrated 19th century French bacteriologist.

anthropo- is a combining form taken from the Greek *anthrōpos*, "a man." This has given us numerous words such as **anthropocentric** (a perspective that places man at the center of the universe); **anthropoid**, "like a man," in reference to certain subhuman primates; **anthropology** (the study or science of man); and **anthropomorphism** (the attribution of human form or character to nonhuman objects, such as classical deities).

antibiotic derives from the Greek *anti-*, "against," + *biotos*, "the means of life." The word has had different meanings through the centuries. The ancients may have used a similar word to mean resistance, in the sense of dealing with the vicissitudes of life. In the 19th century "antibiotic" referred to a belief opposed to the possibility of life, as on other planets. The modern medical use of the word was introduced in 1941 by Selman A. Waksman (1888-1973), who reported finding a strain of actinomyces, an extract of which inhibited the growth of some bacteria. In 1929 Alexander Fleming (1881-1955) first reported an antagonism between certain microorganisms, but it was Selman Waksman who adapted "antibiotic" to the process.

antibody is a word contrived in the late 19th century to include a variety of substances that had been discovered to combat infection and its adverse effects. Among these substances were antitoxins, agglutinins, and precipitins. All of these substances or "bodies" seemed to be "anti" something, so they were called, simply and collectively, "antibodies." Therefore, the original idea was not that these substances were "against the body" but rather that they were "bodies" (for want of a better term) "against" something else. Only later was the word **antigen** contrived as a name for whatever might induce the formation or activity of these antibodies. Today, "antibody" is restricted to the immunoglobulins of the E-type that are elaborated by immunoreactive lymphocytes of the B-type.

antidote is almost direct borrowing of the Greek *antidotos*, which means "an exchange" and comes from a combination of *anti-*, "against," + *dotos*, "what is given." An antidote is administered "against," or in opposition to, a poison.

antigen is a word contrived to name a substance that induces an immune reaction. **Antibody** came first as a collective term for a variety of newly discovered substances that seemed to have a combative or nullifying effect in infection and its concomitants. "Antigen" was devised as a name for whatever stimulated or activated antibodies. The word "antigen" was suggested by the Greek *anti-*, "against," + *gennan*, "to produce." The sense, of course, is not that antigens are "against production." Quite the opposite is true: antigens are conceived to produce or generate whatever is "anti." If this sounds confusing, it may be because immunologists seldom are as devoted to semantics as to science. But then, could a semanticist have done any better?

antihelix is the name given to the prominent ridge at the meatus of the outer ear. This is situated opposite the twisted part of the outer ear and accounts for the name, being derived from the Greek *anti-*, "opposite," + *helix*, "that which is twisted."

antipyretic is derived from the Greek *anti-*, "against," + *pyretos*, "fever," and refers to whatever has the effect of reducing or suppressing fever. The root word is the Greek *pyr*, "fire."

antisepsis was contrived from a combination of the Greek *anti-*, "against," + *sēpsis*, "putrefaction." Today we think of antisepsis as any treatment that renders an object unlikely to be the source or site of infection by pathogenic microorganisms. But the word "antisepsis" actually antedates the promulgation of the germ theory of disease. It was first used in the early 18th century to refer to elimination of anything thought to be putrefactive as a means of combating a plague. Sir Joseph Lister (1827-1912), the celebrated English surgeon, promoted the modern use of antisepsis as a means of reducing infection in wounds. Sir Joseph's surname was taken as the basis for the trade name of a popular mouthwash that is advertised to "kill germs on contact."

antitoxin (*see* **toxin**)

antrum is a Latin word that means "cave or cavity." Its Greek counterpart is *antron*, also "a cave." In anatomy, "antrum" can refer to any cavity or chamber. The maxillary sinus often is called the antrum, and the lower portion of the stomach is referred to as the gastric or prepyloric antrum.

anus is the nether opening of the alimentary canal through which feces are expelled. The Latin *anus* meant the same thing to the Romans. It also meant "ring," in the sense of encirclement. This would seem appropriate inasmuch as the anus encircles the outlet of the bowel.

anxiety is an ancient complaint for which the Romans had almost the same word in the Latin *anxietas*, "trouble, worry." The patient who, as he is being prepared for examination, is found to be wearing suspenders in addition to a sturdy belt to hold up his trousers might be deemed beset by anxiety.

anxiolytic (*see* **sedative**; *also* **tranquilizer**)

aorta is almost a direct borrowing of the Greek *aortē*, the name by which Aristotle referred to the main arterial channel issuing from the heart. But where did the Greeks get *aortē*? Authorities are divided in their explanations. Professor H. A. Skinner cites the Greek verbs *aeirein*, "to lift," or *aortemai*, "to suspend," as possibilities. However, there is a Greek noun *aortēr*, which means "a strap over the shoulder to hang anything on." When viewing an anteriorly opened cadaver, it is easy to see how the aorta might look like a curved strap from which hang the heart, the kidneys, and the abdominal viscera. Thus, the Greeks, who had no knowledge of circulating blood but thought that arteries contained air, may have likened the aorta to a sturdy strap.

APACHE is the acronym for a scheme by which the status of a critically ill patient can be evaluated, usually in the milieu of an intensive care unit. The initials stand for *Acute Physiology And Chronic Health Evaluation*.

aperture comes from the Latin *apertus*, "uncovered, exposed," the past participle of *aperire*, "to reveal, to open." An aperture, then, is an opening through which something can be seen or made evident. The piriform ("pear-shaped") aperture is the opening in the anterior skull through which the nasal passage can be observed. In years past, what we now call laxatives were known even more delicately as **aperients**, the allusion being obvious.

apex is a direct borrowing of the Latin word and means the topmost point of anything. It is said to have originally referred to the peak of a high priest's cap. The plural is **apices**. Thus we refer to the apex of one lung and to the apices of both lungs.

APGAR is an acronym with a triple meaning. First, it stands for a numerical expression, on a scale of 1 to 10, of the condition of a newborn infant based on assessment of heart rate, respiratory effort, muscle tone, reflex irritability, and skin color, taking into consideration observation of *a*daptability, *p*artnership, *g*rowth, *a*ffection, and *r*esolve. Second, the scheme has been adopted as the *American Pediatric Gross Assessment Record*. Third, it is the actual name of its originator,

Virginia Apgar, an American anesthesiologist who first published the concept (*Anesth Analg.* 1953;32:260).

aphakia (*see* **lens**)

aphasia is made up of the Greek *a-*, "without," + *phasis*, "speech," and is used to describe a defect or loss of expression or comprehension of language. It can be a symptom of various destructive brain lesions.

-apheresis is a combining suffix derived from the Greek *aphairesis*, "a taking away," which in turn combines *apo-*, "away," + *hairein*, "to take." In linguistics, apheresis (or **aphaeresis**) occurs when a short syllable has been deleted from a word, as in the use of "most" for "almost." In medicine, the form indicates "a taking away" of whatever precedes the suffix, and its most familiar use is in **plasmapheresis**, the process whereby the plasma component of blood is separated from erythrocytes and other formed elements by centrifugation. Plasmapheresis can be employed to prepare freshly frozen plasma and "packed red blood cells" for transfusion or to remove wanted or unwanted substances in plasma while preserving the cellular content of blood to be returned to the donor.

aphonia is from the Greek *a-*, "without," + *phōnē*, "voice," and means an inability to speak. It refers to a loss of the voice from any cause, as minor as laryngitis or as grave as stroke.

aphrodisiac describes a substance alleged to enhance libido. Aphrodite, the ancient Greek goddess of beauty and sexual love, is said to have sprung from the foam of the sea (Greek *aphros*, "foam"), perhaps as a result of Zeus' dalliance with Dione, one of the female Titans. Aphrodite's counterpart in Roman mythology is Venus, from whose name we get **venereal**, meaning whatever pertains to the act of love.

aphthous refers to ulcers in a mucous membrane, usually in the mouth but also in the lining of other hollow viscera. The Greek *aphthai* ("spotted eruption") was used as a name for thrush, an exudative inflammation of the oral mucosa. *Aphthai* is related to the Greek verb *aptein* which could mean both "to fasten or cling," as does an exudate, and "to kindle or set aflame," a characteristic of inflammation. The Greeks had a great fear of *aphthai* because for them the term also included diphtheria, which they recognized as often fatal to children.

apnea means a suspension of breathing, either voluntary, as in "holding one's breath," or involuntarily, as during sleep or coma. This is just what *apnoia* meant to the Greeks, who derived their word from *a-*, "not," + *pnein*, "to breathe."

apo- is a combining form taken directly from the Greek preposition meaning "away from, far from, apart from, derived from" and is the prefix to a host of Greek words, many of which we have converted to English, e.g., **apocryphal**, **apogee**, **apology**, **apostasy**, **apostle**, and **apostrophe**, among others. Medical terminology is rich in *apo-* words; a sampling follows.

aponeurosis is a thin, wide tendon from which dense connective tissue is broadly splayed into the muscle for which it serves as an attachment. This being so, why does the name sound as if it had something to do with nerves? The answer is that the ancient Greeks could not and did not distinguish between tendons and nerves. Dense, white strands looked all the same to them and were called by the collective term *neuros*. "Aponeurosis" combines *apo-*, "from," + *neuros*, in this case "a tendon."

apophysis as a Greek word means "an offshoot" and was derived by combining *apo-* with *phthysis*, "growth." Apophysis now means a projection from a bone other than an epiphysis (which has a different meaning).

apoplexy is a near borrowing of the Greek *apolēxia*, which meant "a seizure" as a result of being "struck down." The word came from a combination of *apo-* with *plēxē*, "a stroke." The common belief was that anyone seized by sudden disability was "struck down" by the gods. This idea persists in our use of the word "stroke" to refer to the consequence of an abrupt, severe, cerebrovascular disturbance. It is curious, too, that we habitually refer to "cerebrovascular accidents," as if these tragic events were the result of a "falling out" among the heavenly bodies that guide our courses. Incidentally, by knowing the origin and meaning of "apoplexy," one can avoid the fatuous redundancy of speaking of an apoplectic stroke or a stroke of apoplexy.

apoptosis is a neologism that recently has been gaining currency in pathophysiologic circles. The term refers to the dissolution of tissue cells in their natural life cycle, in contrast to premature **necrosis** unnaturally induced. The process of apoptosis involves the fragmentation of cellular components into membrane-bound particles that are then eliminated by phagocytosis or otherwise carried off. The term combines the Greek *apo-*, a prefix denoting separation or derivation, + *ptosis*, "a falling." Incidentally, the word is properly pronounced apo-ptosis, not a-pop-tosis.

apothecary comes closer than one might guess, in its original meaning, to the modern American drugstore with its shelves displaying everything from animal crackers to zippers. "Apothecary" is a near borrowing of the Greek *apothēkē*, "a storehouse," which is a composite of *apo-*, "away," + *thēkē*, "a case or cover," related to *tithēnai*, "to put." It was not until the 17th century that England's "chemists" (as the British call druggists) and grocers formally agreed that henceforth apothecaries would stock only drugs, whereas grocers would limit their trade to foodstuffs. Now, it would seem we have come full circle. The shelves of modern supermarkets are laden with over-the-counter medicaments, whereas drugstores offer almost anything under the sun. By a strange quirk, an apothecary shop today is one that deals exclusively in prescription drugs, eschewing even a soda fountain.

appall is not strictly a medical term, but it has a kind of physiologic origin. It comes from the Latin *ad*, "toward," + *pallere*, "to turn pale." Related is our word **pallor**, a deficiency of color, usually in the face, that can be an adrenergic reaction wherein cutaneous arterioles are constricted, thus causing the skin to blanche. Anything that appalls may be so dismaying as to make one turn pale.

apparatus comes from the Latin *apparare*, "to prepare," and is a combination of *a- (ad)*, "to," + *paratus*, "ready." This brings to mind the motto of the U.S. Coast Guard, *Semper paratus*, "Always ready." From its derivation, then, "apparatus" carries the implication of some arrangement or device "made ready" or prepared for a given purpose. A meaningless device could not properly be called an apparatus.

appetite is an almost direct borrowing of the Latin *appetitio*, "grasping or craving," which, in turn, combines *ad-* (as *ap-*), "toward," + *petitus*, "desire" (*petitus* being the past participle of *petere*, "to seek, attack, or fall upon"). Petulant, impetuous, impetus, complete, and repeat are all similarly derived. (However, the English noun "pet" and the verb "to pet" are not related; their origin is obscure.) Appetite can be a craving for almost anything, though usually we think of appetite in terms of a hearty desire for nourishment. But there are other appetites to serve, some leading to misbehavior. Dr. Henry Janowitz purports that what a man of advancing age claims as increasing virtue is more likely to be only a decline of appetite.

aqua is the Latin word for "water." Some have said that aqua is related to the Latin *aequa*, meaning "smooth or level," the idea being that the surface of water in a bucket or a pond, when not unduly disturbed, is level. But most scholars attribute *aqua* to the postulated Indo-European form *akwā*. Surely the earliest speaking man had a word for water. (The English "water," incidentally, comes from the Anglo-Saxon *waeter*, presumed to have been derived from the Indo-European form *awer*, "wet, or to flow.") Medieval alchemists combined *aqua* with all sorts of romantic terms to describe various liquids: *aqua fortis* ("strong water") was nitric acid; *aqua regis* ("royal water") was a mixture of nitric and hydrochloric acids, so called because it alone could dissolve gold (which would seem a royally extravagant, even if remarkable, feat); *aqua vitae* ("water of life") became a collective term for ardent spirituous liquors. This shows that prevailing attitudes haven't really changed through the years. The Celtic *uisge-beatha* became "whiskey," and the Slavic *voda* ("strong water") became "vodka." The Scandinavians hardly bothered to change the Latin when they named *akvavit*.

aqueduct is borrowed from the Latin *aquaeductus*, which, in turn, is a combination of *aqua*, "water," + *ductus*, "a conduit" (from the verb *ducere*, "to lead"). In anatomy, the name "aqueduct" is given to several channels through various structures, usually for the passage of fluid. For example, the "aqueduct of Sylvius" (memorializing Jacobus Sylvius [1478-1555] who before Latinizing his name was plain Jacque Dubois) is the canal connecting the third and fourth ventricles of the brain and serving as a passage for cerebrospinal fluid. Note that despite its relation to *aqua*, "aqueduct" in English contains an "e" and not a second "a." The classical spelling would be "aquaeduct," but usage has worn away the second "a."

arabinose (*see* **ribose**)

arachidonic is the name of an unsaturated fatty acid that has come into recent prominence as the natural precursor of the ubiquitous prostaglandins, substances now recognized to exhibit important physiologic roles and promising pharmacologic properties. Arachidic acid, the C_{20} saturated fatty acid, was first isolated from peanut oil and named from the Latin *arachis*, "peanut." Arachidonic acid, the C_{20} fatty acid with four double bonds, was thus named to indicate a relation.

arachnoid comes from the Greek *arachnē*, "spider," + *eidos*, "like," and refers to whatever may resemble a spider. The patient with advanced cirrhosis can have a large belly swollen by ascites and spindly arms and legs shrunken by wasting of the flesh. Such a patient is said to have an "arachnoid" habitus. Also, the arachnoid membrane is a delicate, weblike covering of the brain and spinal cord. The Greek word is associated with Arachne, a mythologic Lydian maiden who was so adept at weaving that she presumed to challenge the goddess Athene to a contest of skill. Athene tried to warn her of the consequence of her brashness, but Arachne would not yield. The contest proceeded, and both the maiden and the goddess were incredibly deft in their weaving. From this point, there are two versions of the story. In one, Arachne finally recognizes her folly and is so stricken with remorse that she hangs herself; Athene brings her to life, but as a spider. In the other version, Athene feels threatened and uses her supernatural power to imbue Arachne with such guilt that the maiden hangs herself, whereupon Athene turns Arachne into a spider hanging forevermore from its web, a lasting warning to mortals who might fall into Arachne's error of challenging the gods.

arcus is the Latin word for "bow," and from it came our words "arch" and "archery." **Arcuate** in anatomy describes whatever is bow-shaped. **Arcus senilis** is a bow-shaped or circular cloudy opacity at the periphery of the cornea and is often seen in the eyes of elderly persons.

areola is the diminutive of the Latin *area*, "an open space, courtyard, or park." An areola, then, is "a little space." In anatomic description, an areola is usually a small area set apart by being of different color or texture, particularly around a central point. Hence, the areola surrounding the nipple or the zone of erythema around a pustule qualifies by this definition. Areolar tissue presumably was so named because of the little spaces between the fibers of loose connective tissue.

argentum is the Latin word for silver, coming from the Greek *argyros*, "silver," and *argos*, "white or shining." With a bit of license, these words were abbreviated as the chemical symbol "Ag." The Greek and Latin terms may have originated in the Sanskrit root *radj*, "to shine." **Argyria** and **argyrosis** are terms for the condition wherein silver salts are deposited in tissues of the body. This can be evident as a peculiar, slate-gray cast of the skin and as a dark line of silver pigment at the gingival margin. Years ago this was seen in patients who had consumed large quantities of Argyrol, a proprietary, silver-protein medicament formerly prescribed for sore throats and nervous disorders. An eccentric Philadelphia doctor, Albert C. Barnes, amassed a fortune from the sale of this concoction. Thereby he acquired a world-renowned collection of French paintings that for many years were jealously guarded from public view in his own private museum.

argon is the name of an almost inert gaseous element that, among other uses, has been adapted to devices producing laser beams that lately have been applied to medical purposes. Before this usefulness was discovered, the name "argon" was contrived from the Greek *a-*, "not," + *ergon*, "work." Being inert, argon was thought to do no work.

arm has its analogues in Old Frisian and other Teutonic languages. The Old Norse *armr*

referred to that portion of the upper extremity between the shoulder and the elbow, probably more specifically to the shoulder. The Aryan form *ar* meant "to fit or join." The Latin *armus* refers to the shoulder and upper arm. But the word usually used by the Romans was *bracchium*, from which we take the anatomic adjective brachial, "of the arm," as in the **brachial plexus** (of nerves) and the **brachial artery** and **vein**. (This is not to be confused with the prefix **brachy-**, derived from the Greek *brachys*, "short.")

armamentarium is a direct borrowing of the Latin word meaning "arsenal or armory," thus a collection of weapons. In medicine, a therapeutic armamentarium refers to an assortment of remedies available to combat disease or injury.

ars is cited here because it introduces the maxim *Ars longa, vita brevis*, often quoted by worldly wise professors to weary students. Although the quotation is usually given in Latin, the maxim is attributed to Hippocrates, the famous Greek physician of the 5th century B.C. A literal translation is: "The art is long; life is short." Dr. John H. Dirckx in his book *The Language of Medicine* (2nd edition, New York, NY: Praeger Publishers; 1983), offers what he believes to be a translation more faithful to the spirit of the original: "The craft of healing is so complex that you will scarcely master it in a lifetime." Often one is reminded, "Medicine is both an art and a science." Usually, this is taken to mean that the profession of medicine combines an aesthetic and a practical sense. The Latin *ars, artis*, representing the Greek *technē*, means "a trade, handicraft" (whence "artisan"), whereas the Latin *scientia* implies "knowledge" in the cognitive sense. Dr. Dirckx goes on to point out that though the characterization of medicine as both an art and a science conveys nearly the same meaning now as many years ago, the two key words have virtually exchanged meanings.

arse is a time-honored, if somewhat archaic, word descended from the Teutonic and meaning "the fundament, posterior, or rump" of any animal, including man. Commonly the word is corrupted, through ignorance, by deleting the "r" and "e," then adding an extra "s." This results in a wholly unrelated word that properly designates the long-eared, sure-footed, patient, domesticated mammal *Equus asinus*. To the Romans, the Latin *asinus* meant both "a donkey" and "a fool," which seems a shameful degradation of the faithful beast of burden. The Greek word for donkey was *onos*, and the Latin *onus* means "burden." To avoid mistaking "ass" for "arse," remember this limerick:

> There once was a maid from Madras
> Who had a magnificent ass.
> Not rounded and pink,
> As you probably think—
> It was gray, had long ears, and ate grass.

arsenic comes through the Old French from the Latin *arsenicum* (*arrenicum*) and the Greek *arsenikon* (*arrenikon*), "a yellow ointment." Because ointments containing arsenic were thought to be "strong," some writers relate the term to the Greek adjective *arrenikos*, "masculine or male." Another connection may be with the Persian *zarnika*, wherein *zar* means "gold."

artemisinin (*see* cinchona)

arteriosclerosis is a word introduced by Johann Lobstein (1777-1835), a Strasbourg surgeon, in 1833. It is a combination of the Greek *artēria*, "vessel," + *sklēros*, "hard," + *-osis*, "a condition," thus "a hardening of the arteries."

artery has been handed down through the ages as a word for efferent vessels leading from the heart, but it all began with a misconception. The term is derived from the Greek *artēria*, which, in turn, came from *aēr-*, "air," + *tērein*, "to contain," thus "an air duct." The ancients used *artēria* to refer to the windpipe, but because the efferent vessels from the heart usually were empty when cadavers were dissected, the term *artēria* was applied to these, too. Phlebos, from *phleō*, "I flow," was applied to veins and sometimes to blood vessels generally. Although it soon became apparent, even to the ancients, that efferent vessels carried blood, the term stuck as *artēria leiai*, "smooth artery," in distinction to *artēria tracheia*, "rough artery," which we know simply as the **trachea**.

arthritis comes from the Greek *arthros*, " joint," with the suffix denoting inflammation. **Arthralgia** (+ Greek *algos*, "pain") refers to sore joints. **Arthrodesis** (+ Greek *desmeō*, "I bind") means a procedure designed to immobilize or stiffen a joint. **Arthroplasty** (+ Greek *plassein*, "to form or to fashion") means to reconstruct a joint. Remarkably, the first report of an operative attempt to fashion an artificial joint was recorded in 1826 by John Rhea Barton (1794-1871), an American surgeon (*North American Medical and Surgical Journal.* 1826;3:279). Only recently, with the development of new materials and innovative techniques, has arthroplasty become widely applied.

articulation refers to the joining or juncture of two structures, usually bones, and comes from the Latin *articulus*, "a joint." This, in turn, is a diminutive of the Latin *artus*, meaning "fitted, close, or narrow." Any jointed structure is "articulated." When applied to the act of speech, "to articulate" means to properly join the tongue, palate, teeth, and lips so as to produce intelligible sound.

artificial describes what is made or manufactured as opposed to that which occurs naturally. The term is from the Latin *ars, artis*, "craft" + *factus*, "made." Thus, an **artifact** (or **artefact**) in medicine pertains generally to anything produced or caused to occur by other than natural means.

arytenoid is the descriptive name given to the two opposing cartilages of the larynx. Their pyramidal shape suggests a ladle or cup, whence their name from the Greek *arytaina*, "a pitcher," + *eidos*, "like."

asafetida is nowadays seldom seen (or smelled), but in years past it was not unusual to find children or adults with a little bag containing this substance tied with string about their necks for the purpose of warding off infectious diseases. Asafetida is obtained from the roots of certain plants, originally from Persia, of the order Umbelliferae, which also includes celery and parsnip. The name "asafetida" is from the Persian *aza*, "gum or mastic," + the Latin *foetidus*, "stinking." The name is well deserved. The presumed protective effect, if any, was because persons wearing asafetida bags usually were kept at a distance by others.

asbestosis denotes a condition caused by exposure to asbestos. Presently, asbestos is recognized as a carcinogen, giving rise to mesothelioma in pleural and peritoneal surfaces. The mineral substance got its name from

Greek *a-*, "not," + *sbennumi*, "to quench," i.e., unquenchable. The name is said to have been originally that of a mythical substance which, once ignited, could not be extinguished. In some strange way the reference was reversed when the name was given to a substance that would not burn. In a manner of speaking, one might suppose that whatever could not burn out would also be unquenchable. In any event, asbestos was known as a mineral fiber to the ancients who used it as wicks for lamps and as cremation cloths.

ascaris is a direct borrowing of the Greek *askaris*, the name given to intestinal worms. The origin of this term is obscure, but it might relate to the Greek *asketos*, "fidgety, irrepressible," which would aptly describe a person sorely affected by intestinal worms. The common nematode or roundworm was named *Ascaris lumbricoides* by Linnaeus. This would seem a redundancy inasmuch as *lumbricus* is the Latin word for "worm," often used by the Romans as a term of reproach.

ascites comes from the Greek *askos*, "a pouch or sack," such as that made of leather and used to carry oil, wine, or water. That the fluid-filled abdomen was thought to resemble a wine sack is ironic because we now recognize alcoholic liver disease as the commonest cause of ascites.

ascorbic acid (also known as vitamin C) is a sovereign remedy for scurvy, as its name implies, being from the Latin *a-*, "against," + *scorbutus*, "scurvy" (*see* **scorbutus**). The disease was known to the ancients, but not its cause or cure. A dietary relationship had long been suspected. Jacques Cartier, the 16th century French explorer of North America, is said to have learned from the Indians of Canada how to cure scurvy by making a decoction of spruce needles. But it remained for James Lind (1716-1794), surgeon in His Britannic Majesty's Royal Navy, to prove the ascorbutic properties of certain foods. In 1747 while serving aboard HMS *Salisbury*, Lind gave sailors stricken with scurvy either cider, vinegar, elixir of vitriol (a sulfate), seawater, nutmeg, various cathartics, oranges, or lemons. Evidently he wished to leave no potentially ascorbutic stone unturned. After 6 days, those given citrus fruits miraculously recovered; the others languished. Lind had proved the presence of a potent antiscurvy principle in citrus fruits though the concept of vitamin substances lay far in the future. This probably was the first controlled clinical trial in medical history even though not double-blinded or strictly randomized.

-ase is a suffix used to designate an enzyme. It is a contraction of diastase, a neologism contrived as a name for the first recognized enzyme. This happened to be a substance obtained from malt that was found capable of hydrolyzing starch. The word "diastase" appears to have been coined about 1833 and was borrowed from the Greek *diastasis*, "a separation." This, in turn, is a compound of *dia-*, "through or apart," + *histanai*, "to stand." Thus, the substance found to make the components of starch "stand apart" was called "diastase," and this was later recognized to be an enzyme (a word coined later). With the discovery of a multitude of substances exerting such splitting or "stand apart" activity, "ase" was conceived as being a handy suffix to append to the name of any number of substrates, thereby designating an enzymatic effect.

asepsis comes from the Greek *a-*, "without," + *sēpsis*, "putrefaction." Thus, asepsis pertains when no putrefying agent, such as bacteria, is present. The origin of the term denotes the distinction between asepsis and antisepsis, the latter implying that putrefaction is counteracted.

Asklepios (*see* **Aesculapius**)

Aspergillis is a genus of fungi whose structure was thought to resemble an *aspergillum*, the Latin name for a small brush used by priests to sprinkle holy water. This, in turn, comes from the Latin verb *aspergere*, "to spray."

asphyxia has become a somewhat misplaced term. The word is from the Greek *a-*, "without," + *sphyxis*, "pulse," and should mean "pulseless." Originally the term was applied by the ancients to any condition marked by a diminished or absent arterial pulse, signifying a cessation of the heartbeat. Commonly, in such instances, breathing also had ceased, and the term came to be associated mainly with an absence of respiration. In actual fact, when breathing has been impeded, the heart continues to beat, and a pulse persists for a remarkably long time. Nevertheless, the use of the term "asphyxia" to mean "suspended animation from suffocation" has persisted much longer.

aspirate is a term that, in medical parlance, has been turned around from its original meaning. The Latin *aspirare* means "to breathe or blow upon" (from *ad-*, "toward," + *spirare*, "to breathe"). An aspirate, when the word is used as a noun in phonetics, is the slightly coughed "h" sound and thus preserves the original sense. But in medicine, "aspirate" is used as a verb with two meanings: to remove gas or fluid by suction, and to inhale foreign substances into the respiratory passages. To suck or to inhale are the opposite of "to blow upon," but at least we seem to know what we mean when we talk of "aspirating" joint fluid or when we say a patient "aspirated" gastric contents.

aspirin was originally a trademark that has passed into the common language. "Aspirin," formerly a trademark requiring a capital "A," is the name given by the Bayer company of Germany to its preparation of acetylsalicylic acid (*see* **salicylate**). Salicylic acid was first extracted from the plant *Spiraea ulmaria*, and the principal component of this extract was known by the German term *spiroylige Säure*, later shortened to *Spirsäure*. An "A," to designate "acetyl," was added to "spir," with "-in" as a suffix, and thus "Aspirin" was contrived.

astereognosis is the loss of ability to identify familiar objects by feeling their shape. A patient so afflicted, for example, cannot recognize, with his eyes closed, a key that is placed in his hand. The term is from the Greek *a-*, "without," + *stereos*, "solid, three dimensional," + *gnōsis*, "knowledge, recognition."

asterixis describes the clonic movements, especially of the hands, by patients afflicted with various encephalopathies, but particularly that associated with advanced liver disease. The term comes from the Greek *a-*, "without," + *sterixis*, "a fixed position." The patient with portal-systemic encephalopathy cannot hold his hands in a fixed position. This alternating motion of the hands sometimes is called "liver flap."

asthenia means "weak" and is the opposite of "strong." Thus, the word was derived from the Greek *a-*, "without, lacking," + *sthenos*, "strength." The **asthenic habitus** is that of the thin, frail person. Rather than being content with just "sthenic," we describe the husky, muscular person as **hypersthenic**.

asthma is a direct borrowing of the Greek word for "gasping or panting." Asthma was defined as "sonorous wheezing" by Celsus in the 1st century A.D.

astigmatism comes from the Greek *a-*, "without," + *stigma*, "a point"; hence "no point." In ophthalmology this means "no point of convergence" as a cause of impaired vision. The condition was recognized in the early 19th century and soon after was shown to be corrected by the use of slightly cylindrical lenses. It seems a pity the word is never otherwise used. It would be neat to put down an opponent by saying, "Your argument is astigmatic!"

astragalus (*see* **talus**)

astringent is the property of a substance, when applied to a moist or weeping surface, to dry up a fluid discharge. An example is the use of aluminum chloride in antiperspirants or deodorants. The source of the term is the Latin verb *astringere*, "to tighten, bind, or compress."

astrocyte is from the Greek *astēr*, "star," + *kytos*, "cell," and is the name given to a star-shaped cell found in the supporting tissues of the central nervous system. An **astrocytoma** (+ Greek *-ōma*, "swelling") is a neoplasm arising from these cells.

asylum is a direct borrowing of the Latin word for "refuge or sanctuary." This, in turn, came from the Greek *asylon*, "refuge," which came from a combination of *a-*, "without," + *sylē*, "violence or right of seizure." In ancient Greece certain temples or sacred places had the privilege of protecting from seizure slaves or persons accused of criminal acts. From this, the meaning of "asylum" was extended to any place that offered refuge for persons needing protection or shelter. In years past, in our own country, reference commonly was made to "an orphan asylum" or to "an insane asylum."

atavism refers to "the apparent inheritance of a characteristic from remote rather than immediate ancestors due to a chance recombination of genes or to unusual environmental conditions favorable to their expression" (Dorland). The word is derived from the Latin *at-*, "beyond," + *avus*, "grandfather." Hence, an atavistic expression cannot be blamed on Grandfather, but relates to someone farther up on the family tree.

ataxia comes from the Greek *a-*, "without," + *taxis*, "order or arrangement." The term refers to a lack of motor coordination, particularly that disturbing the gait, a sign of neurologic disorder.

atelectasis comes from the Greek *a-*, "without," + *telos*, "complete," + *ectasis*, "extension or expansion." The term usually is applied to the lungs and refers either to a failure of expansion at birth or to a collapse of previously expanded lung tissue.

atheroma is from the Greek *athērē*, "gruel or porridge," + *-ōma*, "a rising," thereby having the sense of swelling with the consistency of mush. In ancient times the term was used to describe any mushy swelling, such as a sebaceous cyst. Now it refers to the fatty excrescences that accumulate in the endothelium of arteries.

athetosis is a condition marked by involuntary, writhing movements, especially of the hands and arms. Such a sign is seen in patients with various forms of motor disorder due to disturbance in the central nervous system (*see* **chorea**). The Greek *athetos* means "lacking a fixed position" and represents a combination of *a-*, "without," + *tithēnai*, "to bring into position." This last part suggests our word "tether," which comes from the Old Norse *tjōthr* but probably shares a common Indo-European root with the Greek word.

atlas is the name of the first cervical vertebra and also is used to designate a collection of pictorial illustrations. What is the connection? The original Atlas was the name of one of the mythical Titans, descendants of the primordial deities. After a falling out with Perseus, son of Jupiter, Atlas was turned into stone and condemned to carry on his shoulders the weight of the earth and its heavens. A depiction of Atlas bearing the globe became a common adornment of maps, and soon a compilation of maps and other illustrations became known as an "atlas."

Meanwhile, the bone bearing the globe of the head, i.e., the uppermost cervical vertebra, also came to be known as the atlas.

atom is from the Greek *atomos*, meaning "uncut or indivisible," being derived from *a-*, "without," + *temnein*, "to cut." The idea that all matter is composed of particles was accepted by ancient philosophers. The ultimate particle that could not be further divided or cut was the *atomos*. Only in relatively recent times did it become apparent that even the atom was made up of constituent parts, the nature of which remains an active field of investigation.

atopy is a near borrowing of the Greek *atopos*, "out of place." This, in turn is a combination of *a-* as a negative + *topos*, "place." An atopic reaction, such as an allergic dermatitis is "out of place" in the sense of being unusual or affecting only a minority of the population. The basis for atopy is now known to be a peculiar immunopathy.

atresia is derived from the Greek *a-*, "without," + *trēsis*, "a hole." Thus, atresia is a condition wherein there is "no hole," i.e., there should be an opening but there is not. The term was first used in the 17th century. By "atresia" we now refer to a failure of a structure to become hollow or tubular, as in a congenital defect, or to the collapse of a structure once hollow. Atresia, either congenital or acquired, can result, for example, in obstruction of biliary ducts.

atrium was the Latin word for the open area in the center of a classic Roman house. The same word is used anatomically to describe the two smaller chambers of the heart, which consist of open spaces with recessed walls. The atria (Latin neuter plural) of the heart also have been called **auricles**, from the Latin *auricula*, "little ear," presumably because they resembled the floppy ears of a dog. Another quaint name for the inner recesses of the heart is "cockles," likening them to the bivalve mollusks of the family Cardiiae. This name customarily is used in a figurative sense for one's innermost feelings, as when one says, "It warms the cockles of my heart."

atrophy is a close approximation of the Greek *atrophia*, "a want or lack of nourishment," being a combination of *a-*, "without," + *trophē*, "nourishment." The ancient term was used to describe a condition or circumstance where nourishment was lacking for any reason. The modern medical use is to designate the consequence of that condition, as when we refer to atrophy of a muscle. Moreover, the sense of the term has been broadened to include the consequence of causes other than nutritional deficiency, as when we speak of muscular atrophy due to disuse.

atropine is named after Atropos, one of the trio of Fates, all daughters of Themis, who served as counsel to Zeus. According to Greek mythology, these three ladies spun the web of destiny for all mankind. Of the three, Atropos made the final and immutable decision. This explains the derivation of her name from *a-*, "no," + *tropos*, "turning [back]." Atropos usually was depicted as holding shears with which she cut the threads by which all human lives hang. The alkaloid atropine was obtained from a genus of plants well known to be poisonous (*see* **belladonna**). The drug in lethal doses also could sever the thread of life, and so it was named "atropine."

attenuate comes from the Latin verb *attenuare*, "to weaken or diminish." The double "t" is important because it indicates an additive rather than a negative prefix. The Latin verb was derived from *ad-*, "toward," + the adjective *tenuis*, "being thin, delicate, or puny." An attenuated virus is one made weak or nonvirulent by various means.

auditory is from the Latin *audire*, "to hear or give attention to." This, in turn, is derived from the postulated Indo-European form *awēi*, "to become aware or to notice." The same form, through Anglo-French, is heard in the bailiff's cry "Oyez! Oyez!" the call for attention in a courtroom. The auditory or eighth cranial nerve is the pathway by which the sense of sound is conveyed from the ear to the brain.

aura is the Latin word meaning "a breeze, a wind, or an atmosphere." This, in turn, is related to the Greek *aēr*, "breath." Now the word is used both in the sense of a premonitory sign (as a quickening breeze might signal a change in weather) and in the sense of a surrounding evidence (as an atmosphere).

auricle is from the Latin *auricula*, the diminutive of *auris*, "the ear." The external portion of the ear or pinna was given this name because it is only a small part of the ear, the main structure being inside the head. "Auricle" also is used as a name for the floppy appendage of the cardiac atrium, presumably because it looks like a little ear.

auscultation comes from the Latin *auscultare*, "to listen keenly." The Latin word also carried the connotation of obedience to what was heard. Therefore, when we perform auscultation in the course of physical examination, we are obliged to both listen intently and heed what we hear.

autochthonous comes from the Greek *autochthōn* meaning "of the land itself," being derived from *auto*, "self," + *chthōn*, "the earth." Thus, to the Greeks an *autochthōn* was an aboriginal inhabitant. In pathology, whatever is autochthonous is found in that part of the body where it originates, as, for example, an autochthonous neoplasm.

autoclave is a hybrid word contrived from the Greek *auto*, "self," + the Latin *clavis*, "key." The original device was a pressure cooker so constructed that the generated steam tightened the lid. In other words, the autoclave was "self-locking." The term now is used for the chamber in which instruments are sterilized by heat.

autocrine (*see* **paracrine**)

autogenous comes from the Greek *auto*, "self," + *gennan*, "to produce." The term, then, means "self-produced." An autogenous vaccine is produced by using bacteria from the patient for whom the vaccine is being specifically prepared.

autonomic is a combination of the Greek *auto*, "self," + *nōmos*, "law." Accordingly, whatever is autonomic is "a law unto itself." When the concept of the autonomic nervous system was introduced in the early 19th century, it was thought the system was self-controlled and not under the governance of higher centers in the brain. This is no longer held to be true.

autopsy is a misapplied term when used to refer to a postmortem examination. The Greek *autopsia* (derived from *auto*, "self," + *opsis*, "seeing") meant, in fact, "seeing for oneself." According to Professor Alexander Gode (*JAMA.* 1965;191:121) this, for the Greeks, had an even more mystical meaning in the sense of "a contemplative state preceding the vision of God." Galen used *autopsia* to mean "personal inspection." Possibly from this sense came the application of "autopsy," in the early 19th century, to designate a dissection of a corpse, especially with a view to establishing the cause of death. Nevertheless, "autopsy" has little but currency to recommend its use and, if "postmortem examination" is too cumbersome, **necropsy** (Greek *nekros*, "corpse") is the preferred term.

average is not strictly a medical term but often is used in scientific computation to denote the arithmetic mean. The word has a French ring to it and, indeed, it came from the Old French *avarie*. Curiously, *avarie* meant "damage in shipping," and can be traced back to the Arabic *awariyah*, "damaged goods," the Arabic *awar* meaning "blemish." "Average" was first recorded in English about 1500 as a maritime term referring to any expense incurred by loss from damage to goods during transit. Such expense was usually borne evenly among the various parties in the venture. Hence, "average" conveyed the idea of "divided equally."

avulsion comes from the Latin *avulsus*, the past participle of *avellere*, "to pluck, to pull away, to tear off." This, in turn, is a combination of *ab-*, "away," + *vellere*, "to pull." An avulsed nerve is one that is torn away from its supporting structures, as by injury.

axilla is borrowed directly from the Latin. To the Romans, as to us, the axilla was the armpit. Its more remote derivation is uncertain. Axilla may be an abbreviated combination of *axis alae*, "the axle or pole of the wing."

axis is the name of the second cervical vertebra, presumably because the uppermost cervical vertebra (the **atlas**) rotates around the odontoid process of the one below it. The Latin *àxis* means "axle or pole" and is related to the Greek *axōn*, "axis," and can be traced to the Indo-European *ag*, "to move." Axial refers to whatever is located on, around, or in the direction of an axis. Computed axial tomography (better known as **CAT-** or **CT-scanning**; the latter term is preferred by most radiologists, leaving the former to veterinarians) produces images of transverse sections oriented in series along the long axis of the body.

axone is an almost direct borrowing of the Greek *axōn*, "axle." The conducting core of a nerve fiber, encased in a tubular sheath, is the axis of the structure.

azo- is a prefix denoting the presence of nitrogen. Thus, **azotemia** is "nitrogen in the blood" (*see* **nitrogen**). The prefix comes from *azote*, the name given to the newly discovered element by Antoine Laurent Lavoisier (1743-1794), the pioneering French chemist. The story is that Lavoisier placed a lighted candle and a live mouse in a sealed jar. When the candle was extinguished, its flame having consumed all the oxygen, the mouse, too, soon expired. Lavoisier knew that gas remained in the jar and observed that this gas was incapable of supporting life. Thereupon he called the gas *azote*, contriving the name from the Greek *a-*, "without," + *zōē*, "life." Lavoisier was a little off the mark. The Greeks previously had a word *azōtus*, but it meant "ungirt." In this instance, it appears that Lavoisier was caught with his classical pants down.

azygos is the name given by Galen (A.D. 131-201) to the unpaired vein traversing the right thorax. The Greek *azygos* means "unyoked" or "not a pair," and comes from *a-*, "without," + *zygon*, "a yoke."

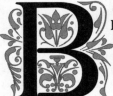**B**acillus is from the Latin *bacillum*, "a small staff or wand," this being the diminutive of *baculum*, "a rod or scepter." The allusion is to the rodlike shape of certain bacteria. When first introduced in microbiology, the term was restricted to straight "little rods," in distinction to **vibrio**, which are wavy forms.

bacitracin is an antibiotic substance produced by the Tracy I strain of *Bacillus subtilis*, an aerobic, gram-positive, sporulating bacillus isolated in 1943 from the contaminated wound at the site of a compound fracture sustained by a young girl named Margaret Tracy (*Science*. 1945;102:376).

bacteria is a neo-Latinized version (in the neuter plural; singular, **bacterium**) of the Greek *bakterion*, "a small rod or staff." In 1853 Ferdinand Cohn (1828-1898), a German botanist, categorized microorganisms as bacteria (short rods), bacilli (longer rods), and spirilla (spiral forms).

bacteriophage (*see* **phage**)

bagassosis is a respiratory disorder caused by inhalation, by susceptible persons, of the dust of *bagasse* (a French word), the husks of sugar cane discarded after the sugar has been extracted. Acute asthmatic bronchitis and even chronic pulmonary fibrosis are hypersensitivity reactions to a fungus (*Thermoactinomyces saccharii*) that lurks in the husks. This is only one of an array of similar occupational hazards, among which are farmer's lung, maple bark stripper's lung, malt worker's lung, and paprika splitter's lung, to name a few.

BAL are the initials of "British anti*lewisite*," an antidote developed during World War II to **lewisite**, a vesicant arsenical war gas concocted at the time of the preceding world conflict (1914-1918) by Winfred Lee Lewis (1878-1943), an American chemist. The antidote, more properly termed **dimercaprol** and evolved through intensive efforts by investigators at Oxford University, was shown to be a potent chelating agent that rendered arsenicals nontoxic. This would be of little more than historic interest were it not for the postwar discovery that dimercaprol was also effective in counteracting the toxic effect of other heavy metals, notably mercury.

balance is the term used for a laboratory scale. The word comes from the Latin *bis*, "twice," + *lanx* (plural *lancis*), "plate," i.e., a two-plate device for comparing known and unknown weights. "Scale" is derived from the Old Norse *skal*, "a bowl," which referred to the container on which objects were lifted for weighing.

balanitis is derived from the Greek *balanos*, "acorn." The Greek word was early used to describe various things that were thought to be shaped like an acorn, such as small pegs, suppositories, pessaries, and the glans penis. The last reference has persisted in balanitis, an inflammation of the glans penis.

ballotte comes through French from the Greek *ballein*, "to throw," and is used in the sense of tossing an object back and forth. In physical diagnosis, **ballottement** is the maneuver whereby a solid mass immersed in fluid, such as the liver in an ascitic abdomen, tends to bounce back when smartly tapped.

balm comes through the French *baume* as a contraction of the Latin *balsamun*, the name of a tree that yielded an aromatic resin that was made into a healing ointment. The Greek *balsamon* meant "a fragrant gum." Anything that soothes or mitigates pain can be used to excess, and perhaps someone sniffed balsamon for its mildly narcotic effect. Hence the word **balmy**, used to mean "silly or eccentric." **Canada balsam** is a resin obtained from the balsam fir and is used to mount sections on slides for microscopic examination. **Embalm** refers to the infusion of balsam by the ancient Egyptians to preserve dead bodies. Though the Egyptians didn't know it, the active ingredient was benzoic acid, and sodium benzoate is even now used as a preservative. Morticians still embalm, but what they now infuse is formalin.

bandage originated with the Indo-European *bhendh*, "to bind," and this led to the Anglo-Saxon *banda*. Through the French this became *bandage*, meaning "that which binds." A bandage to the Greeks was *desmos* and to the Romans, *fascia*.

barber comes from the Latin *barba*, "beard." To the Romans, a barber or shearer was a *tonsor*. From this comes "tonsorial parlor," a highfalutin name for a barbershop. The original barbers also were authorized to use their knife blades for the purpose of therapeutic bleeding, and those so skilled were known as "barber surgeons." Their symbol was a white staff, such as grasped by the patient to mitigate the ordeal; around this was draped the red, blood-stained bandage used to dress the wound. The staff was topped by a basin in which blood was collected. This became the familiar barber pole that still adorns many a barbershop.

barbiturate refers to a derivative of barbituric acid. The name *Barbitursäure* was given in 1863 by Adolf von Baeyer (1835-1917), a German chemist. According to a report collected by Professor H. A. Skinner, Baeyer's synthesis of the substance, from a combination of malonic acid and urea, was aided by the contribution of urine specimens from a Munich waitress named Barbara. If this sounds fanciful, it probably is. Later, "Veronal" was a name given to the hypnotic barbital, presumably in honor of the Italian city of Verona. Did those who bestowed the name remember that Verona was the setting for Shakespeare's *Romeo and Juliet* and the place where the hapless maiden quaffed her (supposedly) fatal sleeping potion?

barbotage refers to the technique in spinal anesthesia wherein a small volume of cerebrospinal fluid is withdrawn by needle from the subarachnoid space, mixed with an anesthetic agent, then reinjected. Occasionally, "barbotage" is used more generally to describe any aspiration and reinjection or flushing procedure, as in gastric lavage. The word is French and comes from *barboter*, "to dabble, as a duck in a pond."

baro- is a combining form derived from the Greek *baros*, "heavy." Barium ore was originally referred to as "heavy earth," and the element was discovered and named in 1808 by Sir Humphry Davy (1778-1829). The density or "heaviness" of barium is attested to by its widespread use, as barium sulfate, in contrast radiography of the gastrointestinal tract. **Hyperbaric** therapy entails use of a special chamber in which patients can be subjected to higher than normal atmospheric pressures or concentrations of oxygen, as used, for example, in the treatment of decompression sickness ("the bends") or carbon monoxide poisoning. The term **bends** is an allusion to the crouching posture assumed by those afflicted with the condition. **Bariatrics** (+ Greek *iatros*, "healing") is a branch of medicine that deals with the study of obesity, its causes, and treatment. **Barometer** (+ Greek *metron*, "measure") is the term for an instrument that measures the "weight" or pressure of atmospheric air.

base in chemistry refers to any substance that can be acted upon by acid to form a salt. More specifically, a base is a negatively charged ion whose donor electrons can bind covalently with a positively charged, acidic ion. The negatively charged ion, then, is the base on which the salt is built. The Greek *basis* is "a stepping," thus a foundation.

beaker is a cylindrical glass container with an open top and pouring spout, a familiar piece of equipment in every laboratory. The name can be traced to the Greek *bikos*, "an earthen wine vessel or jug," which in Vulgar Latin became *bicarium*, "a wine cup," and led to the Old English *biker*, which meant the same.

bedlam is a word describing a scene of confusion and uproar. It is a slurred contraction of Bethlehem, as in the name of the Hospital of Saint Mary of Bethlehem, formerly an asylum in southeast London for the incarceration of persons then called **lunatics**. The hospital was often frequented by onlookers in search of macabre entertainment.

belch (*see* **eructation**)

belladonna is an extract of the leaves and roots of the plant *Atropa belladonna*, sometimes called "deadly nightshade." The extract is capable of producing a potent anticholinergic effect, including dilatation of the pupils. *Belladonna* is Italian for "beautiful lady," and the story is that the drug was taken by ladies of high fashion to induce a limpid look that was deemed attractive. **Atropine**, the name given to a principal alkaloid of belladonna, also has a feminine connection in its derivation from Atropos, one of the trio of mythologic Fates.

belly is descended from an Old Norse word meaning "a bag or sack." The *Oxford English Dictionary* hints that its origin also may have been related to the notion that the belly was the container of the soul. "Bellyache" is used colloquially as both a noun and a verb. When used as a verb, it refers derisively to a common complaint of alleged malingerers. (*see* **abdomen**)

bends (*see* **baro-**)

benign is from the Latin adjective *benignus*, meaning "kind, affable, friendly, or favorable." This, in turn, was derived from a combination of the Latin *bene*, "well," + *[g]natus*, "to be born." A benign person, then, is kind and gentle, presumably because he is "well born." A benign neoplasm came to be thought of as relatively harmless because it was assumed to arise from "well" tissue. Of course, a benign tumor is not always of a favorable disposition.

benzoin is a balsamic resin obtained from certain trees of the genus *Styrax* that grow in the East Indies. It is used as an expectorant and, as the tincture, to make adhesive tape stick fast. Originally, the Arabic term was *luban jawi*, "gum or frankincense of Java." ("Frankincense," incidentally, is from a combination of the Old French *franc*, "superior," + *encens*, "incendiary," as a readily ignitable resin.) Westerners, when introduced to the term *luban jawi*, dropped the "lu," perhaps because they thought it was merely a grammatical article, and the name was further corrupted by the Venetians to *benzoino*. From benzoin was derived **benzoic acid**, the first of a long series of volatile chemical compounds. From benzoic acid, and later from coal tar, was distilled **benzene** (C_6H_6), a solvent of diverse uses. Benzene can be highly toxic, acutely to the central nervous system and chronically to bone marrow. Benzene is not to be confused with **benzine**, a petroleum distillate comprising various mixtures of hexane and heptane. Benzene and benzine do not represent alternative spellings.

beriberi is the Singhalese word for "weak," the duplication being commonly used in Eastern languages for intensification or emphasis. The affliction, now recognized as a polyneuropathy, was endemic in the Far East and resulted from a diet too severely limited to polished rice. Beriberi might be considered a "disease of progress." It was unknown until the invention of a steam-powered mill for the thorough polishing of rice. Now we recognize the deficiency to be mainly that of vitamin B_1. (*see* **thiamine**)

bezoar is derived from the medieval Arabic *badizhar*, which, in turn, comes from the ancient Persian *podzahr*, the name given to the hairball extracted from the rectum of a wild Asiatic mountain goat. The hairball was said to have been prized for its magical efficacy as a universal antidote. Indigestible agglomerations of hair that accumulate in the digestive tract, usually in demented persons who pluck and swallow their own hair, are known specifically as **trichobezoars**, the prefix being the Greek for "hair." Those concretions composed of indigestible plant fibers, such as those from persimmons, are **phytobezoars**, the prefix being the Greek for "plant."

biceps is a Latin word meaning "two-headed" and is derived from *bis-*, "double," + *caput*, "head." Anatomically, the biceps is a muscle with two "heads" of origin. The biceps brachii is in the upper arm; the biceps femoris is in the thigh. Biceps, despite its terminal "s," is singular; there is no such thing as a bicep.

bicuspid refers to a tooth with two cusps or a valve with two leaves. The word comes from the Latin *bis-*, "double," + *cuspis*, "point of a spear." (*see* **cusp**)

bifid is a near borrowing of the Latin *bifidus*, "forked, cloven, or split in two," which, in turn, was derived from *bis-*, "double," + *findere*, "to split."

bifurcate is from the Latin adjective *bifurcus*, "double pronged," being derived from a combination of *bis-*, "double," + *furca*, "fork." The term often is applied to vessels or nerves that divide in their courses. Incidentally, the fork as an eating tool is a relatively recent utensil, when compared with the spoon and knife. The Romans used *furcae* more often to support vines or as yokes applied to the necks of slaves.

bigeminal refers to a cardiac rhythm wherein

heartbeats occur in series of two. The word comes from the Latin bis-, "double," + geminare, "to repeat." Also, in Latin a geminus is a twin and, in the plural, gemini are twins (see **trigeminy**). The Gemini are among the signs of the zodiac (from the Greek zōdiakos, "of or pertaining to animals"). Formerly, it was common to swear "by the Gemini," hence the old expletive "By jiminy!" (though another possible source is Jesu Domini, "Lord Jesus").

bile comes from the Latin bilis, which means "gall or bile" and also "wrath or anger." To the Romans, bilis accounted for two of the four "humors" of the body: yellow bile, black bile, blood, and phlegm. Bilis is said to have been derived from a combination of bis-, "double," + lis, "contention," the idea presumably being that there are two forms of bile that are responsible for two types of temperament. The reason for this may have been the observation of thin, yellow bile emanating directly from the liver, while a more viscid, darker bile was found to be stored in the gallbladder. This had its more modern counterpart in the "A" and "B" bile described by B. B. Vincent Lyon (1880-1953), a Philadelphia gastroenterologist who analyzed bile, obtained by duodenal intubation, for evidence of biliary tract disease. Lyon's "A" bile was thin and yellow; "B" bile, obtained after the gallbladder had been stimulated to contract, appeared darker and more viscid. The purpose was to search extracted bile microscopically for evidence of cholesterol crystals or calcium bilirubinate pigment as a sign of actual or potential stone formation. Today, this would be regarded as a mark of "lithogenic bile."

bilirubin is derived from the Latin bili-, "bile," + ruber, "red." The purpose of the term, apparently, was to distinguish bilirubin from what were thought to be other forms, namely, **biliflavin** (Latin flavus, "yellow") and **biliverdin** (French verd, from the Latin viridis, "green"). When the chemistry of bile was later adduced, there was no need for two words to describe the principal pigment of bile, which, although yellow, was called bilirubin. Biliflavin was abandoned. Biliverdin remains as the designation of dehydrobilirubin or oxidized bilirubin.

biology is from the Greek bios, "life," + logos, "word, reason, or study." The word is of surprisingly recent origin. Such a combined term was not used by the Greeks or, apparently, by anyone else until Ludolf Christian Treviranus (1779-1865), a professor of botany at Bonn, Germany, published his Biology, the Philosophy of Living Nature in 1802. From time immemorial, sages devoted a great deal of study to life and living things, but to them this was "natural philosophy."

biopsy is derived from the Greek bios, "life," + opsis, "vision," thus literally the "viewing of live matter," as in the examination of a tissue specimen obtained from a living organism. This is in distinction to **necropsy**, a "viewing of the dead." In common parlance, "biopsy" is used to refer both to the procedure and to the specimen thus obtained and examined. Only the former is correct, but the latter use probably will gain legitimacy by currency.

bismuth in German is Wismuth which, it has been suggested, relates to the German Wiese, "meadow," combined with Mut, "spirit." The allusion is to the occurrence of bismuth ore in mines as an excrescence or "flowering." There is a contrived New Latin term bisemutum, but this is a 16th century attempt at scholarly transliteration of the German.

black plague (see **plague**)

bladder is said to have originated with the postulated Indo-European root bhel, "blade, bloom, or sprout." This led to the Anglo-Saxon blaedre, "blister," meaning a watery swelling that sprouts from the skin. Thus, blister, bleb, and bladder seem to have a common source.

blast- as a combining form also seems to have originated with the postulated Indo-European root bhel, "blade, bloom, or sprout." This led to the Greek blastos, "germ or offspring." In embryology, the **blastoderm** is the initial mass of cells produced by cleavage of a fertilized ovum. When used as a suffix, "-blast" refers to a primitive cell type from which emerge more highly differentiated cells, as in **myeloblast**. A **blastoma** is a tumor resulting from the "sprouting" of primitive cells.

blephar- is a combining form from the Greek blepharon, "eyelid." Thus, **blepharitis** is an inflammation of the eyelid, and **blephar plasty** is a repair or refashioning of the eyelid.

blood is another word said to have originated with the postulated Indo-European root *bhel*, "bloom or sprout," though the connection is less than certain. It is conceivable that ancient people looked upon the effusion from incised skin as a sort of "blooming." The Old English word was *blōd*, pronounced to rhyme with "food." In the early 16th century the vowel sound was shortened to rhyme with "good," and only later did the spelling change to "blood," the pronunciation coming to rhyme with "flood." A person presumed to be of aristocratic pedigree is sometimes called "a blueblood," despite the fact that his actual blood is as red as anyone else's. Aristocratic Castilians prided themselves on their lineage, in proof of which they pointed to the veins of their arms and hands which, under fair and fine skin, appeared blue. This was in contrast to the venous pattern apparent in persons of supposedly lesser rank whose antecedents had mated with dark-skinned Moors. The Spanish *sangre azul* was, then, taken as evidence of noble birth.

boil as a term for a focal suppurative swelling in the skin is said to have originated with the Gothic *uf-bauljan*, "to blow up." The Old English word was *byl*, and in some archaic dialects "boil" is still pronounced as "bile."

borborygmus is an almost direct borrowing of the word that meant to the Greeks what it means to us: "gut rumbling or growling bowels." The inference that it is a classic example of onomatopoeia, as an echoic word, is inescapable.

bosom (*see* **breast**)

botulism comes from the Latin *botulus*, "sausage." The term refers to a toxic condition first observed in 19th-century Germany and immediately attributed to the eating of contaminated sausage. The poisonous substance was first called "botuline," that is, a derivative of sausage. Not until the end of the century was a bacterial source identified and named *Bacillus botulinus*.

bougie is a direct borrowing of the French word for "taper or candle" and refers in surgery to an instrument used to dilate orifices. The idea is not that candles were used as dilators (though this is possible) but rather that dilators were shaped like candles, being smaller at the tip than at the base. The adjective "tapered" conveys this sense. The French *bougie* was taken from Bejaia, the name of an Algerian port town, long the center of the wax trade and a source of quality candles.

bowel originated with the Latin *botulus*, "sausage," which in Vulgar Latin became *botellus*. This was shortened in French to *boel* and became *bouele* in Middle English. The external appearance of the intestine, indeed, suggests that of a sausage. The fact that sausages were originally encased in segments of animal bowel, usually that of sheep, is merely incidental. The Romans had a perfectly proper name for the bowel, *intestina*.

bowleg (*see* **valgus**)

brachy- is a combining form taken from the Greek *brachys*, "short." **Brachydactylia** (+ Greek *daktylos*, "finger") is an abnormal stubbiness of the fingers and toes. **Brachygnathia** (+ Greek *gnathos*, "jaw") is evident as a pronounced recession of the mandible. "Brachy-" is not to be confused with **brachial** as a reference to the arm or with **brady-**.

brady- is a combining form taken from the Greek *bradys*, "slow."

bradycardia is a slower than normal rate of heartbeat (brady- + Greek *kardia*, "heart").

bradykinin was discovered as a substance resulting from the action of snake venom on plasma globulin. When injected into experimental animals, the substance caused lowering of blood pressure and slowly developing contraction of the gut. Because of this slow response by the gut, Rocha de Silva and his associates (*Am J Physiol.* 1949;156:261) named the substance bradykinin (brady- + Greek *kinein*, "to move"), now known to be a polypeptide.

bradyphrenia is a condition marked by excessive fatigability of mental and psychomotor action (brady- + Greek *phrēn*, "mind"), such as seen in cases of epidemic encephalitis.

brain is said to have its origin in the Old Teutonic root *bragno[m]*, leading to the Old English *braeg[e]n*. Although this may have a tenuous relation to the Greek *bregma*, "the top of the head," it should come as no surprise that there is no classical term, handed down through the ages, for the brain as an organ. The ancients had only a vague and uncertain concept of the brain's function. Oddly, they tended to place the seat of emotions in more mundane structures, such as the kidneys, spleen, and liver.

breast is a distant relative of the Middle High German *bruistern*, which meant "to swell up." Similarly, **bosom** is attributed to the Sanskrit *bhasman*, "blowing, as a bellows." **Buxom**, on the other hand, was once spelled "bughsom," derived from the Old English *būgan*, which meant "to bow or bend." Hence, in the old days, a "buxom bride" was much admired as one who gave promise of being pliant and obedient. Later, the meaning changed to approach that of "blithe" and still later to "full of health and vigor." To have arrived at its present meaning, buxom must have suggested to someone that generously proportioned female breasts connote vim and vitality.

bronchiectasis (*see* **ectasia**)

bronchus is a dissimulated borrowing of the Greek *bro[n]gchos*, by which the ancient Greeks referred to conduits of the lung. This may, in turn, have been derived from the Greek *brechein*, "to be moistened," in the sense that the bronchial lining is always moist.

brucellosis is a disease named after Sir David Bruce (1855-1931), an English army surgeon who identified the cause of undulant, or Malta, fever in 1887. Bruce found the infecting bacteria, *Bacillus melitensis* (the latter term being Latin for "Maltese"), in the spleens of British soldiers who died of undulant fever on the Mediterranean island of Malta. The stricken soldiers had contracted the disease by drinking contaminated goat's milk.

bruise comes from the Old French *bruiser*, "to break, smash, or shatter." When we refer to a hefty hulk of a fellow capable of "taking the place apart" as a "bruiser," we are using the term in the original sense.

bruit comes through the French from the Latin *brugitus*, "a rumbling." This, in turn, may have been derived from the Latin *rugire*, "to roar." The *Oxford English Dictionary* suggests that the initial "b" may have been added for an echoic effect.

bruxism is a classical term for gnashing the teeth and is derived from the Greek *brychein*, "to grind or gnash the opposing rows of upper and lower molar teeth." **Gnash** is of Old Norse descent and probably began as an imitative sound. Habitual bruxism or gnashing of the teeth can cause dental damage and may contribute to the temporomandibular joint syndrome.

bubo comes from the Greek *boubon*, which was variously used to refer to the groin or to swelling in the groin. An association between pestilential fever and glandular swelling in the groin was recognized as early as the 1st century A.D. Reaching an epidemic scale and more than decimating the population of Europe in the Middle Ages, the disease became known as the **bubonic plague**. The causative organism was known as *Pasteurella pestis* until 1970; thereafter, it was classified as *Yersinia pestis,* commemorating its discovery in 1894 by Alexander Yersin (1863-1943), a Swiss bacteriologist then working in Hong Kong. (*see* **plague**)

buccal, in reference to the inside of the cheek, is said to have originated in the Hebrew *bukkah*, "empty, hollow." The Latin *bucca* means "cheek" and also "a loudmouthed person." We still use "cheek" to describe a person who exhibits undue arrogance. The homonym, "buckle," first meant the fastening of a helmet's chin strap lying along the cheek. The Latin *buccina* (from the Greek *bukanē*) means "trumpet." The **buccinator** muscle gives tonus to the wall of the cheek and is essential to blowing a horn. However, a buccaneer, though he may be a bold fellow with "cheek," takes his name from the French *boucanier*, originally "one who grills meat on a frame," a practice first observed among natives of the West Indies who were suspected of cannibalism and later adopted by seafarers who were more than suspected of piracy. The popular meaning of the French *boucan* is "rowdy."

buffer as a term for any substance in solution that serves to maintain a given pH when an acid or alkali is introduced is said to have originated indirectly, about the turn of the century, from the writings of Søreh P. L. Sorenson (1869-1939), a Danish chemist.

Actually, Sorenson wrote in French and used the word **tampon**, which can refer to either a plug or a pad. This was translated through the German into English as "buffer," in the sense of "warding off a blow."

bulimia means "excessive or exaggerated appetite." The word comes from the Greek *bous*, "ox," + *limos*, "hunger." The Greeks often used an allusion to the ox to describe whatever was huge or monstrous. In this same manner we allude to the horse in our use of "horseradish" or "horselaugh." At the risk of mixing our animals, we might say that bulimia results in "eating like a horse."

bulla in Latin was "a bubble, stud, or knob," hence any rounded protrusion, particularly that which was hollow or cystic. The **ethmoid bulla** is a rounded protrusion of the ethmoid bone into the lateral wall of the nasal cavity, enclosing an air cell or sinus. Also, blisters on the skin or blebs on the pleura are called bullae.

bunghole is a vulgar term for the anus. The same word more properly refers to the small opening in the cover through which a cask or barrel is filled or emptied. The "bung" was the stopper by which the hole was plugged.

bunion comes from the Italian *bugnone*, "a lump." This, in turn, is probably derived from the Greek *bounos*, "hill or mound," which may be of Cyreniac origin. (*see* **hallux**; *also* **valgus**)

burking is an eponymic addition to the English language, seldom used today but nevertheless of interest to medical students. As the study of human anatomy became widespread and essential to the instruction of doctors-to-be, cadavers became increasingly difficult to procure. With no legal provision for dissectable subjects, the practice of body snatching and grave robbing flourished. Two proficient procurers in Edinburgh were named Burke and Hare. When corpses were in short supply, Burke undertook to ignore the distinction between the quick and the dead by murdering those poor persons assayed to be worth more dead than alive. Robert Knox, then professor of anatomy at Edinburgh, made insufficient inquiry into the provenance of specimens delivered to him and became an innocent victim of these nefarious acts which, when discovered, ended the careers of Burke, Hare, and Knox. Meanwhile, the practice had become a cause for concern throughout Britain and came to be called "burking." The wicked business ended when the procurement of legitimately dead bodies for dissection was legalized by Warburton's Anatomy Act of 1832.

burp (*see* **eructation**)

bursa is a direct borrowing of the Medieval Latin word for "bag or purse." This came from the Greek *bursa*, "a hide or wineskin." In medical parlance, a bursa is a sacklike structure containing a viscid fluid that serves as a shock absorber and lubricant for bony joints. The English word **bursar** is similarly derived and designates "the one who holds the purse."

buttock refers to one of the two gluteal prominences of man or animals and is a diminutive of butt, meaning the thick stump or end of anything. In Old English, -ock was a diminutive suffix, as in "bullock," meaning "a small bull," or "hillock," meaning "a small hill."

butyric is from the Greek *bouturos*, "butter," which, in turn, was derived from a combination of *bous*, "ox," + *turos*, "cheese." It happens that cheese was known before butter, and the Romans considered butter useful as a salve or source of oil for lamps but not as a food. Butyric acid was originally discovered in rancid butter.

buxom (*see* **breast**)

**achexia** is from the Greek *kakos*, "bad," + *hexis*, "condition or state." Cachexia describes the grossly debilitated condition of a patient with advanced disease or malnutrition. Such a patient is, indeed, in a bad state.

cadaver is a direct borrowing of the Latin for "corpse" and, in turn, is derived from the Latin *cadere*, "to fall, perish, be slain, or be sacrificed." A cadaver, obviously, is the body of a person who has perished. But why, then, are not all dead bodies so called—why are only the bodies used for anatomic dissection called cadavers? Perhaps the answers lie in the Latin sense of "to fall, to be sacrificed." Often, though not always, the body laid on the dissecting table is that of an unfortunate person who has "fallen" in life's struggle and at whose death the mortal remains are unclaimed and unburied, and hence deemed suited for "sacrifice" to the learning of medical students.

caduceus is a winged rod adorned by two serpents entwined in a double-helix array. As such, it became the symbol of Mercury, the swift messenger of the gods and, in his own right, the god of science and commerce. Also, Mercury was the patron of travelers, rogues, vagabonds, and thieves. By some misconception, the caduceus became the insignia of the U.S. Army Medical Corps. The proper symbol of medicine is the staff of Aesculapius, which is a coarse rod entwined by a single serpent. Why the serpent? To the ancients, the serpent embodied renewal of youth and health because it periodically shed its skin and emerged to all appearances as a transformed creature. For a further exposition, the interested reader is referred to W. J. Friedlander's *The Golden Wand of Medicine, a History of the Caduceus Symbol in Medicine* (New York, The Greenwood Press; 1992).

caesarean section (*see* **cesarean section**)

café au lait is French for "coffee mixed with warm milk." In medicine the phrase is used to describe the light brown color of circumscribed areas of melanin pigment in the skin that, in some cases, may be evidence of a neurofibromatosis syndrome.

caffeine is an alkaloid present in coffee, tea, cola, cocoa, and other beverages. The term is from the French *café*, "coffee," to which the suffix "-ine" was added to indicate a derivative thereof. "Coffee," in turn, is said to have originated in the Arabic *qahwah*, pronounced in Turkish as "kahveh." It has been further suggested that the root word was the Arabic *qahiya*, "to have no appetite," the inference being that the beverage was thought to be a remedy for a lack of appetite. (*see* **coca-**; *also* **theophylline**)

-caine (*see* **coca**)

calamine is a preparation of zinc oxide with just a dash of ferric oxide that is usually put up as a lotion and used as a topical astringent and mildly antiseptic agent. In the ancient world, zinc ores were known as *lapis calaminarus,* an alliterative rendition of "stone of Cadmus." The ore was first found near Thebes, the city supposedly founded by the legendary Cadmus who, incidentally, is reputed to have brought from Phoenicia the basis for the original Greek alphabet. In Greek the ore was called *kadmeia*, "earth," whence "cadmium."

calcaneus is a name for the heel bone (also called **os calcis**) and comes from the Latin *calx*, "limestone." This, in turn, is related to the Greek *chalix*, "gravel or cement," and to the Arabic *kalah*, "to burn." Lime (calcium oxide) is formed by heating limestone (calcium carbonate). Actually, calcaneus came not from the classical Latin but from the Late Latin of monkish scribes. Apparently, something about the heel bone suggested a lump of chalk, which comes from the same source as **calcium**.

calculus in Latin means "a pebble," presumably being the diminutive of *calx*, "limestone." Pebblelike stones forming in the biliary or urinary tracts were and are quite naturally referred to as "calculi," even when their content is other than calcium. Because pebbles were used in counting at one time, we now have our verb "calculate" and its various derivatives, including "calculus" as the name for that branch of mathematics employing highly systematized algebraic notations.

calf as a term referring to the rounded, muscular back of the lower leg comes from the Anglo-Saxon *cwealf*, which meant the same and is postulated to have originated in the Indo-European *gelbh*, "to bunch up." When the muscles extending the foot contract, they appear to "bunch up." Incidentally, a quite distinct root word *guelbh*, "womb" (and later, "cub"), is said to have led to the Anglo-Saxon *cealf*, meaning the offspring of an animal, especially a cow.

calisthenics (sometimes spelled with two "l"s) are being prescribed more often these days and, presumably, for what was intended when the word was introduced in the mid-19th century, viz., physical exercises conducted in girls' boarding schools. The word was concocted by combining the Greek *kallos*, "beauty," + *sthenos*, "strength."

calix is Latin for "cup or pot," being related to the Greek *kylix* which means the same. This is not quite the same as the Latin *calyx*, from the Greek *kalyx*, "the covering of a bud or flower." However, in anatomic parlance, calix (plural **calices**) and **calyx** (plural **calyces**) are used more or less interchangeably when referring, for example, to the cup-shaped collecting system of the upper urinary tract.

callus is a near borrowing of the Latin *callum*, "thick skin," probably related to the Greek *kalon*, "dry or seasoned wood." (*see* **corpus**)

calm is an attitude often helpful in caring for the sick or injured. Oddly, our word "calm" originated in the Greek *kauma*, "a burning heat, as of the sun." This eventually became the Old French *calme* and had taken the meaning of "the time of day when the flocks (and presumably their shepherds) are at rest." Incidentally, the Spanish *siesta* comes from the Latin *sexta* and indicates "the 6th hour." This means noon and the time any sensible person takes a nap.

calorie is said to have its origin in the Indo-European root *kāl*, "gray, brown, or warm," whence the Latin *calere*, "to be warm." From this came the French *chaleur*, "heat," and then the English **nonchalant**, meaning "cool or not hot." Incidentally, the Latin *caldarius*,

"warm water," led to the French *chaudière*, "boiler," and to our "chowder." A French chauffeur was originally a stoker and only later a driver of a motorcar. A calorie (spelled with a lower case "c") is the French unit of heat and is defined as the amount of heat required to raise the temperature of 1 gram of water through 1° Celsius. The biomedical unit now in general use is the Calorie (with a capital "C"), also known as the **kilocalorie** (abbreviated kCal) which is 1000 times greater, i.e., the amount of heat required to raise the temperature of 1 kilogram of water by 1° Celsius.

calvarium comes directly from the Latin word for "a bald scalp" or "the dome of the skull." More familiar to lay persons is the name "Calvary," given to "the place of the skull" at the outskirts of Jerusalem where Jesus was crucified in the year that became A.D. 33. Another name for the same place is Golgotha, which is Aramaic and also means "skull."

calyx is an almost direct borrowing of the Greek word for the covering or cap of a bud or flower, being derived from the verb *kalyptein*, "to cover or conceal." This is the sense in which "calyx" is used in botany. Whether the calyx of the renal pelvis was fancied as a bud of a flower or represents a variant spelling of the Latin *calix* is uncertain.

campto-, campylo- are combining forms taken from the Greek *kamptēr*, "a bend or angle," and *kampylos*, "bent or curved." **Camptodactyly** (+ Greek *daktylos*, "finger") is a fixed flexion of one or more fingers. **Campylognathia** (+ Greek *gnathos*, "jaw") is a deformed lip or jaw. **Campylobacter** (+ Greek *baktērion*, "a little rod") is a genus of small, curved, gram-negative bacteria that only recently have been recognized to cause disease in man. A species so implicated is *Campylobacter fetus*, formerly known as *Vibrio fetus*, so named because the organism was earlier identified as a cause of abortion in cattle, sheep, and goats. The subspecies *jejuni* is occasionally found to cause enteritis. Another supposed subspecies, *Campylobacter pylori*, recently associated with chronic gastritis, has been found, on the basis of its genome, to be not a Campylobacter at all but has been assigned a new genus,

Helicobacter (Greek *helix*, "a spiral or coil").

canal comes from the Latin *canalis*, "a pipe, conduit, or gutter." A **canaliculus**, as the diminutive, is "a little conduit." Both terms have been applied in anatomy to a variety of pipelike structures.

cancellous refers to a latticelike configuration of bone and is a near borrowing of the Latin *cancellus*, "a grating or latticework." Incidentally, a canceled check or ticket is rendered nonnegotiable by inscribing scratch marks or making perforations, as a lattice.

cancer is taken directly from the Latin word for "crab." The ancients also used the word in reference to malignant tumors. The allusion, doubtless, was to the manner in which invasive neoplasms tenaciously grasped the tissues in which they grow. Also, Galen (A.D. 131-201) observed, "Just as a crab's feet extend from every part of the body, so in this disease the veins are distended, forming a similar figure." In Old English, any chronically inflamed unduration, particularly about the mouth, was called a *canker sore*, probably because the Latin word was pronounced "kanker." **Chancre**, as the French term for the lesion of primary syphilis, also was derived from the Latin *cancer*.

Candida albicans is a species of yeastlike fungus that can infect human tissue. The disease it produces in the mouth or throat is known as **thrush** (a term of obscure origin). The genus in which the fungus is classified was known formerly as *Monilia*, from the Latin *monile*, "necklace," perhaps because of its strandlike growth pattern. *Candida albicans* would seem a redundancy, inasmuch as *Candida* comes from the Latin *candidus*, "gleaming white," and *albicans* is from the Latin verb *albicare*, "to make white." An explanation might be that the growth of the fungus itself is white, and the infection produces a characteristically white, gelatinous exudate on mucosa surfaces.

cannabis is both the Greek and the Latin word for "hemp." This word is related to *canna*, "a reed." Hemp (*Cannabis sativa*), a member of the mulberry family of plants, often grows in marshy areas and this, presumably, is its association with reeds. The tough fibers of the hemp stalk can be fashioned into rope or twine. A coarse fabric from this material was referred to as "cannabaceous," hence our word "canvas." It is said the dried flower clusters and leaves of the plant can be smoked, as marijuana (the origin of this term is as elusive as the smoke). (*see* **hashish**)

cannula is the diminutive of the Latin *canna*, "a reed," and came to mean any slender, tubular instrument. The double "n" distinguishes this from "canal," though a cannula could be inserted in a canaliculus.

canthus is the Latin derivation of the Greek *kanthos*, "the corner of the eye," which is exactly what it means now. Because the Greek word also meant the iron binding of a cartwheel, it is likely that the ancients may have applied *kanthos* to the entire margin of the eyelid.

capillary comes from the Latin *capillus*, "a hair of the head," being derived from *caput*, "head," + *pilus*, "a hair." This use of "capillary" to designate an exceedingly fine tubular vessel was, of course, unknown to the ancients but has been attributed to Leonardo da Vinci in his 15th century writings, though its function as a connection between the arterial and venous channels was yet not understood. (*see* **hair**)

capsule is from the diminutive of the Latin *capsa*, "box," hence "a little box." In this sense, "capsule" can refer to any encompassing structure or to the small container used for a dose of medicament.

caput is the Latin word for "head, top, or summit." This, in turn, is related to the Greek *kara* and *kephalē*, having the same meaning. In anatomy the term is applied to anything having the shape or position of a head. **Caput Medusae** refers to a collection of dilated veins around the umbilicus, consequent to portal venous hypertension. The mythical Medusa was once a voluptuous maiden whose crowning glory was her blond tresses. By captivating Neptune Medusa incurred the wrath of Minerva who, in a rage, turned Medusa's hair into writhing serpents and transfigured the poor girl into a hideous Gorgan. So frightful was the sight of the transformed Medusa that whoever looked on her was turned into stone. It was the heroic Perseus who succeeded in beheading Medusa, whereupon he presented the trophy to Minerva, who emblazoned the figure of Medusa's head on her breastplate.

carbohydrate is a hybrid term combining the Latin *carbo*, "charcoal," and the Greek *hydor*, "water," thus designating substances composed of carbon, hydrogen, and oxygen (the last two in the proportion found in water).

carbuncle is the diminutive of the Latin *carbo*, "coal or charcoal." The allusion is to "a little, live coal." To the Romans, *carbunculus* referred to the red gemstone garnet. For a focal, inflamed swelling in the skin and subcutaneous tissue to be called "a carbuncle" seems natural. Interestingly, **anthrax**, producing a similar lesion, is so called from the Greek word for coal.

carcinoid tumors, found usually in the gastrointestinal tract but occasionally elsewhere, are so called because, when first described in the early 19th century, they appeared to resemble cancerous neoplasms but were thought benign in their limited growth and lack of adverse effects. Hence, the name was contrived by combining "carcin-" (from "carcinoma") + "-oid" (from the Greek *eidos*, "like"). However, in 1954 Jan Waldenström and his Swedish colleagues, among others, demonstrated a peculiar syndrome of cutaneous flushing and endocardial lesions in patients whose carcinoid tumors had metastasized from the small intestine to the liver. Such tumors were found to secrete toxic amounts of serotonin and various vasoactive peptides.

carcinoma is supposed to have originated with the Indo-European root *kar, karkar*, "hard." From this came the Greek *karkinos*, "crab," presumably because of the crustacean's hard shell. In Hippocratic writings, *karkinos* is used to refer to any firmly indurated, nonhealing ulcer, whereas *karkinōma* (the suffix designating "a swelling") indicated a malignant tumor. Not until the 19th century was "carcinoma" restricted to malignant neoplasms of epithelial origin.

cardiac is said to be traceable to the Indo-European root *kered*, which meant "heart," as does the Greek *kardia* in Hippocratic treatises. The term also has been applied to structures near the heart, especially the most proximal portion of the stomach at its junction with the esophagus. In such usage the adjective "cardial" rather than "cardiac" would help avoid confusion.

cardinal has come to be an adjective that describes anything of prime importance. In medical diagnosis, reference is made to "cardinal" symptoms or signs. The Latin *cardo* means "a hinge" and *cardinalis* is "whatever pertains to a hinge." This was also taken to mean "that which something hinges upon," hence important. "Cardinal" also is the title given to a prelate of the Roman Catholic church whose eminence is second only to that of the Pope. From the brilliant red vestments worn by these high church officials comes the use of "cardinal" as a color and, in turn, as the popular name of our North American finch whose plumage is of that brilliant color.

caries is the Latin word for "decay or rot" and has been applied to such foci in teeth and bones. We can be grateful for the term. One would prefer to avoid dental caries, but to have "tooth rot" would be devastating.

carina is Latin for "keel of a boat" and has been borrowed by both plant and animal anatomists to refer to any projecting ridge. For example, the carina of the trachea is the semilunar ridge marking the bifurcation leading into the mainstem bronchi.

carminative refers to any medication given to allay indigestion, particularly that to relieve gas, belching, and flatulence. The newer physiology has validated the old empiric use of certain carminatives. For example, peppermint was long included in prescriptions for its carminative effect. Now it is known that peppermint tends to relax the lower esophageal sphincter, thus allowing eructation of troublesome stomach gas. The mints provided at the exit of a restaurant, therefore, serve a rational purpose, though it is unlikely the maître d' ever heard of the lower esophageal sphincter. The origin of "carminative" is uncertain. Some say it may have been derived from the Latin *carmen*, "a song, lyric poem, or ritual formula." Others contend it is more likely to have come from the Latin *carminare*, "to card wool," the allusion being to the effect of clearing out the adventitious substances causing dyspepsia.

carotid is taken from the Greek *karotides*, an ancient term for the principal arteries in the neck leading to the head. The Greek *karotikos* meant "stupefying," as apparently it was known that sustained pressure on the arteries of the neck caused insensibility. "To garrote," originally a Spanish technique for inflicting capital punishment by tightening an iron collar around the neck of the condemned, can be similarly traced to the Greek *karotikos*. On the other hand, "karate," a term for one of the martial arts, cannot. This comes from a Japanese word meaning "empty hands," thus signifying that in karate no weapon is used other than the bare hands.

carotid body (*see* **glomus**)

carpal is from the Greek *carpos*, "wrist." The Indo-European root has been postulated as *k[w]erp*, "to twist." For centuries, the eight carpal bones were only numbered; it was not until the early 18th century that they were given individual names. Generations of medical students have learned to recall these names by a mnemonic device: "Never (navicular) lower (lunate) Tillie's (triangular) pants (pisiform); Grandma (greater multangular) might (lesser multangular) come (capitate) home (hamate)."

carphology is not the study of anything, as the ending might suggest, but rather it is a condition wherein a gravely ill patient involuntarily picks at the bedclothes. Recognized since Galen's time as an ominous sign, the symptom was known to Shakespeare. In *Henry V* (Act II, scene iii) Mistress Quickly gives a knowing account of the death of Falstaff: "For after I saw him fumble with the sheets...I knew there was but one way." Carphology (which probably should be spelled "carpholegy" but isn't) is a combination of the Greek *karphos*, "dry twig," + *legein*, "to collect."

cartilage is from the Latin *cartilago*, "gristle." The Greek word for cartilage is *chondros*, and this provides **chondro-**, the usual combining form applied in anatomic terms to cartilaginous structures.

caruncle is a near borrowing of the Latin *caruncula*, the diminutive form of *caro*, "flesh." Hence, *caruncula* means, literally, "a little bit of flesh." The term is applied to various fleshy projections from mucous membranes. An example is the **lacrimal caruncle**, the small red body at the inner canthus of the eye.

cáscara sagrada is Spanish and means "sacred bark." In the usual English pronunciation, the accent is on the second syllable of "cascara," whereas in Spanish the accent is on the first syllable. The source of the substance is *Rhamnus purshiana*, better known as "the buckthorn tree." The tree was held sacred by the ancient Greeks for reasons that are not now clear. Not until the 13th century is there a record of an extract from the bark being used as a cathartic in Europe. The cathartic property comes from its content of anthraquinones.

casein comes from the Latin *caseus*, "cheese." Casein now refers to the protein of milk, a particularly valuable source of nourishment inasmuch as it contains all the essential amino acids. **Caseous** is an adjective that can describe anything of a cheesy consistency, as in "caseous tuberculosis."

castor oil formerly was called **oleum ricini**, and its active cathartic ingredient is now known as **ricinoleic acid**. The oil is expressed from the seeds of *Ricinus communis*, also known as "the castor bean" or "palma Christi," probably because the appearance of the bean was likened to the scarred palm of Christ. The Latin *ricinus* referred to "the sheep tick," and apparently the castor bean was thought to resemble this small creature. An explanation of "castor" is uncertain. It is not related to the Latin word for "beaver," and castor oil is not to be confused with **castoreum**, a substance obtained from certain glands of the beaver and used as a base for perfume. Rather, it has been suggested that "castor oil" was a confused expression of "Christi oil."

castrate comes from the Latin *castrare*, "to prune, to cut off," and specifically "to remove the testicles." Women are said to be castrated when the ovaries are removed. The Indo-European root word may have been *kes*, "a knife, or to cut."

catabolism is a borrowing of the Greek *katabolē*, "a throwing down." This, in turn, is a combination of *kata*, "down," + *ballein*, "to throw." Thus, catabolism is a throwing or tearing down of body tissue.

catacrotic (*see* **dicrotic**)

catalepsy is an almost direct borrowing of the Greek *katalēpsis*, which was used by Hippocrates to designate any abrupt seizure or sudden incapacitating sickness. The Greek word is derived from *kata*, "down," + *lambanein*, "to get hold of." The term is used now to indicate a state of unresponsive rigidity.

catalyst is from the Greek *katalysis*, "a dissolving," a word used by ancient writers in the sense of "dissolution or breaking down." The components of *katalysis* are *kata*, "down," + *lysis*, "a loosening or setting free." The term "catalyst" for a substance causing a chemical change but not in itself entering the reaction was proposed by Jons Jakob Berzelius (1779-1848), a Swedish chemist, in the early 19th century. The word has since also been used figuratively as a metaphor for whoever or whatever serves to expedite an action, as in "He was a catalyst for change."

catamnesis (*see* **mnemonic**)

cataract is probably from the Greek *kataraktēs*, "something that rushes down." This could apply to the rapid descent of water in a stream or to the dropping of a gate or window grating. In reference to an opacity in the ocular lens, the allusion presumably is to the closure of a window. Another explanation is that the term for the ocular lesion comes from the Greek *katarraptēs*, "to cover over by stitching or patching," and that "catarapt" was mistakenly converted to "cataract."

catarrh is from the Greek *katarroia*, "a running down." The Greek *katarrein*, "to flow down," combines *kata*, "down," + *rhein*, "to run or flow." The Greeks used *katarroia* to refer to any supposed humor that had formed in excess and was discharged by the body. Ordinary nasal catarrh or "runny nose" was attributed to a flow of fluid from the recesses of the head into the nose. "Catarrh" also was once used loosely to refer to any inflammation, especially that implying congestion. Infectious hepatitis was formerly called "catarrhal jaundice."

catatonia is a near borrowing of the Greek *katatonos*, "a stretching down," that combines *kata*, "down," + *tonus*, "that which tightens or stretches." Hippocrates is said to have used the verb *katateinein* in the sense of "to stretch for the purpose of setting a bone." The word now refers to a manifestation of schizophrenia wherein the patient exhibits a stubborn negativism, often with stuporous rigidity alternating with impulsive excitement.

catgut is a suture material that never was made from the gut of a cat. Rather, it originally was fabricated from the intestine of sheep. Why, then, the cat? Probably this was a transliteration of "kit," an old word for a fiddle, the strings of which were made from gut. "Kit," in turn, probably came to be used as a contraction of the Greek *kithara*, "a lyre, harp, or lute." From this also came the name of the familiar guitar.

catharsis is a direct borrowing of the Greek *katharsis*, "a cleansing." Originally, the term "cathartic" was applied to all medicines supposed to cleanse or purify, thus ridding the body of disease. Later it was restricted to purgative agents. The late Willard Espy observed that the given name Catharine is taken from the same Greek source, meaning "pure." His arch comment: "Whether you trace cathartic to Catharine or back to the original Greek depends, I suppose, on how, if a woman, you feel about yourself, or how, if a man, you feel about women."

catheter was used by the Greeks, as *kathetēr*, to refer to any instrument that was inserted for a purpose, such as a plug or pessary. The word came from the Greek *kathiemai*, "to send down or to sound," as a probe. The ancients used a hollow metal tube as a means of emptying the urinary bladder, and this tube they called a *kathetēr*.

cation (*see* **ion**)

Caucasian as sometimes used to designate a person whose skin appears white, or nearly so, has a curious origin. According to Professor Alexander Gode (*JAMA.* 1963;185:574), the association of "Caucasian" and "white" goes back to 1781 when a German anthropologist, Johann Friedrich Blumenbach (1752-1840), proposed on the basis of his craniometric researches a five-fold division of mankind into whites (Caucasians), blacks (Negroes), yellows (Mongols), browns (Malaysians), and reds (Amerindians). Blumenbach called the whites "Caucasians" because what he regarded as the ideal white man's skull was most nearly represented in his collection by a specimen from the southern Caucasus, a mountain range between the Caspian and Black Seas in the eastern portion of the Republic of Georgia. Even today all too often in case reports one finds a white man called "a Caucasian male." This is a pseudoscientific pomposity.

cauda is the Latin word for "tail." The **cauda equina** (Latin *equus*, "horse"), the array of sacral and coccygeal nerves emanating from the tapered end of the spinal cord, is so called because it resembles a horse's tail. The **caudate lobe** of the liver extends downward from the posterior surface as a sort of tail of the liver.

causalgia is a combination of the Greek *kausis*, "burning," + *algos*, "pain." The term refers to a burning pain, especially in an extremity, associated with atrophic skin changes owing to peripheral nerve injury.

caustic comes from the Greek *kaustikos*, "capable of burning," in the sense of whatever is capable of inducing a corrosive burn. Incidentally, the Latin *encaustium*, a term for the technique of fixing fast the wax colors in paintings, was shortened in Old French to *enque*, which then became the English "ink."

cautery comes from the Greek *kautērion*, "a branding iron," and, indeed, the focal application of heat, a sort of branding, is what we do today when we cauterize anything. In the past a distinction was made between "actual cautery" and "potential cautery." In actual cautery, searing heat was delivered to an area by an instrument made hot in a flame. A potential cautery was effected by a caustic substance that, when applied to a surface, produced coagulation by chemical reaction, often generating heat, and usually attended by a burning sensation.

cecum is spelled **caecum** by purists and is taken from the Latin *caecus*, "blind." It refers to the *cul de sac* (French for "bottom of the sack") of the proximal colon just below the entrance of the ileum. The cecal sac is "blind" in that its lumen leads nowhere. An earlier term for this appendage of the colon was the Greek *typhlos*, "blind," from *typhos*, "smoke," used in the sense of smoke obscuring vision or shutting out light. An old term for inflammation of the cecum was **typhlitis**; inflammation of the vermiform appendix was **perityphlitis**.

-cel- is a combining form that can be attributed to either of two Greek words which, while distinct, have somewhat related meanings: *kēlē*, "a rupture or hernia," and *koilos*,

"hollow, as a cavity." In the Anglicized forms, the "k" is made "c" (except in "keloid"), and the Greek *koil-* is usually spelled "coel-." Here is where the confusion begins. **Hydrocele** is sometimes misspelled "hydrocoele."

celiac, as it is usually spelled in American writings, actually comes from *koilos*, which is why purists insist on spelling it "coeliac," and they are right. Some people think it is a pedantic affectation to use "coel-" for "cel-," but there is more to it than that; these are different derivatives. The "celiac" artery and plexus are so named because they serve the contents of the abdominal cavity; thus, the spelling should be **coeliac**.

cell is from the Latin *cella*, its earliest meaning being "a place to hide and store grain, fruits, oil, or wine." The origin of our common word "cellar" is thus evident. Later, *cella* came to refer to any relatively small, confined space, and it is in this sense that it was applied to the basic organic unit of life that we recognize now as a cell.

cellulose is derived from *cellula*, "a little cell," perhaps in the sense of "a little part of a cell." This is the substance that forms the exoskeleton of plant cells.

centigrade is a French word derived from the Latin *centum*, "one hundred," + *gradus*, "a step or degree." In 1742 the Swedish scientist Anders Celsius (1701-1744) proposed an eminently sensible scheme of dividing the span in temperature from the freezing to boiling points of water into 100 degrees (0°-100°), thus providing a centigrade scale. It is only a coincidence that the initial "C," used to designate temperature readings from such a scale, stands for both "centigrade" and **Celsius** (who, of course, is not to be confused with Celsus, the renowned 1st century A.D. Roman encyclopedist). Thus, on the centigrade scale, the normal body temperature is 37°C, this having now supplanted the formerly familiar 98.6°F. The "F," as everyone knows, is the initial of Gabriel Daniel **Fahrenheit** (1686-1736), a German instrument maker who was born in the then-Prussian city of Danzig but lived most of his life in England and Holland. Fahrenheit is credited with making the first thermometer using mercury, rather than an alcohol-water mixture, as the fluid medium.

In calibrating his new thermometer, Fahrenheit set at 0° the temperature registered in a batch of saline and ice, presumably thinking nothing could be colder; he wished to avoid minus figures. He set the freezing point of pure water and ice at 32° and what he thought was the normal body temperature at 96° (a slight miscalculation). All of this seems arbitrary, but one must be mindful that Fahrenheit lived and worked before a decimal metric system was generally adopted. Fortunately, the centigrade or Celsius scale is now coming into almost universal medical use, although the laity in the United States insists on clinging to the Fahrenheit scale to indicate ambient temperatures.

centrifuge comes through the French from the Latin *centrum*, "center," + *fugere*, "to flee." **Centrifugal** refers to the motion of anything away from the center. Conversely, **centripetal** (Latin *petere*, "to seek") refers to the motion of anything toward the center.

cephalic comes from the Greek *kephalē*, "head." An exception in usage, however, is the "cephalic" vein, which courses along the outer aspect of the upper arm. In Arabic, according to Professor H. A. Skinner, this vein was called *al-kifal*, "the outer," and by mistaken translation this became "cephalic." This may have led to the erroneous notion that bleeding induced from the cephalic vein, a favorite procedure employed by barber surgeons, would draw blood from the head. Note that there is no corresponding cephalic artery (excepting, perhaps, the **brachiocephalic**, or innominate, artery, a trunk serving both the right arm and the head).

cerebellum is so called as the diminutive of the Latin *cerebrum*, "the brain." Hence, the cerebellum is "the little brain," which indeed it appears as it lurks beneath the posterior portion of the ponderous cerebrum. The distinctive function of the cerebellum in coordinating muscular action was not recognized until early in the 19th century.

cerebrum is the Latin word for "brain." The Romans used the same word variously to refer to the head, skull, understanding, and a hot temper.

ceruloplasmin is an alpha-2 globulin in serum that transports copper. The name is a hybrid concoction of the Latin *caerulus*, "azure," +

the Greek *plasma*, "anything molded, as a pervasive substance." The reference to a blue color relates to the reaction for copper in qualitative analysis. In another usage, the locus caerulus is a pigmented eminence ("blue spot") in the superior angle of the floor of the fourth ventricle.

cerumen is from the Latin *cera* and the Greek *keros*, both meaning "wax." But the Romans used no such word for the waxy accumulation in the external auditory canal. To them it was *sordes aurium*, "the dirt of the ear."

cervix is Latin for "neck," particularly the nape or back of the neck. In anatomy, "cervix" is used to describe the narrow or necklike portion of a structure, as in the uterine cervix. From the Latin noun comes the adjective **cervical**, which can describe anything pertaining to any sort of neck.

cesarean section (or **caesarean section**) is the procedure whereby an infant is removed from the uterus by incising the anterior abdominal wall of the mother. In ancient times this was regularly undertaken upon the death of a child-bearing woman near term. Julius Caesar, or more likely one of his antecedents, was said to have been born in this manner, hence the eponym.

cestode is from the Latin *cestus*, "girdle or belt." This, in turn, is said to have come from the Greek *kestos*, "stitched or embroidered," especially as a girdle might be so fabricated or decorated. In medicine, "cestode" refers to any tapeworm of the phylum Platyhelminthes (Greek *platy*, "flat," + *helmis*, "worm"). Such a long, flat worm made up of segmented proglotids might have been thought to resemble an embroidered belt.

chalazion is the diminutive of the Greek *chalaza*, which meant both "hail," referring to pellets of ice, and "a small pimple or tubercle." The relation between the two meanings is somewhat obscure. In any case, "chalazion" is now used as the term for an inflamed swelling of a Meibomian gland in the margin of the eyelid. The gland was so named after Heinrich Meibom (1638-1700), a German anatomist.

chancre is a French word meaning "ulcer," coming from the Latin *cancer*, "crab," probably because chronic ulcers often are hard and indurated like a crab's shell. In modern times, "chancre," both in French and in English, has come to refer to the venereal sore of primary syphilis. (*see* **cancer**)

chancroid is the lesion caused by infection with *Hemophilus ducreyii*. It somewhat resembles a chancre but was recognized as a different disease.

charlatan is a derogatory term applied to a physician or quasimedical practitioner held in disrepute because he makes claims for remedies that lack efficacy. The word is borrowed from the French, who adapted it, in turn, from the Italian *ciaclare*, meaning "to babble, to prattle, or to chatter." Thus, a charlatan is one who talks a good game but can't produce. The allusion is similar to that which gave rise to "quack."

charley horse is a term commonly used to describe pain and stiffness, usually in thigh muscles and especially that consequent to athletic stress. The explanation is said to be that Charley was the name customarily given to an elderly, often partially lame horse that was retired from more strenuous service and reserved for family use.

cheek is said to go back to the Anglo-Saxon *ce[a]ce*, "the jaw." Later, the Middle English *cheke* referred to the fleshy part of the jaw or jowl. Sometimes the fleshy roundness of the fundament is called "the cheek of the buttocks," but this is a long way from the jaw.

cheilosis (*see* **perleche**)

chelation is a chemical reaction whereby a metallic ion is sequestered and bonded firmly with at least two nonmetallic ions in the receptor molecule. The product is a highly stable heterocyclic ring compound, and the metal, so bound, is prevented from exerting any potentially deleterious effect. An example is ethylenediaminetetraacetic acid (EDTA), which has a marked avidity for calcium. Another example is penicillamine, an effective chelator of copper, mercury, and lead. The term is taken from the Greek *khēlē*, "claw."

chemo- is a combining form taken from the Late Greek *chemeia*, which had a meaning similar to "chemistry," albeit consonant with the primitive science then known to the ancients. The origin of the Greek word is obscure. Some authorities have contended that it relates to a similar word that was an arcane name for Egypt and also meant "black." It seems that conjuring chemical substances was early referred to as "the Egyptian or the black art." Passing into Arabic, the prefix "al-" was added, and the word became **alchemy**. Much of the medieval preoccupation with seeking a transmutation of base metals into gold was known by this term. After the 16th century, the "al-" was dropped. Modern chemistry is said to date from 1661 when Robert Boyle (1627-1691), an English natural philosopher, established a distinction between chemical elements and compounds.

chemotaxis (+ Greek *taxis*, "an orderly arrangement") is the movement of an organism or cell in response to a chemical concentration gradient.

chemotherapy (+ Greek *therapeia*, "treatment") is a term first used by Paul Ehrlich (1854-1915), the German bacteriologist (who shared the Nobel Prize for medicine and physiology in 1908), in reference to the effects of chemical agents on living cells, including microorganisms. Ehrlich's concept of selective chemical destruction of infecting organisms led to his discovery of arsphenamine, an arsenical compound then better known as **Salvarsan**, as a treatment for syphilis and other treponemal infections. Salvarsan was designated by Ehrlich as "606" because it was the product of his 606th experiment in his search for such a compound. Today, "chemotherapy" is thought of principally in regard to chemical agents to combat cancer.

cheno- is a combining form taken from the Greek *khēn*, "goose." Chenodeoxycholic acid, a bile acid first obtained from goose gall, was developed as a medication for the dissolution of gallstones. **Urso**deoxycholic acid, first obtained from the bile of bears (Latin *ursus*, "bear"), has similar properties and now is more often used for this purpose.

Cheshire cat syndrome refers more to the physician than the patient and was the term used by Dr. E. G. L. Bywaters (*Postgrad Med.* 1968;44:19) to describe his plight at being confronted by a trio of patients exhibiting all the signs of polyarteritis nodosa but not, in fact, having the disease. The allusion is to the befuddlement of Alice in Wonderland at seeing the grin without the cat. Should one address oneself to the grin, thought Alice, or wait until the features of the cat were more clearly discernible? Should one treat the patient who appears to have a suggestive sign of disease, mused Bywaters, or withhold treatment until unmistakable evidence of the disease is in full array?

chest comes from the Greek *kistē*, "a box." In Old English, the word was variously spelled *cist*, *ciest*, *cest*, and finally chest.

-chezia is a combining form taken from the Greek *chezein*, defined delicately in scholarly dictionaries as "to ease oneself." What it really means is "to defecate." **Stool**, another euphemism, is used both as a verb for the act and as a noun for the product. The reference, of course, is to the perch one uses for the purpose. **Dyschezia** is difficult defecation, and **hematochezia** is the passage of visible, relatively fresh blood through the anus. This is distinct from **melena**, which is "black stool" containing altered blood.

chiasma is a Greek word meaning "crossed, like the letter 'X' (chi)," hence, the optic chiasma, a decussation or crossing of the two optic nerve tracts in an X configuration.

chicken pox is said to be so called not because the disease was thought to come from the familiar fowl but to distinguish its typically mild course from that of the more grave small pox. The distinction between the two diseases was first established by William Heberden (1710-1801), an English physician. "Chicken" has been used otherwise to connote weakness or pettiness, as in "chicken-hearted" and "chicken feed," the latter when deriding a paltry sum of money (as government officials are wont to do when considering anything less than a billion dollars).

chilblain is a combination of "chill" + "blain," i.e., a blain caused by exposure to cold. *Blain* is an archaic English word meaning an inflammatory swelling or sore, often ulcerated, on the surface of the body. What used to be called "chilblains" now would be known as a necrotizing angiitis due to cryoglobulinemia.

chimera is an almost direct borrowing of the Greek name for a mythic monster having a lion's head, a goat's body, and a dragon's tail. The fire-breathing *chimaira* was among the unpleasant creatures that inhabited the infernal regions of Pluto's domain. In medicine, a chimera is "an individual organism whose body contains cells derived from different zygotes, of the same or different species, occurring spontaneously as in twins (blood-group chimeras), or produced artificially as an organism that develops from combined portions of different embryos or one in which tissue or cells of another organism have been introduced" (Dorland).

chiropody (*see* **podiatry**)

chiropractic is a system of therapeutics based on the contention that disease results from neural dysfunction and that this can be corrected by manipulation of the spinal column and adjacent structures. The word is concocted of the Greek *cheir*, "hand," + *praktikos*, "fit for doing." The term thus emphasizes the manipulative aspect of treatment. Presumably an outgrowth of osteopathy, the concept was vigorously promoted by Daniel David Palmer (1845-1915), an aptly named Iowa grocer who in 1910 published *The Science, Art, and Philosophy of Chiropractic*. Shortly thereafter, he established the Palmer School of Chiropractic at Davenport, Iowa. There are now 15 colleges of chiropractic in the United States and Canada, and the system they teach has gained a substantial following. Mainstream physicians recognize the efficacy of "laying on of hands," but in doing so they are much less vigorous than chiropractors.

chirurgeon (*see* **surgery**)

chloroform is so called because it is a compound of **chlorine** (named in 1810 by its discoverer Sir Humphry Davy from the Greek *chloros*, "green," because of its color as a gas) and formyl ($CHCl_3$). Its use as a surgical anesthetic agent was first demonstrated in 1847 by Sir James Simpson (1811-1870), an obstetrician of Edinburgh. This was the year following the initial public demonstration of ether in Boston. Chloroform became popular, especially in Britain during the ensuing century, in part because it was administered successfully to Queen Victoria during childbirth. With increasing recognition of its hepatotoxic and cardiodepressant effects, and because better agents became ailable, its use in anesthesia eventually was abandoned.

cholagogue (Greek *cholē*, "bile," + *agein*, "to move or lead") describes an agent such as cholecystokinin that effects the passage of preformed bile into the duodenum, mainly by stimulating contraction of the gallbladder. This action is distinct from that of a **choleretic** agent, such as represented by certain bile salts, that stimulates the formation of bile by the liver cells.

cholecyst- is not used as a word by itself, but its various combinations come from the Greek *cholē*, "bile," + *kystis*, "bladder." Thus, **cholecystectomy** is "a cutting out of the gallbladder," **cholecystography** is "a recording or picture of the gallbladder," and **cholecystokinin** is a substance that "moves" the gallbladder, i.e., causes it to contract.

choledochus is a Latinized name for the common bile duct that is, by itself, seldom heard. It is derived from the Greek *cholē*, "bile," + *dochē*, "a receptacle." **Choledocho-**, however, is a familiar combining form used to indicate whatever may pertain to the common bile duct.

cholelithiasis (*see* **lithotomy**)

cholera is a direct borrowing of the Greek name for a disease characterized by intense vomiting, diarrhea, and consequent debility. Whether such cases so called by the ancients included those that would be identified as cholera today is uncertain. Several possible derivations of the Greek *cholera* have been proposed. One is that the word combined *cholē*, "bile," + *rhein*, "to flow," the allusion being that acute vomiting and diarrhea reflected a profuse discharge of body "humors," including bile. Another holds that "cholera" relates to the Greek *cholos* or *cholades*, "the intestines," to which *rhein*, "to flow," was added. In its epidemic form, the disease often was called "Asiatic cholera," at least by Europeans. It was Robert Koch (1843-1910), the German bacteriologist, who discovered in 1883 the *Vibrio cholerae* as the infectious cause of the disease. Cholera epidemics in America, as late as the 19th century, were frequent and devastating in summer seasons as far north as New York.

choleretic incorporates the Greek *cholē*, "bile," and designates an agent that augments the flow of bile by stimulating the formation of bile by the liver cells. This is distinct from the action of a **cholagogue**.

choleric describes the temperament of a person who is hot-tempered or irascible and is taken from the Greek *cholē*, "bile," in the belief that one easily angered is troubled by an excess of "yellow bile," a component of the quartet of ancient "humors."

cholesterol was formerly known as "cholesterin" and is a complex alcohol often occurring as a fatlike, pearly substance. Because it was first recognized as a constituent of gallstones and thought to represent solidified bile, its name was made up of the Greek *cholē*, "bile," + *stereos*, "solid." The ending "-ol" was later substituted for "-in" to indicate its chemical structure as an alcohol. A **cholesteatoma** (adding the Greek *ōma*, "swelling") is a waxy concretion of which cholesterol is a principal component.

chondro- is a combining form signifying cartilage and is taken from the Greek *chondros*, which, as an anatomic term, meant "cartilage or gristle." Actually, the Greek *chondros* generally referred to cereal grains which, when cooked, formed gruel. Apparently, to the Greeks, cartilage resembled a thick gruel. A **chondroblast** (from the Greek *blastos*, "germ or seed") is a precursor of the **chondrocyte**, the cell-producing cartilage. **Chondrodystrophy** is a disturbed growth of cartilage resulting in achondroplasia, literally a lack of proper form in cartilage and a cause of dwarfism. (*see* **cartilage**)

chord is an almost direct borrowing of the Greek *chordē*, "a string of gut used in musical instruments or as a bowstring." The Greek word can also refer to sausage. The "ch" from the initial Greek letter chi is preserved in musical and most anatomic terms, such as **chorda tympani** (the latter word from the Greek *tympanon*, "a drum") and **chordae tendinae** (the latter word from the Greek *tenein*, "to stretch"). The "h" is dropped in the spelling of "cord," a kind of thin rope.

chorea is manifested by convulsive twitchings and movements that suggest a grotesque dance. The word is derived from the Greek *choreia*, "dancing, especially by a group or chorus." The symptom in older days was known as Saint Vitus' dance. Saint Vitus was a Roman lad who was martyred together with his tutor Modestus and his nurse

Crescentia during the persecutions of the Emperor Diocletian in the 3rd century A.D. During the 15th and 16th centuries it became the custom for children to dance around statues of Saint Vitus in supplication of good health. The dancing often reached a peak of frenzy, and Saint Vitus' name came to be applied to the involuntary writhing movements of chorea, which in the past was usually associated with childhood acute rheumatic fever. Now we speak of **athetosis** (Greek *athetos*, "not fixed"), a writhing symptom of various conditions, most of them associated with lesions in the caudate nucleus and putamen.

chorion is a direct borrowing of the Greek word for "skin or leather." In Hippocratic writings, the word was used to refer to membranes, particularly those that enclose the fetus.

choroid describes the rich vascular plexus that invests the pia mater of the brain and projects into the third, fourth, and lateral ventricles, effusion from which produces the cerebrospinal fluid. The choroid plexus is so called because of its resemblance to the vascular **chorion**. The **choroidea** (or simply "the choroid," as it is usually called) is the thin, vascular coat investing the eyeball between the retina and the sclera.

chrom- is a combining form taken from the Greek *chrōma*, which means "the surface of the body," particularly the color or complexion of the skin, and hence has a relation to "color" generally. The element **chromium** is so called because its compounds are highly colored. **Chromaffin** (the latter portion coming from the Latin *affinis*, "a close relationship") is a term applied to cells that stain readily with, or have an affinity for, various chromium salts. **Chromatin** and **chromosome** (+ Latin *soma*, "body") were so named because they appear as nuclear inclusions deeply stained by dye applied to sections of tissue examined microscopically.

chronaxy is the interval between application of a stimulus and the excitation of a neural element. The term is a combination of the Greek *chronos*, "time," + *axia*, "value or measure."

chronic comes from the Greek *chronos*, "time." A distinction between illnesses that are abrupt, sharp, and short-lived ("acute") and those that are protracted in time ("chronic")

was made in early Hippocratic writings.

chrysotherapy is derived from the Greek *chrysos*, "gold," + *therapeia*, "treatment," and means just that: the use of gold salts as medicaments. Such therapy is prescribed, for example, for selected patients with rheumatoid arthritis.

chyle is from the Greek *chylos*, "juice or fluid." Professor H. A. Skinner points out that in ancient Greek *chylos* and *chymos* had almost identical meanings. Both meant "juice," but *chymos* referred more to natural juices, whereas *chylos* referred to processed juices, such as decoctions wherein a juice was formed by boiling. In reference to the contents or products of the digestive tract, the two Greek words often were confused. However, their respective derivatives, chyle and **chyme**, are clearly distinguished in modern physiology. Since the discovery of the lymphatic channels, chyle has been recognized as a product of digestion represented by the fat-laden lymph transported from the small intestine. Chyme is the semifluid content of the alimentary tract, representing a mixture of ingested food and various digestive juices.

cicatrix is the Latin word for "scar." This is an example of a classical, polysyllabic word having no real advantage when compared to a simple, well-known word. To call the mark of a healed wound a cicatrix instead of a scar may be thought impressive, but it is rather pompous.

-cide is a suffix adapted from the Latin *-cida*, a combining form that denotes "a cutter or a killer." The Latin *-cida*, in turn, is derived from the verb *caedere*, "to strike down or slay." The suffix appears in a number of current terms, e.g., **amebacide**, **bacteriocide**, **fungicide**, **viricide** (or **virucide**)—and, of course, in **homicide**.

cilium is the Latin term that refers to the edge of the eyelid. The word may have come from the Greek *kylix*, "a cup," the allusion being to the eyelid as a cup for the eyeball. An alternative origin is from the Greek *kylisma*, "a place to roll in." In either case, only much later was **cilia**, as the neuter plural, used to refer to eyelashes. It is in this same sense that the term was then applied to the fine, hairlike processes emanating from the surfaces of certain cells, such as those of the respiratory epithelium. The ciliary body and muscle of the eye were so called because their plicated appearance suggested that of eyelashes. The Latin word for eyebrow is *supercilium*; from this we have our adjective **supercilious**, meaning haughty or disdainful, as expressed by raising the eyebrows. (*see* **hair**)

cinchona is the name given to the bark of a tree indigenous to South America. The chief alkaloid in an extract of cinchona is **quinine**, and thereby hangs a tale. The early Spanish invaders of Peru learned of a "fever tree" whose bark, when pulverized and brewed as a beverage, effected miraculous cures of "the fevers and the tertians," by which was meant the febrile rigors of malaria that typically occurred at intervals of three days. A persistent, though unsubstantiated, legend is that the brew was given to the acutely ill Condessa Anna del Chinchon, or perhaps it was her husband the Conde, the Spanish viceroy in Peru, who was laid low by fever. On her (or his) prompt recovery, the Conde introduced the wonder drug to Europe, where it confirmed its reputation by curing the ague. The drug was then variously known as "the Countess' powder," "the Peruvian bark," "the Jesuits' bark" (because members of that religious order were the principal importers), and "the cardinal's bark" (because the eminent Cardinal de Lugo in Rome was among its promoters). Carl von Linné (1717-1783), also known as Linnaeus, the famous Swedish botanist and taxonomist, gave the genus of rubiaceous trees bearing the bark the name *Cinchona* in honor of the countess, though in doing so he misspelled her name. A more recently isolated antimalarial drug is **artemisinin**, derived from the herb *Artemisia annua*. This genus, which includes the sagebrush and the wormwood, was named in honor of Artemisia of Caria, a 4th century B.C. woman botanist who took her name from Artemis, the Greek goddess of the hunt and the moon.

cingulum is the Latin word for "belt or girdle," coming from the verb *cingere*, "to encircle or gird." The cingulum of the brain is a band of association fibers that almost surrounds the corpus callosum. From the same source comes "cinch," the band that secures the saddle of a horse.

circadian is a neologism presumably concocted from the Latin *circa*, "around," + *diem*, "a day." It is used to refer to events occurring within a 24-hour period, as in a circadian rhythm exhibited by certain regularly repetitious phenomena in living organisms.

circinate is from the Latin *circinare*, "to make round." The term is used to describe various more or less circular anatomic structures or whatever may resemble a coil.

circle is derived from the Latin *circulus*, the diminutive of *circus*, and therefore "a little ring." The Latin *circus* is closely related to the Greek *kirkos*, "a circle or ring." The circle of Willis, named for Thomas Willis (1621-1675), an English physician and anatomist who has been accorded the title of "father of neurology," is a remarkable circular arterial anastomosis at the base of the brain, linking the internal carotid arteries from either side with the midline basilar artery posteriorly.

circulation is from the Latin *circulare*, "to make a circle." Galen (A.D. 131-201), the celebrated Greek physician, came close to comprehending the circulation of blood but was confused because he lacked knowledge of the capillary link between arteries and veins. It remained for William Harvey (1578-1657), the English physician, to establish the physiologic concept of continuously circulating blood. Harvey described his convincing experiments and reasoning therefrom in his monumental *De Motu Cordis* ("On the Motion of the Heart"), published in 1628.

circum is the Latin preposition meaning "around or about." From this, used as a combining form, we get a host of medical words, including **circumcision**, "a cutting around," usually in specific reference to the prepuce; **circumflex**, "to bend around"; **circumscribe**, literally "to write around" but figuratively "to delimit"; and **circumvallate**, "walled around."

cirrhosis was so named by René Théophil Hyacinthe Laënnec (1781-1826), the distinguished French physician. In describing the scarred livers of alcoholics, Laënnec was impressed by their abnormal color and related this to the Greek *kirrhos*, "tawny," a dull, yellowish-brown. Thus, "cirrhosis" as a name has nothing to do with fibrosis, even though fibrosis is a feature of the disease.

Unfortunately, "cirrhosis" is commonly confused with other words of similar sound, such as "sclerosis" or "scirrhous," which are quite unrelated. Also, it should be kept in mind there is only one cirrhosis, and that relates to the liver. There is no such thing as "cirrhosis of the heart" or any structure other than the liver. To say "cirrhosis of the liver" or "hepatic cirrhosis" is redundant.

cisterna is the Latin word for "reservoir" and is related to *cista*, "a box or chest." Thus, the **cisterna chyli** is a dilated segment in the lumbar region of the lymph channel that becomes, above, the great thoracic duct. Incidentally, this name was disputed as inaccurate because the Roman cisterna actually had no incoming or outgoing channels, but the use of "cisterna chyli" was so well established that it defied change. The **cisterna magna** is an enlargement of the subarachnoid space between the cerebellum and medulla oblongata, where cerebrospinal fluid collects.

clap is a vulgar but venerable term for gonorrhea, appearing in English literature as early as the 16th century. A popular and probable explanation is that the word comes from *Le Clapier*, the medieval name for a district of Paris that was a haven for prostitutes. The French name means "rabbit warren," the allusion being obvious. A common French term for brothel was *clapise*, a shortened form of which became attached to the disease often acquired therein.

claudication is a symptom of arterial insufficiency in the legs and is commonly misunderstood to refer to pain. The term is from the Latin *claudicare*, "to be lame or to limp." Ischemia in an exercising muscle can cause pain but also impairs contraction, thus causing lameness. "Intermittent claudication" was originally described in horses going lame with exercise and then recovering with rest. Incidentally, the Roman emperor Claudius, who ruled from A.D. 41-54, was so named because he limped, presumably from a birth defect; he also stammered.

clavicle comes not from the diminutive of the Latin *clavis*, "key," as is frequently suggested, but rather from the Latin *clavicula*, meaning "tendril," the shoot from the stem of a vine by which the plant gains support. The thin, curved bone connecting the sternum and the scapula suggests the tendril of a vine.

climacteric now refers to that time in life when procreative powers cease. The Greek *klimakterikos* was "the step in a stair or the rung of a ladder," hence a point of change at which one went either up or down. The ancient Greeks considered that five climacteric periods marked changes in one's life, the critical years being usually calculated as multiples of seven, that is, at the 7th year, the 21st year, the 49th year, the 63rd year, and the 77th year. The decline in procreative power was thought to be marked by the 49th year.

clinic comes through the French *clinique*, "at the bedside," from the Greek *klinē*, "a couch or bed." Late Latin writers used *clinicus* to refer to medical instruction given at the bedside as contrasted to abstract lectures and disputations. Nowadays, "clinic" is used to mean (*a*) a gathering of students for instruction in practical aspects of any endeavor (there are "clinics" devoted to sports and computers, among other things); and (*b*) a place for assembly of patients, particularly (and contradictorily) those who are ambulatory and not confined to bed, in contrast to those in a hospital. **Clinical** refers to those aspects of a medical problem determined by direct contact with patients rather than from laboratory testing, and a **clinician** is a medically trained person primarily concerned with the care of patients, in distinction to an academician or a laboratory worker. The **clinoid** processes are the bony projections that demarcate the pituitary fossa and resemble the four posts of a bed. (*see* **sella turcica**)

clitoris is an almost direct borrowing of the Greek *kleitoris* and is said to be related to *kleis*, "a door latch," the clitoris being likened to a "latch" on the vagina.

cloaca is the Latin word for "drain or sewer." In biology, a cloaca is, aptly, a common ampullary terminus of both the alimentary and urinary tracts, such as normally characteristic of birds, reptiles, amphibians, many fishes, and a few mammals. In human pathology, a cloaca is an anomaly.

clone is a term adapted to biomedical use relatively recently in reference to a group of genetically identical cells descended from a single common ancestor. "Clone" also is used as a verb to denote the establishment of such a strain of cells. The meaning of the word, a near borrowing of the Greek *klōn*, "a twig," has been extended to denote any exact duplicate.

Clonorchis designates a genus of Asian liver flukes. The name is composed of the Greek *klōn*, "branch," + *orchis*, "testicle." Organisms of this genus have branched testes. The most common species is *Clonorchis sinensis*, the latter term referring to its Chinese origin.

clonus is from the Greek *klonos*, "any violent motion or tumult." The ancients used this term to describe epileptic convulsions. Now, in medicine, clonus refers to rapidly alternating rigidity and relaxation, such as may occur at the ankle joint. This is in contrast to a tonic, or sustained, contraction of a muscle.

Clostridium designates a genus of anaerobic, spore-forming bacteria commonly infecting ischemic or necrotic tissues. The name comes from the Greek *klōstēr*, "a thread or yarn." The microorganism most commonly found in gas gangrene, *Clostridium perfringens*, is so called from the Latin *perfringere*, "to break up," presumably because it elaborates necrotizing enzymes. *Clostridium difficile*, an opportunistic invader in injured or ischemic bowel, is so called simply because it is so extremely difficult to culture.

clot is an Anglo-Saxon word meaning "a coagulated mass," and is related to "clod," as a lump of earth, and to the German *Klotz*, "a lump or block," as of wood.

clue (*see* **labyrinth**)

clyster (*see* **enema**)

coagulation is from the Latin *coagulare*, "to curdle." To the Romans a *coagulum* was curdled milk.

coarctation is derived from the Latin *coartare*, "to press together," hence its application to a stricture, particularly in a major blood vessel such as the aorta.

coca is said to be the Spanish spelling of the Peruvian Indian name *cuca*, given to a shrub growing on the eastern slopes of the Andes mountains, but the word may have been derived from the Aymara *kkoka*, which has the same meaning. In pre-Columbian times, it was known that the leaves of this plant, when chewed, yielded a euphoric sensation, thus inuring the user to a harsh life. When the active principle of coca leaves was isolated in the mid-19th century, the alkaloid was called **cocaine**, the "-ine" suffix indicating a derivative. This name should be pronounced in three syllables, as "koh-kah-een." Alas, it proved too easy to say "koh-kane." When synthetic analogs were developed, it was imagined that -**caine** was a suffix denoting a local anesthetic property, and there followed a host of misnomers, to wit, "procaine," "lidocaine," "benzocaine," "hexylcaine," *ad erratum*. It is said that the original recipe for the Coca-Cola beverage, concocted in 1886 by John Styth Pemberton, an enterprising Atlanta, Georgia, druggist, included a pinch of coca leaves. If so, this could have accounted for the drink's early popularity. The Coca-Cola company de-cocainized its coca leaves in 1906, the year of the Pure Food and Drug Act. "Coca" is, of course, not to be confused with "coco" or "cocoa"; all are quite different. The coconut (often misspelled "cocoanut") is the fruit of the coconut palm, its hollow center a serous fluid, its meat often shredded for use in flavoring or decorating various baked goods, and its tough outer covering used to make mats. **Coco** is from the Portuguese word for "grimace"; three depressions at the nut's base give the appearance of a scowling face. **Cocoa**, as the familiar breakfast beverage, is a transliteration of *cacoa*, derived from the Nahautl Indian name for a small evergreen tree, *Theobromo cacoa*, that grows in Central and South America and yields seeds which, when dried and pulverized, provide cocoa and chocolate. The brew contains the xanthines **theobromine** and **caffeine**. *Theobroma*, the name contrived by Linnaeus in 1737 for the genus of plants bearing cocoa beans, is thought to be taken from the Greek *theos*, "god," + *brōma*, "food," thus "a food for the gods," but the "theo-" may be a Latinized form of "tea."

coccus is from the Greek *kokkos*, "a kernel or berry." Giving this name for the rounded forms of bacteria is said to have been suggested in 1874 by Theodor Billroth (1829-1894), the celebrated Viennese surgeon. The **gonococcus** is the microorganism of the species *Neisseria gonorrhoeae* and is so called from the Greek *gōnē*, "seed, as in semen," because of the mistaken belief that the urethral discharge resulting from infection by this organism was an abnormal flow of semen. Albert Ludwig Siegmund Neisser (1855-1916) was a German physician. The **staphylococcus** is so named from the Greek *staphylē*, "a bunch of grapes," because that is the way the microorganisms tend to cluster. The **streptococcus** occurs in short chains, hence its name from the Greek *streptos*, "twisted, as in a chain or necklace."

coccyx is from the Greek *kokkyx*, "the cuckoo bird." The ancients gave this name to the rudimentary tail vertebrae of man because of their resemblance to the bill of a cuckoo. The coccyx was at one time called "the whistle bone" because of its anatomic relation to the source of flatus.

cochlea is the Latin word for "snail," coming from the Greek *kochlias*, "a small spiral shell." The structure of the inner ear closely resembled that of a snail's shell.

code is a near borrowing of the Latin *codex* (or *caudex*), "the trunk of a tree, a block of wood, a book, or a ledger." The early Romans used a wax-smeared board on which to inscribe letters or numbers. The English noun can mean "a systematic set of rules" or "a system of symbols used to convey messages requiring secrecy or brevity." In the verb form, "to code" has recently acquired a meaning peculiar to medical practice, i.e., to invoke a predetermined procedure to resuscitate a patient in cardiac or respiratory arrest. The anguish of Hamlet's soliloquy "To be or not to be" is paraphrased in hospital wards as "To code or not to code" when considering the prospect of patients in peril.

codeine is from the Greek *kodeia*, "the head of a poppy," thus alluding to the source of the alkaloid. The ending "-ine" denotes a derivative. The name was conferred by Pierre-Jean Robiquet (1780-1840), a French physician, in 1832.

coeliac (often spelled **celiac** by Americans) disease, one feature of which is abdominal distention, now refers specifically to primary intestinal malabsorption as it occurs in children or adults and once was known as "nontropical sprue." *Coeliaca* was used by the ancients to describe any condition marked by swelling of the belly. (*see* **celiac**; *also* **-cel-**)

coelom is the proper spelling of what often is written as **celom** when referring to the primitive body cavity of the embryo. (*see* **-cel-**)

cohort occasionally appears in medical reports as a designation for a group of subjects employed in clinical investigation. The Latin *cohors* in military parlance was 1 of 10 divisions of a Roman legion, approximately equivalent to a modern battalion (about 500 soldiers).

colchicine is an alkaloid long known to be useful in the treatment of gout and more recently found effective in preventing attacks of familial recurring polyserositis. The term is taken from *kolchikon*, the Greek name for the meadow saffron or autumn crocus, the original herbal source of the alkaloid. The Greek name came from Colchis, the district south of the Caucasus mountains where the plant grew.

cold turkey is a vernacular way of referring to the total, abrupt cessation of a drug, especially a narcotic. The expression alludes to the "gooseflesh" or "duck bumps" that appear in the skin of persons withdrawing from addiction to opiates. The nodular appearance is that of the skin of a plucked, uncooked, cold turkey.

colic is a cramping abdominal pain caused by spasmodic contraction of the smooth musculature of the abdominal viscera, commonly observed in infants. Presumably, colic originally was thought to arise in the colon.

collagen is a combination of the Greek *kolla*, "glue," + *gennaō*, "I produce." The name, contrived in the 19th century, refers not to any phenomenon that occurs in living tissue but rather to the early observation that dense connective tissue, when boiled in a pot, yields a gluey gelatin.

colliculus is a diminutive of the Latin *collum*, "neck," that in anatomy has been applied to a variety of small elevations or necklike structures, e.g., the colliculus of the arytenoid cartilage.

colloid combines the Greek *kolla*, "glue," + *eidos*, "like" and describes, literally, "a gluelike substance." The term was proposed in the 19th century to distinguish the two main classes of soluble substances, the first being the crystalloids. Glue or gelatin was cited as an example of the second type, to which the name "colloid" was given.

collum is the Latin word for "neck," hence our word "collar." The use of the Latin word is retained in anatomy as a reference to the neck as, for example, in musculus longus colli, the "long muscle of the neck."

coloboma is the Greek word for "a mutilation," being related to *kolobos*, "curtailed or docked." In medicine the term applies particularly to congenital defects or fissures in the uveal tract of the eye.

colon as a term for the large intestine is from the Greek. But from which Greek word? There are three candidates. *Kolon* meant "the large intestine" to the Greeks and may have come from *kolos*, "curtailed or stunted," thus alluding to the observation that the large intestine is only about one-third the length of the small intestine ("large" and "small" referring, of course, to the caliber of the two segments rather than to their length). A different Greek word, *kōlon*, meant "a limb" in the sense of a member of the body. Perhaps the jointed configuration of the large intestine, as in its ascending, transverse, and descending segments, suggested a limb, such as an arm or leg. Finally, *koilia* meant "the hollow of the abdomen." The reader can choose and be as right (or wrong) as any expert. As a combining term, **colo-** yields **colostomy**, literally "a mouth of the colon"; **colotomy**, "a cut in the colon"; and **colectomy**, "the removal or cutting out of the colon."

colors often are included in biomedical terms of classical origin. These root forms are used ([L] = Latin, [Gr] = Greek):

alb-, "white" (L)
anthrac-, "black (as coal)" (Gr)
argent-, "silver" (L)
argyr-, "silver" (L)
ater-, "dull black" (L)
auro-, "golden" (L)
azu-, "blue" (L)
beryl-, "pale- or sea-green" (Gr)
caerul-, "blue" (L)
candid-, "bright white" (L)
chlor-, "green" (Gr)
chrom-, "colorful or tinted" (Gr)
chrys-, "golden" (Gr)
cirrho-, "tawny yellow" (Gr)
cneco-, "pale yellow" (Gr)
coccin-, "scarlet" (L)
croce-, "saffron, yellow" (L)

cyan-, "dark blue, blue-green" (Gr)
erythro-, "red" (Gr)
flav-, "yellow" (L)
fulv-, "light brown" (L)
fusc-, "dark brown" (L)
iodo-, "violet" (Gr)
leuko-, "white" (Gr)
luteo-, "yellow (as mud)" (L)
mela-, "black" (Gr)
niger-, "glossy black" (L)
pelio-, "livid, dull gray-blue" (Gr)
phaeo-, "dusky, gray, or brown" (Gr)
purpur-, "purple" (L)
rhodo-, "red" (Gr)
rubeo-, "red" (L)
spadix-, "chestnut brown" (L)
violo-, "violet" (L)
virido-, "green" (L)
xantho-, "yellow" (Gr)

colostrum is the Latin word for "the first milk secreted by the mother's breast after childbirth" and was so used by the Romans. It may be related to the Greek *kolos*, in the sense of "unfinished." However, the Greek word for colostrum was simply *protogala*, from *proto-*, "first," + *gala*, "milk."

colpo- is a combining form usually relating to the vagina and taken from the Greek *kolpos*, "any fold, cleft, or hollow." Thus, **colporrhaphy** (+ Greek *rhaphē*, "suture") is a repair of the vagina; **colposcopy** (+ Greek *skopein*, "to observe") is an inspection of the vagina; and **colpotomy** (+ Greek *tomē*, "cutting") is an incision of the vagina.

coma is an almost direct borrowing of the Greek *kōma*, "a deep sleep." In Hippocratic writings the word was used also for lethargy, but its modern medical meaning is restricted to a state of profound unconsciousness.

comedo is the Latin word for "glutton," derived from the verb *comedere*, "to eat up." How does this relate to the use of the word in reference to a plugged sebaceous gland in the skin, commonly called "a blackhead"? According to one explanation, the plugged sebaceous gland, when squeezed, exudes a wormlike fragment of waxy material, and apparently the ancients thought this was the remains of a small worm that had burrowed into the skin to devour flesh. The plural is **comedones**.

comes is the Latin word for "companion" and

denotes an artery or vein that accompanies a nerve trunk, as in vena comes. The plural is **comites**, as in venae comites.

commensal describes an organism that lives on or within another organism to its own benefit and with no harm to the host. An example would be an enteric parasite that derives its sustenance by residing in the gut yet causes no symptoms or signs of illness in its host. The term combines the Latin *com-*, "together," + *mensa*, "table," indicating that the parasite and the host dine amicably at the same board.

commissure designates the site where corresponding parts are joined. The palpebral commissure is where the upper and lower eyelids join, as at the "corners" of the eye. Neural commissures are where paired, lateral bundles of nerve fibers cross, usually in the midline of the brain or spinal cord. The term is an almost direct borrowing of the Latin *commissura*, "a joining together," being a combination of *com-*, "together," + *mittere*, "to send."

complaint is that which the patient presents to his doctor. The word is derived from a combination of "*com-*," as an intensive, + *plangere*, "to wail or to lament." Originally, the Latin verb *plangere* meant "to beat the breast or head as a sign of grief." So the patient who, in anguish, puts his hand to his head and wails, "Oh, doctor, what a pain!" is literally complaining.

complement is a slight contraction of the Latin *complementum*, "that which fills a void." This, in turn, comes from the verb *compere*, "to fill up." The term was given its biomedical sense by Paul Ehrlich (1854-1915), the famed German immunologist and bacteriologist, to designate the substance necessary to complete certain hemolytic reactions. At the turn of the century, Jules Jean Baptiste Vincent Bordet (1870-1961), a Belgian, and Octave Gengou (1875-1957), a Frenchman, showed that other substances could "fix" complement, thus preventing an otherwise expected hemolytic reaction in sensitized red blood cells. This became the basis for a variety of widely used diagnostic "complement fixation tests." In general usage, there is an important distinction between "complement" and "supplement," whether used as nouns or verbs. A complement is whatever it takes to make up the whole of anything, to supply a lack, to make the whole complete. A **supplement** is also an addition, but not necessarily to the point of completion or for the purpose of making up a lack. For example, a supplemental publication added to a volume of a journal or to a textbook can be an addition to a whole, with no intent of correcting a deficiency.

complexion is derived from the Latin *com-*, "together," + *plectere*, "to plait or to braid." Ancient philosophers thought in terms of four elements or basic attributes: "fire" being hot and dry, "air" being warm and moist, "earth" being cold and dry, and "water" being cold and moist. How these attributes were "woven together" would determine a person's visage, appearance, or complexion.

concha is the Latin word for almost any crustacean, particularly its shell. The word is related to the Greek *ko[n]gchē*, "a cockleshell." The ancients used these terms to describe various shell-like cavities in anatomy. In modern nomenclature, the **conchae** are small bones of the inner nasal passages and the hollows of the external ear.

concoction describes the result of mixing ingredients (or, figuratively, words) and is derived from the Latin *concoquere*, "to boil together," which itself is a concoction of *con-*, "together" + *coquere*, "to cook." Thus, originally the key element was heat. Later, the meaning was extended to include any means of mixing, no matter how contrived. Medications that are mixtures of two or more ingredients are sometimes called "concoctions." **Decoction** is similar but more restricted and more emphatic in the use of heat, being a combination of *de-*, "down," + *coquere*. To decoct is to boil down. Both terms retain a pertinence to pharmacology.

condom is now openly publicized as a means of ensuring "safe sex." The term is attributed alternatively (*a*) to the Latin verb *condere*, among its meanings being "to conceal, hide, or suppress," or (*b*) as an eponym immortalizing an 18th-century English physician whose name may have been Condon, or something similar, and who is said to have prepared a prototype of the device using an inverted cecum of a sheep.

condyle is derived from the Greek *kondylos*, "a knuckle or knob." Its later use, in anatomy, was restricted to the rounded articular surfaces of various bones.

condyloma has the same origin as **condyle** but came to be used to describe the warty excrescences around the anus or genitals, usually associated with venereal disease.

conjunctiva is the feminine of the Latin adjective meaning "connecting or joining together." In anatomy the modified noun "membrane" is implied but not used when referring to the covering membrane that connects the globe of the eye with the eyelid.

conniventes (*see* **plica**)

constipation is derived from the Latin *constipare*, "to crowd together," being a combination of *con-*, "against," + *stipare*, "to cram or stuff." To the Romans, *constipare* meant "to pack anything tightly." It was not until the 16th century that the derived word was applied to the state of a dilatory bowel stuffed with inspissated feces. **Obstipation** (Latin *ob-*, "in front of") is used to describe intractable constipation to the point of no bowel movement at all, as may occur with complete obstruction.

consumption is an archaic term for any wasting disease, notably tuberculosis. It comes from the Latin *consumere*, "to use up." The acute, fulminant form of disseminated miliary tuberculosis was known, of yore, as "galloping consumption."

contagion is from the Latin *contingere*, "to touch closely." The Indo-European root is said to have been *tag*, "to seize," a word we still use in similar context. A **contagious** disease is one that might be transmitted by close touch with someone or something so contaminated.

contaminate is from the Latin *contaminatus*, "polluted, impure, or degraded." This, in turn, is derived from a combination of *con-*, "together," + *tangere*, "to touch or meddle with."

contrecoup is French for "counterblow." The reference is to traumatic lesions, especially of the cranium or its contents, that occur on the side opposite where a blow was struck.

control when used in research reports refers to a neutral subject or procedure against which an experimental counterpart is compared. Used thus, "control" comes close to its derivation from the Latin *contra*, "opposite to or facing against," + *rotula*, "a little wheel," in the sense that the little wheel is a roll or a ledger. Therefore, a "counter roll" would be a ledger for checking or verifying accounts. Charles Darwin (1809-1882) spoke of "controlled experiments" in 1875, although it was naval surgeon James Lind, as noted in a previous entry (*see* **ascorbic acid**), who earlier undertook what was probably the first controlled clinical investigation when he proved the efficacy of citrus juice in preventing scurvy.

contusion is from the Latin *contudere*, "to crush, pound, or bruise." In the 15th century reference was made in Middle English to a *counteschown*, the lesion resulting from being smitten with a staff or falling.

convalescence comes from the Latin *convalescere*, "to grow strong or to regain strength." This had its origin in *con-*, as an intensive, and *valere*, "to be strong or vigorous." Convalescence, then, is a period during which vigor, lost by injury or illness, is regained.

convolution (*see* **gyrus**)

convulsion is from the Latin *convellere*, "to tear away or wrest." Related forms of the term have been used through the ages to describe intermittent muscle spasms, usually involuntary, causing violent agitation of the limbs and trunk.

copper gets its name from that of the island of Cyprus. To the Romans, *aes* was a crude metal, including copper and its alloys, such as bronze. A major source of supply was Cyprus, and copper became known as *aes Cyprium*, then simply *cyprium*. The switch to *cuprum* came from Kupros, the Greek name for Cyprus. *Cuprum* accounts for "Cu" being the chemical symbol for copper.

copro- is a combining form denoting a relationship to feces. It comes from the Greek *kopros*, "dung." **Scato-**, derived from the genitive of the Greek *skōr, skat-*, also refers to dung or excrement. Whatever is scatologic is an expression relating to excrement or excretory function.

coprolalia is a term for scatologic raving ("copro-" + the Greek *lalia*, "babble"), as observed in certain cases of dementia.

coprophagy is the ingestion of excrement ("copro-" + the Greek *phagein*, "to eat"), a practice common to certain forms of animal life and occasionally observed as aberrant behavior in severely demented persons.

copulate comes from the Latin *copulare*, "to couple or to join, as with a bond." The term is now restricted almost solely to sexual intercourse.

cor is the Latin word for "heart" but also means "the seat of feelings." Cor is used as a component of numerous medical terms, such as "cor biloculare" and "cor pulmonale." Moreover, the Latin word has a host of English offspring, such as **core**, **cordial**, **accord**, **concord**, **record**, **courage**, **encourage**, and **discourage**. Cordial, by the way, was once used to designate a medicament supposedly exerting a beneficial effect by stimulating the heart, an example being "blackberry cordial." The popularity of these purported remedies doubtless owed to their content of alcohol. We still refer to certain spirituous liqueurs as "cordials."

coracoid is from the Greek *kōrax* (the "x" here representing the letter xi, not chi), "a crow or raven." The coracoid process of the scapula is a strong, curved, bony eminence that overhangs the shoulder joint, somewhat in the shape of a crow's beak.

corium is the Latin word for "skin or hide" and refers specifically to the zone of dense connective tissue underlying the epidermis. The corresponding Greek word is *chorion*, borrowed directly as the embryologic term for the outermost covering of the developing zygote, serving both nutritive and protective functions.

corn is the common name given to those annoying, often painful, knotty excrescences in the skin of the toes, usually caused by undue friction or pressure by too tight shoes. The term relates to the Latin *cornu*, "horn or hoof." This use of the word bears no relation to "corn" as a cereal grain, which is of Old Teutonic origin.

cornea is the feminine form of the Latin adjective meaning "horny" and refers, in anatomy, to the thin but tough, transparent structure forming the anterior part of the fibrous tunic of the eye.

cornu is Latin for "horn or hoof," referring especially to the dense substance of which these structures are composed. The cornu Ammonis is another name for the hippocampus major, given because it resembles a ram's horn, the symbol of Jupiter of Ammon.

coronary is from the Latin *corona*, "crown." The corresponding Greek word appears to be *choronos*. "Coronary," then, refers to anything resembling a crown, or that which surrounds or encompasses, as a garland. Apparently, someone thought this was the configuration of the coronary arteries as they festooned the heart. Some confusion has arisen because the Greek *korōne* meant "a sea crow." The same word was used to refer to the heel of a bow where a notch secured the bowstring. It was from allusion to such a notch that the **coronoid** processes of the ulna and mandible were so named.

coroner is a title taken from the Latin *corona*, "crown." In olden days, a coroner was an officer of the English crown. Among his duties were looking into and recording the deaths of the king's subjects. In many American jurisdictions, the title of coroner has been superseded by "medical examiner," whose principal charge remains the investigation of sudden, unnatural, or suspicious deaths. One wonders why, in this republic, we have taken so long to give up the title of "coroner."

corpus is the Latin word for "body, matter, or substance," and hence it has had wide application in anatomy. The plural is **corpora** and the genitive is **corporis**. The **corpora Arantii**, the nodules of cartilage in the semilunar valves of the heart, were described by Guilio Aranzi (1530-1589), an Italian anatomist. The **corpora mamillaria**, two small rounded protuberances at the base of the brain, were so named because of their fancied resemblance to the female breasts. The corpus luteum of the ovary is, literally, "a yellow body," the term incorporating the Latin *luteum*, "mud-colored." The **corpus callosum** of the brain is so called from the Latin *callosus*, "hard or thick-skinned." From this same Latin source come **callus** and **callous**, noun and adjective, respectively.

corpuscle is an almost direct borrowing of the Latin *corpusculum*, the diminutive of *corpus*, hence "a little body."

corrugate comes from the Latin *corrugare*, "to wrinkle." The corrugator muscles are those that wrinkle the skin. To the Romans, *nares corrugare*, "to wrinkle the nose," meant a sign of disgust, as the action still does to us.

cortex is the Latin word for "bark, shell, hull, or rind," all in the sense of an outer covering. In anatomy, the cerebral cortex is the outer layer of the principal part of the brain; the renal cortex is the outer portion of the kidney; and cortical bone is the dense outer part, in contrast to the inner marrow. Corticosteroid describes a substance found in the adrenal cortex.

corticosteroid (*see* **steroid**)

coryza is an ancient and now somewhat pompous word for "a cold in the head." It is said that the Greek *koryza* was derived from *kara*, "head," + *zeein*, "to boil." The allusion, apparently, was to the runny nose, which suggested an effluent of a nasty humor.

cosmetic comes from the Greek *kosmein*, "to arrange or adorn." Thus, cosmetic surgery can be thought of as a rearrangement of certain anatomic features for the purpose of adornment. As such, its cost is excluded from coverage by most health insurance schemes.

costal is an adjectival derivative of *costa*, the Latin word for "rib" and, figuratively, for "side or wall." The combining form **costo-** and the adjective "costal" refer to whatever may pertain to a rib or ribs. The same source yielded our words "coast" and "coastal."

cough is a word of uncertain origin, but almost surely it must have begun as an echoic expression of just what it represents, that is, a forceful expression of air from the lungs and bronchial tree. A similar origin can be postulated for **croup**, by way of the Danish *hropja*, the common name for a condition, usually observed in infants and children, wherein the bronchi become congested and partially obstructed, thus giving rise to a barking cough, hoarseness, and stridor.

coumarin (*see* **warfarin**)

cowpox (*see* **vaccine**)

coxa is the Latin word for "hip," which, in turn, is said to have come from the Sanskrit *kaksha* of the same meaning. The Latin *coxa* led to the French *cousin* and thence to our word "cushion."

cranium is the Latin word for skull and is related to the Greek *kranion*. Generally, the term refers to the skull minus the mandible, that is, the major portion that serves principally as the brain case. Craniotomy (+ Greek *tomē*, "a cutting") is an ancient and venerable operation for cutting an opening in the skull. The old belief was that this provided a sure means of allowing the escape of evil spirits.

crazy has no medical significance but still is a word often used and heard. Its origin has been traced to the Old Norse, whence came the Middle English *crasen*, "to crack or break." Words that may be related are "crackle" (full of cracks) and "crash." Another word that, regrettably, has been spoken in hospital corridors by doctors and nurses who should know better is **crock**, a pejorative reference to complaining patients whose examination seems to yield no challenging diagnosis or opportunity for effective treatment. Extended to man, this use of "crock" seems to go back to the term applied in rural England to an old or barren ewe or an old and decrepit horse. Whatever its origin, "crock" has no place in proper medical nomenclature. Even more deplorable is the similar use of **gomer**, an acronym for "Get out of *my* emergency room!"

cream as a vehicle for dermatologic medicaments is said to have had its origin in the Indo-European *ghreir*, "to smear or rub." The Greek *chrisma* means "anything smeared on, such as a scented unguent." The Greek *christos* means "anointed"; hence "the Christos" or "Christ" was "the anointed one." The Anglo-Saxon *crisma*, through French, became "cream."

creatinine is the anhydride of **creatine**, both words derived from the Greek *kreas*, "flesh or meat." The two nitrogenous substances were first discovered in meat extracts.

cremaster is an almost direct borrowing of the Greek *kremastēr*, "a suspender." The ancient anatomists gave this term to the muscles that suspend the testicles in the scrotum. The **cremasteric fascia** invests the spermatic cord.

crena is the Latin word for "notch or cleft" and is so used in certain anatomic terms, such as **crena ani** for the cleft between the buttocks. More familiar is the adjective **crenated**, as used to describe red blood cells whose surface membranes appear notched or burrlike.

crepitus is the peculiar sound or tactile sensation of gas, usually air, that has infiltrated soft tissues, as in subcutaneous emphysema. The term is a direct borrowing of the Latin *crepitus*, "a rattle or a crackling sound." The noun, in turn, relates to the Latin verb *crepare*, "to make rattle or to chatter noisily."

cretin is from the Old French *chrêtien*, which literally meant "a Christian," but became a somewhat contemptuous term applied to certain benighted human beings who were looked upon as hardly more than brutes. As a consequence of persecution in France, a group of adherents to Arianism, judged to be a heretical sect, sought refuge in remote valleys of the Pyrenees. Because of a chronically deficient diet, notably lacking in iodine, children of these people often were born with stunted bodies and minds. Philippus Aureolus Theophrastus Bombastus von Hohenheim (1493-1541), better known as Paracelsus, a celebrated Swiss physician, was the first to recognize the relation between goitrous parents and cretinous children. A cretin, we now know, is a victim of the congenital, juvenile form of **hypothyroidism**, **myxedema** being the condition in adults.

cribriform is a combination of the Latin *cribrum*, "a sieve," + *forma*, "likeness." The **cribriform plate** of the ethmoid bone and the **cribriform fascia** of the thigh are so called because of their numerous perforations.

cricoid comes from the Greek *krikos*, "a ring," being a variant of *kirkos*, "a circle." The **cricoid cartilage** was so named because it resembled a signet ring. The **cricopharyngeus muscle** encircles the lowermost portion of the hypopharynx.

crisis is derived from the Greek *krinein*, "to decide or judge," particularly in the sense of choosing or separating. Thus, a crisis occurs when an acutely ill patient appears to be on the verge of either survival or death. In effect, it can be said that a judgment is thus made between the quick and the dead. The ancients observed that there were critical days in the course of various acute diseases, especially those marked by fever. Fevers are said "to break" either by crisis, i.e., rapidly, as though a prompt decision had been rendered; or by lysis, i.e., gradually resolving. A related word is "criterion," a direct borrowing of the Greek *kritērion*, "a standard by which a judgment is made."

crista is the Latin word for "a tuft or ridge on the head of a bird, or the plume on a helmet," thus leading to the English "crest." The crest-like ridge of the ethmoid bone projects into the cranial cavity like a cock's comb, hence it is called the crista galli (Latin *gallus*, "a cock or rooster").

crock (*see* **crazy**)

crotch is a vernacular term for the region where the legs come together. It is also used in the sense of a fork or a point of division. The crotch of a tree is where its limbs divide. The origin of the word is obscure. It may have come from the Middle English *croche*, which meant "a shepherd's crook or crosier." This, in turn, probably came from the Old Scandinavian *krokr*, "hook." From this also was derived our word "crouch," meaning to assume a "hooked" position. A word probably related is **crutch**, the implement used to aid the lame and originally fashioned from the crotch of a tree.

croup (*see* **cough**)

cruciate describes whatever is crossed and is taken from *crux*, the Latin word for "cross." The cruciate ligaments, as in the knee, are so named because they cross each other. A related word is "crucial" in the sense of decisive, the reference being to the choice one must make when arriving at a "crossroad."

crud is a slang expression occasionally heard in medical circles to refer to illnesses that are annoying but trivial and which defy accurate diagnosis. In another sense, "crud" is an incrustation of refuse or of heavy, sticky snow unsuited to skiing. "Cruddy" can describe anything despicable. The origin of the word is unknown, but it may be a transliteration of "curd," the coagulum of soured milk.

crus is the Latin word for the leg, more specifically the shin. The term also is associated with the Latin *crux*, "cross," perhaps because *crus* was considered the perpendicular leg of a cross. In any event, crus is used in anatomy to describe various formations in the shape of V or X. The crus of the diaphragm is the crossing of muscles at the esophageal hiatus. **Crural** refers to the leg or whatever appears shaped like a leg.

crutch (*see* **crotch**)

cryo- is a combining form used in reference to freezing. The term is taken from the Greek *kryos*, "icy cold."

cryophilic (cryo- + Greek *philos*, "affinity") describes organisms that thrive at cold temperatures.

cryoprecipitate (cryo- + Latin *praecipitare*, "to cast down") is a particulate sedimentation induced by exposure to cold.

cryotherapy (cryo- + Greek *therapeia*, "treatment") is the use of freezing temperatures as a means of inducing degeneration and necrosis in diseased tissues.

crypt is taken from the Latin *crypta*, "an underground passage or gallery," that is related to the Greek *kryptos*, "hidden." The crypts of Lieberkühn, named for Johann Nathaniel Lieberkühn (1711-1756), a German anatomist, are the lumens of glands, which form passages in the intestinal mucosa.

cryptogenic means, literally, "of hidden origin." Often the word is used as a modifier in a supposedly diagnostic term but really is only a pseudosophisticated way of saying, "We really don't know where this condition comes from."

cryptorchidism (which should be spelled **cryptorchism** but usually isn't) refers to an undescended testicle that remains "hidden" in the abdomen.

CT-scanning (*see* **axis**)

cubitus is the Latin word for "lying down" and is related to *cubitum*, "the elbow." A favorite Roman posture was to rest on the elbows when reclining. Even now we speak of a patient lying on his left side as being in "the left lateral decubitus position," though it would be simpler to merely say he was lying on his left side. To stray further, *cubitus* also was a word the Romans used for sexual intercourse. Hence, a **concubine** is a person someone lies with, the intent being amorous dalliance. (*see* **decubitus**)

culdo- is a contrived combining form taken from the French *cul de sac* (*cul*, "bottom," + *de*, "of the," + *sac*, "sack") and, in gynecology, is used to refer to the vagina.

culdocentesis (+ Greek *kentēsis*, "a puncture") is the aspiration of the recto-uterine space by needle puncture of the vaginal wall.

culdoscopy (+ Greek *skopein*, "to inspect") is the visual examination of the female pelvic structures by means of an endoscope inserted through the posterior vaginal fornix.

culture is a near borrowing of the Latin *cultura*, "a tilling of the soil for the purpose of raising crops." This is closely related to the Latin *cultus*, which had a variety of meanings, all having to do with raising up, training, refinement, and the like. In referring to bacterial culture, one adheres closely to the original Latin meaning.

cuneiform describes whatever is wedge-shaped and is taken from the Latin *cuneus*, "wedge." The term is used to describe several of the small bones in the wrist and foot. A wedge-shaped lobule of the occipital lobe of the cerebrum is called the **cuneus**.

curare is the toxic essence of *Strychnos toxifera* and several other tropical American plants. The poison, applied to the tips of arrows, was concocted by Indians of the Macusi tribe, who called the plant source *urari-yé* and the poison *urari*. Curare in its refined form has been used as a paralytic agent in anesthesia and other circumstances requiring complete muscular relaxation.

cure comes from the Latin *cura*, "care, concern, or attention." The current use of the word seemingly sprang from a belief that proper and sufficient "care" was tantamount to "cure." Would that this were so! The familiar admonition to "Cure occasionally, relieve often, console always" comes from the ancient French aphorism "*Guerir quelquefois, soulanger souvent, consoler toujours.*"

curette is the French word for "scraper" and is related to the verb *curer*, "to clean out." **Curettage** or **curettement** are adopted from the French and refer to the operation of scraping a wound or other lesion for the purpose of cleansing.

curie (*see* **radium**)

curriculum is the Latin word for a "race course" and is related to the verb *currere*, "to run." This explains why the student often regards a curriculum as a "rat race." In academic terms, a curriculum is a "running account" of an established course of study. A **curriculum vitae** is an account of a career or "life's race."

cusp comes from the Latin *cuspis*, "a pointed end, as of a spear." The term is used in anato-

my to refer to the pointed extremity of anything, such as the cusp of a tooth or the cusp
of a valve. **Bicuspid** means "two-pointed"
and may refer to a tooth or a heart valve.
Tricuspid refers to the heart valve with three
points.

cutis is the Latin word for "skin." The Greek
kytos referred to any hollow vessel. Indeed,
the skin can be considered as the vessel containing the body and, overall, is the largest
organ of the body. **Cutaneous** describes
whatever relates to the skin. The diminutive
cuticle refers to "the little skin," such as that
emanating from the perionychium.
Incidentally, "cute" in the sense of attractive-
ly perky is unrelated; "cute" is an apheresis
of "acute," meaning "sharp."

cyanosis comes from the Greek *cyanos*, "dark
blue." This is the color assumed by the skin
and mucous membranes when deprived of
oxygenated blood.

cyclops as a term for a particular ocular
anomaly is borrowed from *Kyklōps,* the
name given by the Greeks to a mythical
race of lawless, giant shepherds who
inhabited Sicily. Their most striking feature
was a single, large, rounded eye situated in
the middle of the forehead. The name
came, literally, from *kyklos*, "a circle or
ring," + *ōps*, "eye." Medically, a cyclops is a
monster born with a single, centrally

placed eye.

cyclothymia is a condition marked by recurring, wide swings in mood from elation to
depression. The term is contrived from a
combination of the Greek *kyklos*, "a circle," +
thymos, "mental state or mood."

cyst is derived from the Greek *kystis*, "a bladder,
bag, or pouch," this being related to the verb
kyō, "I hold." In anatomy, the term "cystic"
can refer to any sort of bladder or cavity.

cystine is an amino acid so named because it
was first discovered as a hydrolytic product of
protein in urine, where it crystallized as a
concrement in the bladder.

cystocele describes a protrusion of the urinary
bladder into the vagina. The term combines
the Greek *kystis*, "bladder," + *kēlē*, "hernia."

cyto- is a combining form, also appearing as
-cyte, indicating whatever pertains to a cell.
It is derived from the Greek *kytos*, "hollow, as
a cell or container." In combination, "cyto-"
can describe all sorts of cells. **Anisocytosis**
(Greek *an*, "not," + *iso*, "the same") describes
a group of cells, normally regular, that vary
markedly in size. **Poikilocytosis** (Greek *poiki-
los*, "varied") describes a condition wherein
cells are of markedly abnormal shape. A
karyocyte (Greek *karyon*, "a nut or kernel") is
a nucleated cell, particularly an early nor-
moblast or an erythrocyte that normally
would not harbor a nucleus.

Dacry- is a combining form that refers to tears or to tearing, as in weeping (both words pronounced with a long "e"). The term is an almost direct borrowing of the Greek *dakry*, "a tear." Thus, **dacryadenitis** is an inflammation of the lacrimal gland.

-dactyl- is a combining form referring to a finger, or sometimes a toe, and is derived from the Greek *daktylos*, "finger." **Syndactyly** (Greek *syn-*, "together") is the condition wherein adjacent digits are joined by a congenital web.

dandruff is usually plainly evident as a condition; as a word, its origin is obscure. The first syllable may relate to an archaic English dialect word for small scales of skin, hair, or feathers. The second syllable probably comes from the Old Norse *hrufa*, "scab." **Dander** seems to be a contraction of "dandruff." In any case, dandruff is likely the most frequent diagnosis evident by periodic physical examination of healthy persons.

dartos is the name, as in tunica dartos, given to a layer of smooth muscle fibers intermingled with the fascia enveloping the testicles in the scrotum. It is a borrowing of the Greek word for "that which is flayed."

data is the plural (a point not always remembered by American speakers and writers) of the Latin *datum*, "a thing given," the neuter past participle of *dare*, "to give." In science, data are assembled as facts, statistics, or the like; one rarely encounters datum in reference to a single fact or statistic, but such use would be entirely proper.

deadly (*see* **mortal**)

deaf in Middle English was spelled (and pronounced) *deef*. So, the old-timer who pronounces the word to rhyme with "reef" is not being comical; he is being archaic. The original Indo-European root probably was *dheubh*, "dull to perception." Curiously, our adjective "absurd" bears a relation to deafness. The Latin *absurdus*, "senseless or silly," is a combination of *ab-*, "from," + *surdus*, "deaf, unheeding."

debridement is a French word that combines *dé-*, "not," + *brider*, "to bridle," thus literally an "unbridling." Originally, the term was used for the process of cutting constrictive bands but later, in surgery, came to refer to the cutting away of injured or necrotic tissue.

deceased is a delicate way of saying "dead." Not only is it delicate, it is used almost invariably as a passive verb. No one with a civil tongue speaks of "deceasing" himself or anyone else. "Deceased" comes from the Latin *decedere*, "to go away, to depart." This is akin to referring to death as "a passing away." **Demise** is a delicate noun for death. Its origin is somewhat tortuous but probably goes back to the Latin *demittere*, "to drop, to send down." A worthy suggestion might be to leave "deceased" and "demise" to persons given to unctuous speech, such as morticians. "Dead," even though a four-letter word, is perfectly respectable.

deci- is a combining form that is a contraction of the Latin *decimus*, "a tenth." The decimal system is a numeration based on tenths. A deciliter (abbreviated as "dL") is $\frac{1}{10}$ of a liter, or 100 milliliters.

decidua relates to the Latin verb *decidere*, "to fall away." **Deciduous** trees are those from which the leaves fall away in the chill of autumn, and deciduous teeth are those shed by youngsters in the normal course of development. In medicine, "decidua" is the name given to the mucosa of the uterus that "falls away" after parturition. The **menstrual decidua** is the hyperemic endometrium that is shed in the normal menstrual cycle. A **decision**, in common parlance, is reached after all other options or possibilities are discarded. The late Dr. Chester Jones, long an esteemed clinician at the Massachusetts General Hospital, is often quoted as saying, "If you can't make a diagnosis, make a decision."

decoction (*see* **concoction**)

decrepit describes whatever is infirm or broken down by age or hard use. The word is an almost direct borrowing of the Latin *decrepitus*, "broken down," which, in turn, combines *de-*, "from," + *crepare*, "to make rattle or creak."

decubitus is from the Latin verb *decumbere*, "to lie down," and is related to the Latin *cubitum*, "the elbow." The Romans habitually rested on their elbows when reclining. Decubitus is a reclining position, usually further specified as, for example, "the left lateral decubitus." A **decubitus ulcer** is a bedsore, the consequence of pressure necrosis in a dependent part from lying in one position too long. Some related words are **cubicle** (a small chamber in which to lie down), **cubbyhole** (a small place to lay anything), **incumbent** (a state of lying in or occupying), and **concubine** (one who lies with another). (*see* **cubitus**)

decussation is from the Latin verb *decussare*, "to divide crosswise," i.e., in the form of an "X." The decussation of the anterior pyramids of the medulla oblongata is the crossing of fibers from one side to the other to form the lateral spinothalamic tracts.

defecate (*see* **feces**)

degenerate comes from the Latin *degenerare*, "to disgrace, to fall short of, or to be inferior to one's ancestors." The derivation is from *de-*, "down from," + *genus*, "the race." In biology, a degenerated cell is one that has deteriorated in structure or function when compared with its normal counterparts of the "race."

deglutition is a combination of the Latin *de-*, "down," + *glutire*, "to gulp." Now the term is used in the gentler sense of simply swallowing. A related word is "glutton."

dehiscence can describe any abnormal gaping or splitting of tissue but most often is applied to separation of one or more layers of a partially healed wound or incision. The term is taken from the Latin *dehiscare*, "to part, divide, gape, or yawn."

dehydrate is a relatively recent hybrid term contrived from the Latin *de*, "out of," + the Greek *hydor*, "water." Whoever or whatever is dehydrated has been deprived of water.

delirium is said to have been first used by Aurelius Cornelius, better known as Celsus, the celebrated Roman encyclopedist of the 1st century A.D. The term is from the Latin *de-*, "away from," + *lira*, "a furrow." Whoever is mentally confused or incoherent cannot plow a straight furrow and may be said to have strayed from the groove.

deltoid refers to the shape of Δ (delta), the fourth letter of the Greek alphabet. Hence, in anatomy it can describe anything triangular in configuration. The deltoid muscle at the shoulder is more or less triangular.

delusion comes from the Latin *deludere*, "to dupe or deceive." The Latin *ludere* means "to play or to amuse oneself," and a *ludio* was an actor. One who suffers delusions is being misled by imaginary circumstances.

dementia is the Latin word for "madness" and comes from a combination of *de-*, "out of," + *mens*, "the mind." Whoever is demented is out of his or her mind. In a now outmoded classification, one form of mental derangement was known as **dementia praecox**, the second word being the Latin for "premature" (and the source of our word "precocious"). *Praecox* (Latin *prae-*, "before," + *coquere*, "to cook") thus literally means "uncooked" or "half-baked." What was formerly called dementia praecox, because it was often observed in younger persons, is now recognized as **schizophrenia** or one of its variants.

demise (*see* **deceased**)

demulcent comes from the Latin *demulcere*, "to stroke lovingly or to caress," a combination of *de-*, "down," + *mulcere*, "to pet or to soften." The Romans used *demulcere* particularly for the soothing stroking of horses. In medicine, a demulcent is a soothing drug, especially one topically applied to allay the irritation of inflamed surfaces.

dendrite means "branched like a tree" and is derived from the Greek *dendron*, "tree." In anatomy the term refers particularly to the branching protoplasmic processes of nerve cells. In botany, a rhododendron (Greek *rhodon*, "rose") is an evergreen tree bearing rose-colored flowers, and a philodendron (Greek *philos*, "loving") is a climbing plant with evergreen foliage that clings to trees, so called because it has an affinity for or "loves" trees.

dengue is the name of an acutely painful, febrile illness endemic in the West Indies, the Middle East, India, and the South Pacific. It is also known as "breakbone fever." Its victims often exhibit contortions because of intense muscle and joint pains. One explanation is that the name originated in the Swahili word *ki-dinga*, "a sudden cramp or seizure." Another explanation relates to the Spanish *denguero*, which means "affected or finicky." Slaves in the West Indies were said to have called the disease "dandy fever," presumably because of the affected gait or postures of persons so afflicted.

dental is taken from the Latin *dens*, "tooth or tusk," and refers to whatever pertains to teeth. The Latin *densus* means "hard, compact." **Dentin** is the principal substance of a tooth, surrounding the pulp and being covered by enamel. **Dentate** means "arranged like teeth"; the serrated mucocutaneous border at the anus is a dentate line.

depilatory refers to an agent, usually applied as a cream, that removes unwanted hair. The word is derived from the Latin *de-*, "away," + *pilus*, "hair."

depressor (*see* **levator**)

dermis comes from the Greek *derma*, "the skin." A related Sanskrit word is *dartis*, "leather or hide." When used alone, dermis refers to the corium or dense layer of connective tissue underneath the stratified squamous epithelium of the skin. More often, **derm-** is a combining form contributing to a host of terms pertaining to the skin, such as **dermatology** (the science of the skin), **dermatitis** (inflammation of the skin), **dermatome** (an instrument for slicing the skin), **dermatographia** (a condition wherein gentle stroking induces a localized swelling that appears as a "writing" on the skin), and many others.

desiccate comes from the Latin *desiccare*, "to dry up or to drain," this being derived from a combination of *de-*, "away," + *siccus*, "dry." The **sicca** syndrome is characterized by excessive dryness of the normally moist membranes of the eye and mouth. The French *sec*, "dry," particularly as it refers to wines lacking sweetness, is a related word.

desmo- is a combining form taken from the Greek *desmos*, "a band or fetter." Consequently, "desmo-" has come to refer to dense fibrous or connective tissue.

desmoid describes a scirrhous connective tissue neoplasm (e.g., one that is "tightly bound"), such as can occur in persons afflicted with Gardner's syndrome.

desmoplasia (desmo- + Greek *plassein*, "to form or mold") is a pervasive growth of fibrous tissue, particularly that investing certain neoplasms.

desquamation (*see* **squamous**)

detritus is the past participle of the Latin *deterere*, "to rub off or to rub away." Detritus, then, is that which is rubbed away and refers, as a medical term, to debris collected in or around degenerating or necrotic tissue. (*see* **trituration**)

detrusor comes from the Latin *detrudere*, "to push down or to dislodge." The detrusor muscle of the urinary bladder serves to aid in the expulsion of urine.

dexter is the Latin word for "right," as opposed to "left." As the combining form **dextr-**, it has been incorporated in numerous anatomic terms designating the right-sided component of various bilaterally symmetric structures. Because a majority of persons are naturally more facile with their right hands, **dexterity** has come to mean "skill or deftness." A related word, as previously mentioned, is **adroit**.

dextrin is an intermediate product of the hydrolysis of starch and is so called because of its **dextrorotary** ("turning to the right") effect on polarized light.

dextrose is a colorless, crystalline hexose that exhibits a **dextrorotary** property. More specifically it is D-glucose, the "D" standing for "dextro-." (*see* **glucose**)

dhobie itch has been sometimes used as a nickname for tinea cruris, a pruritic fungus infection of the groin. *Dhobie* is the Hindustani word for "a washerman." More specifically and properly, "dhobie itch" refers to a contact dermatitis caused by hypersensitivity to the marking fluid (bhilawanol oil) used by native laundry workers in India.

dia- is a busy combining form taken from the Greek preposition *dia*, which has many meanings, including "through, throughout, thoroughly, completely, across, and opposed to." It appears as a prefix in many truly Greek words and also has been used to lend a classical tone to many newly concocted words.

diabetes is a direct borrowing of the Greek word meaning both "a siphon" (*dia*, "through," + *banein*, "to run or pass") and "a compass," i.e., the device used to draw circles. Areteus the Cappadocian, a famous Greek physician of the 2nd century A.D., explained that *diabētēs* as a disease was so called because its victims, exhibiting polyuria, "passed water like a siphon." The common sort of diabetic urine is laden with sugar, hence the second part of "diabetes **mellitus**" is the Latin word for "sweetened with honey." The urine of patients with "diabetes **insipidus**," on the other hand, though voluminous, is lacking in sugar and therefore tasteless or insipid. To the Romans, *insipiens* meant "foolish," as derived from *in-*, "lacking," + *sapientia*, "taste or sense." The Latin *sapor* means "taste" in the concept both of flavor and of refinement, much as we use the English word.

diagnosis is a direct borrowing of the Greek *diagnōsis*, but to the Greeks this meant specifically "a discrimination, a distinguishing, or a discerning between two possibilities," in the sense of resolving or deciding. The word combines *dia-* in any or almost all of its meanings + *gnōsis*, "knowledge" when applied to the discernment of disease as it affects a given patient.

dialysis is a direct borrowing of the Greek word for "a loosening of one thing from another." It is almost exactly in that sense that "dialysis" is used in medicine as "a process of separating crystalloids or colloids in solution by the difference in their rates of diffusion through a semipermeable membrane" (Dorland).

diapedesis (dia- + Greek *pēdan*, "to leap") was used by ancient writers to refer to serous oozing from small blood vessels. In modern medical parlance, diapedesis refers to the escape of blood corpuscles through the discontinuous endothelium of intact vessels, particularly as this occurs in response to inflammation.

diaper refers not to the shape or function of the familiar "three-cornered pants" but to the fabric and its color. The word combines *dia*, "thoroughly," + the Greek *aspros*, "white." In ancient times the fabric was a pure linen of fine texture that was pristinely white.

diaphoresis is a Greek word used by ancient writers for "profuse sweating." It includes the Greek *phorein*, "to convey." Diaphoresis is still used as a rather pompous medical synonym for "sweating."

diaphragm is a near borrowing of the Greek *diaphragma*, "a partition," this being a combination of *dia-*, "across," + *phragma*, "a fence or wall." Certain ancient writers ascribed great significance to the muscular diaphragm separating the chest from the abdomen, some even attributing to it powers of the mind. This explains the naming of the **phrenic** (Greek *phrēn*, "the mind") nerve that supplies the diaphragm, possibly because the diaphragm sits atop the spleen and kidneys, organs once thought to be the seat of emotions.

diaphysis incorporates the Greek *physis*, "growth." Originally, the term referred to "the bursting of a bud" or "the point where a branch grew from a stalk." Later, in anatomy, "diaphysis" came to be applied to the shaft of a long bone, particularly as a growth center, in distinction to the epiphysis.

diarrhea is an almost direct borrowing of the Greek *diarrhoia*, "a flowing through," which incorporates the Greek *rhein*, "to flow." The ancients used the term, as we do, in reference to excessive, watery evacuation from the bowel.

diastase is a word coined in the 19th century as the name for a substance (later identified as an enzyme) capable of breaking down or separating starch into its component sugars. It was derived from the Greek *diastasis*, "a standing apart." Because diastase was thought of as the prototype of an enzyme, the last three letters, "-ase," came to be a suffix designating an enzymatic property. (*see* **-ase**)

diastasis is still used in its original Greek meaning when applied to a separation of the abdominal muscles, as in diastasis recti.

diastole is a direct borrowing of the Greek word meaning "a distinction or difference" and is a combination of *dia-*, "apart," + *stellein*, "to put." With separation there is the idea of introducing or expanding a pause between two circumstances or events. It is in this sense that "diastole" came to be, in physiology, the name for the period of relaxation and dilatation of the heart muscle between systolic contractions.

diathermy is a contrived term incorporating the Greek *therma*, "heat," intensified by the prefix "dia-," thus referring to "penetrating heat."

diathesis is a Greek word meaning "an order of

arrangement," particularly in the sense of "a disposition." Ancient writers conceived that certain persons, because of their make-up or temperament, were particularly disposed to certain diseases. We use the term in much the same way when we refer to a predisposition as, for example, in "hemorrhagic diathesis."

dichotomy is taken from the Greek *dikhotomos*, "divided," this being a combination of *dikha*, "in two," + *tomē*, "a cutting." A dichotomy, then, results in two equal parts or a pair. In biology the term refers to branching equally to become a pair. Used figuratively, "dichotomy" means a division into two usually contradictory parts or opinions.

dicrotic is derived from the Greek *di-*, "two or twice," + *krotein*, "to strike." The term has been applied to a doubly peaked pulse wave. **Anacrotic** (Greek *ana-*, "upward") means the secondary impulse is on the ascending limb of the pulse wave; **catacrotic** (Greek *kata*, "down") means the secondary impulse is on the descending limb.

dicumarol (*see* **warfarin**)

diet comes from the Greek *diaita*, "a way of living or a mode of life." Originally, the term was used for a hygienic regimen generally and only later it was restricted to a mode of eating considered conducive to good health. Incidentally, this is quite distinct from "diet" meaning "an assembly or parliament," which is taken from the Latin *dies*, "day," implying that a formal meeting is held on an appointed day.

digastric is the name of a muscle in the anterior neck that depresses the mandible and elevates the hyoid bone. It is so called because it has two bellies. Its name comes from the Greek *di-*, "two," + *gastēr*, "belly." Obviously, this muscle, despite its name, has nothing to do with the stomach.

digestion is derived from the Latin *digerere*, "to arrange, sort out, or distribute." Medieval chemists used the term in the sense of "dissolving." In the 17th century a device was introduced whereby bones could be softened by cooking under pressure; this was called a "digester." The early physiologists borrowed the term in the belief that ingested food was treated in the stomach in a manner similar to digestion as carried out in the chemist's laboratory. As it turned out, they may have

been closer to the mark than they might have guessed.

digit is a contraction of the Latin *digitus*, "a finger or a toe." A **digitation** is a fingerlike process, and to **interdigitate** means to appear as interlocking fingers. "Digit" as a term for a number came from the custom of counting on one's fingers. Inasmuch as we normally have 10 fingers, this accounts for the decimal system of numbering and for the metric system based on 10. (*see* **finger**)

digitalis comes from the Latin *digitus*, "finger." The allusion is to the tubular blossoms of the plant whose dried leaves, when pulverized, provide the drug. The shape of the flower suggests the empty finger of a glove. In part, this explains the plant's common name, "the foxglove." But why the "fox"? No one really knows. By curious coincidence, "digitalis" was proposed as the Latinized name for the plant in the 16th century by a German botanist, Leonhard Fuchs (1501-1566). *Fuchs* is German for "fox." Apparently, he chose *digitalis*, a Latin way of saying "pertaining to the finger," because the common German name for the plant is *Fingerhut*, which means, literally, "a finger hat" or thimble. But we are still left wondering why the foxglove was so called as early as the 11th century.

dilate is a verb meaning "to enlarge or expand" and is taken from the Latin *dilatare* meaning the same and derived from *dis-*, "apart," + *latus*, "wide." Often in medical parlance and writing **dilation** and **dilatation** are used more or less interchangeably. The instrument used to dilate is commonly called a **dilator**; one almost never hears reference to "a dilatator." According to Fowler's *Modern English Usage*, "dilation" and "dilator" are wrongly formed from the Latin (the first "-at-" being part of the word and not contributing to the suffix "-tion," indicating an action). Therefore, we are instructed to always use "dilatation" in reference to either the procedure or its result and "dilatator" for either the instrument of the operator. To consistently use "dilatation" won't be difficult; but the venerable Fowler's notwithstanding, it is doubtful "dilatator" will play in Peoria.

dimercaprol (*see* **BAL**)

diopter originated in the Greek *dioptra*, an

instrument used for accurately measuring heights and angles. "Diopter" later was adopted as a name for the unit of refracting power of lenses, the standard of 1 diopter being a focal distance of 1 meter.

diphtheria got its name from the Greek *diphthera*, "a prepared hide or leather." The allusion is to the parchmentlike membrane in the throat characteristic of the disease. Diphtheria was known to the ancient Greeks and feared because of the high rate of mortality among children, but they did not call it by that name. To them it was "the Egyptian disease" or "the Syrian ulcer," yet another example of blaming a malady on someone else.

diplo- is a combining form taken from the Greek *diploos*, "double or two-fold."

diplococcus describes a bacterium that looks like a pair of tiny berries (diplo- + Greek *kokkos*, "berry").

diploidy is the normal state of having paired sets of homologous chromosomes in somatic cells. (*see* -ploid)

diplopia was contrived as a combination of "diplo-" + the Greek *opsis*, "vision." This term for disunited visual images first appeared in print in the early 19th century.

dipsomania is the result of combining the Greek *dipsa*, "thirst," + *mania*, "madness." The term first appeared in English in the mid-19th century to describe "a frenzy to drink," specifically referring to alcoholic beverages and was considered a form of insanity.

disease comes from the Old French *desaise*, a combination of *des-*, "away from," + *aise*, "ease." In its early use, the term referred to any tribulation that disturbed one's ease. Only later did "disease" acquire its restricted medical sense.

disk is a near borrowing of the Greek *diskos*, "a circular, flat stone," which the Greeks were much given to hurl. Sometimes the *diskos* had a hole in the center, either to swing it by a strap or to use it as a *quoit* (a doughnut-shaped object to toss at a peg). "Disk" or "disc" now refers to any circular, platelike structure as, for example, the intervertebral disk.

disoriented is an adjective describing a person who has lost a sense of direction or relation to surroundings. The term comes from a combination of the Latin *dis-*, "deprived of," + *oriens*, "the rising sun or the direction of east," the latter being a present participle of *oriri*, "to rise." To say a person is "disoriented" is the equivalent of saying, "He doesn't know which end is up."

dispensary comes from the Latin *dispensare*, "to weigh out." Originally, the term was applied to a place where medicinal agents were measured and distributed. Later, it came to mean a place where the sick or injured were treated but not confined as inpatients. In the past, outpatient departments often were called "dispensaries."

dissect is from the Latin *dissecare*, "to cut apart," this being a simple combination of *dis-*, "apart," + *secare*, "to cut." An anatomic dissection, then, is "a cutting apart" of a body or a part thereof for the purpose of identifying and examining its components. The Latin verb *resecare* means "to cut back, trim, curtail." Thus, a surgical **resection** is an operation wherein an organ is "cut back" or removed in whole or in part.

disseminate (*see* semen)

distal (*see* proximal)

distill is derived from the manner in which vapor from a heated liquid is condensed and collected, drop by drop. The word is a combination of the Latin *de-*, "from," + *stilla*, "a drop." To **instill** originally meant "to introduce something drop by drop."

diuresis is made up of a combination of the Greek *dia-*, "thoroughly," + *ourein*, "to urinate." There is a distinction between stimulating the excretion and flow of urine from the kidney as compared to stimulating contraction of the urinary bladder so as to cause its evacuation. By common acceptance, a diuretic agent is understood to be that which promotes the formation of urine by the kidney. An example, among others, would be chlorothiazide. On the other hand, bethanechol, which induces smooth muscle contraction, is a bladder evacuant, not a diuretic.

diurnal (*see* journal)

diverticulum is a direct borrowing of the Latin word for "a bypath or small wayside shelter," coming from the verb *divertere*, "to turn aside." The "culum" implies the diminutive and indicates that a diverticulum is subsidiary to the main channel. It is important to remember that "diverticulum" is the Latin neuter singular and that "diverticula" (not "diverticuli" or "diverticulae") is the neuter plural, a point that many careless speakers and writers seem to ignore.

dizzy (*see* **vertigo**)

doctor is taken from the Latin *docere*, "to teach." In years past, "doctor" was a title of courtesy and respect bestowed on a learned man. Later, it became associated with the title of the highest academic degree. Meanwhile, "doctor" acquired, chiefly among speakers of English, a specifically medical connotation. Probably this was because, of all learned scholars, only members of the medical faculty became familiar figures to the public at large. In no other language than English are practitioners of medicine commonly referred to as teachers. (*see* **-iatros**)

dolicho- is a combining form derived from the Greek *dolichos*, "long." Thus, **dolichocephalic** refers to a long head, and **dolichocolon** to an unusually long and redundant large intestine.

doll's eyes are so called in medical parlance because in patients with certain types of metabolic coma, notably in hypoglycemia and hepatic encephalopathy, moving the head from side to side will elicit abrupt movement of the eyes to the opposite side. This is suggestive of the mechanical movement of doll's eyes. The typical movement is a sign of cortical depression with intact brainstem connections.

-dontal (*see* **tooth**)

dope comes from the Dutch *doop*, meaning "a sauce or viscous liquid." It became applied to narcotics because while raw opium is being processed, it becomes a thick liquid when heated. Later, any substance having a numbing or stupefying effect became known as "dope." By extension, a person afflicted with a narcotic effect was called, in slang, "a dopehead" or simply "a dope." But there is more to the vagaries of this little word. Unscrupulous racehorse promoters found they could often ensure the outcome of a race by giving a drug to the mount preselected to win. Anyone privy to this illicit information was said to have "the inside dope." Soon, any worthwhile intelligence came to be called "the dope."

dopamine is an immediate metabolic precursor of epinephrine and norepinephrine, hence important in central sympathomimetic actions. Sometimes called by its nickname **dopa**, it has nothing to do with "dope." It is merely a somewhat unfortunate acronym for 3,4-dihydroxyphenylethylamine.

Doppler describes a recordable effect of sound or ultrasound waves when they emanate from or are directed at a moving object. The technique has been applied to medical diagnosis, especially in determining the extent and direction of blood flow. The term is taken from the name of Christian Doppler (1803-1853), an American mathematician, who was the first to explain why, for example, the pitch of a locomotive whistle is higher when the train is approaching the listener than when the train is speeding away.

dorsum is Latin for "back." Thus, the dorsum of the hand or foot is the "back" of that part, opposite the palm or sole. The adjective **dorsal** is understood to pertain to the back of any part, but especially to the back of the thorax. The dorsal vertebrae are the thoracic vertebrae. "Dorsal" also is used to mean "posterior," as in the dorsal roots of the spinal nerves. Incidentally, to endorse a check is to sign one's name to the back of the document.

dose is said to have had its origin in the postulated Indo-European root *dō*, "to give." A descendant is the Greek *dosis*, "that which is given." A related word is the Latin *donare*, "to bestow," and from this we derive "donate." A dose, then, is the "giving" of a specified amount of a medicine.

douche is the French word for "a shower bath" and can be traced to the Latin *ductus*, the past participle of *ducere*, "to lead." A douche, then, is a stream of water or watery solution directed to a body part or cavity for the purpose of cleansing.

dram is an almost forgotten unit of measure. It came originally from the Greek *drachmē*, a coin approximately equivalent to a Roman *denarius*. The coin also was used as a weight and later a "drachma" or dram became $\frac{1}{8}$ ounce as an apothecary's weight (but $\frac{1}{16}$ of an avoirdupois ounce). Before adoption of the metric system, a dram of fluid was commonly taken to be 1 teaspoonful (nearly equivalent to 5 milliliters), the symbol on a prescription being written as "℥." The fluid ounce was written as "f. ℥," intended to be translated as 2 tablespoons (approximately equivalent to 30 milliliters). Reference to teaspoons and tablespoons as prescribed doses of liquid medicines was necessary because these units of measure were the only ones available in most households. **Ounce** comes from the Latin *uncia*, "a twelfth," this being $\frac{1}{12}$ of a Roman *libra* or pound (hence the abbreviation "lb" for pound). If all of this seems confusing, it is. One must keep in mind the differences between liquid and dry measurements and between Roman and English custom.

draught is often and alternatively spelled **draft**, especially in the United States, and always pronounced as "draft," though a Scotsman might utter a guttural sound before the "t." It is an old word that can be traced to the Old Norse *draga*, "to pull, carry, or drag," and is related to the Latin *trahere*, "to draw." At one time "draught" meant a dose of medicine as it would be "drawn off" from a larger container. Occasionally, an old-timer will speak of taking "black draught," a purgative that included senna, magnesium sulfate, and extract of licorice.

dropsy is now an archaic term for a condition wherein the body tissues are swollen by an accumulation of excess fluid. Its use in English comes, through the French *hydropsie*, from the Greek *hydrops*, which meant the same thing. *Hydōr* is the Greek word for water of any kind. In former times, "dropsy" often was used as a diagnosis in itself. Now we refer to edema, ascites, or anasarca as more descriptive signs, and we require a designation of the underlying cause, such as congestive heart failure or cirrhosis, as the diagnosis. This enhanced perception accounts for the disuse of "dropsy."

drug is a word that tends to be avoided by etymologists because its origin is obscure. The Middle English *droge* and the Old French *drogue* both referred to chemical substances variously used as medicaments or dyes. A related word is the Dutch *droog*, "dry," including any desiccated substance, such as

herbs. An alternative postulate is that "drug" may have come from the Middle Low German *droge*, as in droge vats, "dry or drawn casks," the droge being later, perhaps mistakenly, applied to the former contents.

duct is a contraction of the Latin *ductus*, "a drawing or a leading," which is related, in turn, to the verb *ductere*, "to draw, to lead, or to escort." However, Latin authors never used *ductus* when they referred to a conduit for fluids. Rather, they used *canalis*, "a pipe or gutter."

duodenum began as the Greek *dodeka-daktulon*, "12 fingers," the idea being that the proximal, retroperitoneal portion of the small intestine is about 12 finger-breadths long. This came to be translated, through the Arabic, as the Late Latin *duodenum*. In classical Latin this would have been *duodecim*, "12" (from *duo*, "two," + *decem*, "ten"). In German, the duodenum is *der Zwölffingerdarm*, "the 12-finger intestine."

dura mater is the name for the tough, outer membrane encasing the brain and spinal cord. It is composed of the Latin words *dura*, "hard or tough," and *mater*, "mother." This makes little sense until one knows that the Latin *dura mater* is a literal translation of its precedent, the Arabic term which meant "strong mother" (in the sense of "protector") of the brain.

dys- is an inseparable combining form, originating in the Greek, that confers a bad sense on whatever word it is hooked onto. "Dys-" conveys a meaning of defective, difficult, ill, or painful. There are a host of medical terms beginning with "dys-." Some of them are closely related to Greek words. Incidentally, "dys-" is not to be confused with "dis-," a prefix borrowed from the Latin and meaning "apart, asunder, deprived of." Some "dys-" words are more tortuously contrived. An example is **dysfunction**, to refer to anything that goes wrong.

dyschezia (*see* **-chezia**)

dyscrasia is an almost direct borrowing of the Greek *dyskrasia*, "a bad mixture of humors, a bad temperament"; the Greek *krasis* means "mixture or make-up." The term originally referred to any diseased condition but now, for some obscure reason, is restricted to hematology, as in "blood dyscrasias."

dysentery is the condition of a painful gut, usually attended by diarrhea. The Greek *dysenteria* (+ *enteron*, "intestine") means "a bowel complaint."

dysgeusia combines "dys-" + Greek *geusis*, "taste" and is a pompous way of saying "a bad taste in the mouth."

dyslexia joins "dys-" + Greek *lexis*, "diction" to designate an impaired ability to read or write words, a familial disorder more frequent in boys. (*see* **alexia**)

dyspareunia comes from the Greek *dyspareunos*, "ill-mated," but now means painful sexual intercourse. The Greek *pareunos* (*para-*, "beside," + *eunos*, "bed") means "lying beside."

dyspeptic describes a nondescript digestive malaise. The term was contrived by combining "dys-" + Greek *pepsis*, "digestion."

dyspnea relates to the Greek *dyspnoia* (+ *pnoia*, "breathing"), and both mean "difficult or labored breathing." To detect subtly labored breathing, try breathing along with the patient. You may be surprised how dyspnea thereby becomes evident.

dystrophy is an abnormal growth or development, from whatever cause. The term combines "dys-" + the Greek *trophē*, "nourishment."

Ear is from the Old Norse *eyra* and is related to the Latin *auris* and the Greek *ous*, all of which mean "ear." The Greek *akouein*, "to hear," is a forerunner of **acoustic**, the adjective describing whatever pertains to hearing. The acoustic nerve is the eighth cranial nerve, also known as the auditory or the vestibulocochlear nerve. The Latin *auris* gives **aural** and the combining form **auri-**, both of which pertain to hearing or the ear, except for the **auricle** ("little ear") of the heart, a sort of nickname for the atrial appendage, so called because it was thought to resemble the floppy ear of a dog. The Latin *auris* is not to be confused with the Latin *aura*, "a breeze or atmosphere," or the Latin *aurum*, "gold."

eburnation comes from the Latin *ebur*, "ivory," and thus means a conversion to the appearance of ivory. In eburnation, bone becomes abnormally hard and as dense as ivory. In dentistry, it refers to a condition wherein exposed dentin assumes an ivorylike look.

ecchymosis is from the Greek *ekchymesthai*, "to pour out," which combines *ek-*, "out," + *chymos*, "juice." The juice, of course, refers to blood, and *ekchymōsis* was used in Hippocratic writings to refer to the escape of blood from rupture of small blood vessels and the consequent infiltration of surrounding tissues (*see* **purpura**). An ecchymosis to lay persons is a **bruise**. This less sophisticated term, as might be expected, comes from the Anglo-Saxon *brȳsan*, "to break."

echinococcus is derived from a combination of the Greek *echinos*, "a hedgehog or a sea urchin" (the allusion being to the prickly or spiny surfaces of such animals), + the Greek *kokkus*, "berry." The name was suggested by the numerous, spiny hooklets seen in the minute, berrylike scolex of the larval form of the parasite. (*see* **hydatid**)

echography is a method of diagnostic imaging, also known as **ultrasonography**. The image is produced by the "echo" of high-frequency, ultrasound waves as they encounter body tissues of varying densities. In Roman mythology, Echo was the name of a lovely nymph whose one failing was that she talked too much. One day Juno, Queen of Olympus, was searching for her errant husband Jupiter whom she suspected was cavorting with one or another of the nymphs. By her prattling, Echo detained Juno, thus allowing the nymphs to escape. Juno was so incensed by the ploy that she cursed Echo by depriving her of the use of her tongue, except in reply. Juno's harsh sentence on poor Echo: "You shall still have the last word but no power to speak first!" So it is the "reply" to ultrasound waves that creates the image in echography.

echolalia is a stereotypic repetition of words or phrases by one person in response to those spoken by another. For example, "How are you?" is met not by the expected answer but by an echoic "How are you?" Echolalia often is a symptom of autism and certain forms of schizophrenia. Echolalia also is observed as a phase in an infant's learning of a language. The term combines "echo-" + the Greek *lalia*, "talk."

eclampsia is derived from the Greek *eklampein*, "to shine forth suddenly, to flash." In the 18th century, "eclampsia" was coined as a reference to scintillating flashes of light in the visual field of a victim subject to sudden convulsions of any sort. Later, the term was restricted to the symptom as it was observed in an adverse course of pregnancy. Still later, the term was applied to the entire syndrome of toxemia of pregnancy, including hypertension, edema, and renal impairment that lead, in some cases, to convulsions and coma.

eclectic is a term once applied to a certain style of medical practice. In bygone days, eclectic medicine involved selecting those methods of treatment deemed best from a variety of cults, rather than slavishly following the dictates of any one system. In more recent times, eclectic physicians were those inclined to select single remedies, particularly those of botanical origin, for specific maladies. Today, what is called **holistic** medicine can be said to be eclectic. The term comes from the Greek *eklektikos*, "selective."

ecology would seem to have been only recently conceived, but in fact the word was introduced in 1869 by Ernst Heinrich Haekel (1834-1919), a German zoologist and votary of classical Greek. The word was then half-forgotten until recently revived to find a place in almost everyone's vocabulary. "Ecology" was derived from the Greek *oikos*, "house or place to live," + *logos*, "a treatise or study," and taken to mean the science of the habitat of living things, particularly as that habitat is affected by its environment.

écorché is an anatomic representation of the body or a portion thereof with the skin removed to reveal the underlying musculature, a depiction familiar to all medical students. The term is French, the past participle of *écorcher*, "to flay, as to strip off the skin," from the Latin *excorticare* that means the same.

ectasia is the condition of being dilated, expanded, or distended. The term is an almost direct borrowing of the Greek *ektasis*, "an extension or dilatation." It can also be a combining form, as in **bronchiectasis** (Greek *bronchus*, "windpipe"), a dilatation of the intrapulmonary air passages usually associated with chronic suppurative infection. "Ectasia" can also describe dilatation, expansion, or distention of blood vessels, the iris of the eye, or glandular ducts. "Ectasia" is not to be confused with "ecstasy," which is taken from the Greek *ekstasis*, "to be mindlessly distracted."

ectoderm is derived from the Greek *ektos*, "outside," + *derma*, "skin." The term refers to the outermost germ layer of the embryo from which the skin and its appendages originate. The other two layers are the **entoderm** (from the Greek *endon*, "within or inner") and the **mesoderm** (from the Greek *mesos*, "middle"). The triad of germ layers was conceptualized by Robert Remak (1815-1865), a German embryologist and neurologist.

-ectomy is a combining form and means "a cutting out." It combines the Greek *ek*, "out," + *tomē*, "a cutting." Preceded by the name of

almost any anatomic structure, it forms a word for the surgical removal of that structure. An example is "appendectomy."

ectopia is a transliteration of the Greek *ektopis*, "displacement," a combination of *ek*, "out of," + *topos*, "place." The word was not used by the Greeks as a medical term but is said to have been given by Robert Barnes (1817-1907), an English obstetrician, as a name for an extrauterine pregnancy. Ectopic can describe anything "out of place," i.e., in a location other than its normal habitat.

ectropion is a near borrowing of the Greek word for "an everted or turned-out eyelid." It is related to the Greek *ektropē*, "a turning out or aside." An inverted, or turned-in, eyelid is an **entropion**.

eczema is an almost direct borrowing of the Greek word for "anything thrown off or out by heat" and is derived from a combination of *ek*, "out," + *zeein*, "to boil." To the ancients, a skin eruption was a "boiling over" of the body "humors." Formerly used to refer to almost any vesicular or scaly rash, "eczema" now is usually restricted to immunopathic eruptions. In this sense, the term may be reverting to the original concept of unruly humors.

edema comes from the Greek *oidēma*, "a swelling." The original Greek is more favored in the British spelling of "oedema" than in the American version. In ancient writings, the term was applied to any tumorous condition but later was restricted to swelling in tissues resulting from the accumulation of fluid.

efferent (*see* **afferent**)

effervescence is derived from the Latin *effervescere*, "to boil over," which combines *e-*, *ef-*, "out or from," + *fervescere*, "to become boiling hot." Now the term describes any liberation of gaseous bubbles from a fluid, hot or cold. A **seltzer** is a naturally effervescent spring water of high mineral content. Taking liberty with this strict definition, the makers of a familiar, over-the-counter headache remedy dubbed their product Alka-Seltzer, which is notably effervescent but hardly natural. Seltzer is a truncated version of the German *Selterserwasser*, named for its origin in the village of Selters near Wiesbaden.

effete means "exhausted or worn out" and

comes from the Latin *effeta*, "spent, as from bearing young" and combines *e-* (*ef-*), "from," + *fetus*, "breeding." The term accurately describes the woman who has become exhausted from childbirth, but in general usage "effete" has acquired a sense of decadence.

effluent (*see* **flux**)

ego is the Latin "I," the first person singular pronoun. In psychiatry, the ego is purported to be "that portion of the psyche that possesses consciousness, maintains its identity, and recognizes and tests reality" (Dorland).

egophony is Greek and is spelled "aegophony" by purists. It is a combination of *aix*, "goat," + *phonē* "a voice or sound." The auscultatory sign is a bleating sound heard just above collections of pleural fluid and is best elicited by having the patient voice the letter "a" as in "bake"; the resulting egophonous sound comes through the stethoscope as "e" in "beet" (or "bleat").

ejaculate (*see* **inject**)

elbow is derived from the Anglo-Saxon *eln-boga*, literally "the arm-bending." The related Latin word is *ulna*, "elbow or arm," the name given to the larger of the two bones in the forearm and whose proximal end forms the prominence of the elbow.

electron is a slight transliteration of the Greek *elektron*, the name given by the Greeks to the substance amber, the yellow-brown, translucent, fossil resin that was found capable of gaining a negative electric charge when rubbed. An interesting analogue is found in Arabic, in which amber is *kahraba*, and a closely related form means electricity. The ancient Greeks were aware that rubbed amber exerts an attracting force, but it remained for William Gilbert (1544-1603), an English physician and natural philosopher, to use the term **electrified** to describe this form of magnetism.

element is descended from the Latin *elementum*, "a rudiment, beginning, or first principle." To the ancients, there were four *elementa* of all matter: fire, air, water, and earth. The origin of the Latin word is not known but, because *elementum* could also refer to one of a series, the suggestion has been made that it might have come from a euphonious recitation of the three letters "L," "M," and "N," as "el" +

"em" + "en," just as we refer to our rudimentary "ABCs."

elephantiasis is the name given to a sign of disease marked by thickened, corrugated skin. The obvious allusion is to the hide of the elephant, which is a pachyderm (from the Greek *pachys*, "thick," + *derma*, "skin"). The Latin name for the animal is *elephantus*, and the Greek name was *elaphus*. Some say there may be a relation to the Hebrew *aleph*, sometimes given as *eleph*, which is the first letter of the Hebrew alphabet and also the symbol for an ox, signifying anything huge. (*see* **filariasis**)

ELISA is an acronym that conveniently designates a type of immunoassay that defines certain antigens and antibodies. The term is taken from *Enzyme-Linked ImmunoSorbent Assay*.

elixir to the pharmacist is a fluid, usually a mixture containing alcohol and water with coloring and flavoring added that serves as a vehicle for a medicinal agent. An example is "elixir of phenobarbital." Most authorities trace "elixir" to the Arabic *al-iksir*, literally "a dry powder" but more specifically an essence that was sought by alchemists to turn base metals into gold. Therefore, to medieval practitioners of the arcane arts, "elixir" had the connotation of magic. When the goal of alchemy proved too elusive, the search continued for an *elixir vital*, a potion intended to ensure eternal youth. This, too, remains undiscovered. On a more prosaic note, we are reminded that there is a Latin adjective *elixus*, meaning "wet through and through, soaked," and this seems more in keeping with the pharmacologic "elixir" as we know it. But somehow that faint aura of magic still clings to the term "elixir."

emaciation (*see* **macerate**)

embalm (*see* **balm**)

embolism comes from the Greek *embolos*, "a wedge or plug," which combines *en*, "in," + *ballein*, "to throw or cast." An embolus, then, is something "thrown in." Rudolf Virchow (1821-1902), the famous German pathologist, is said to have suggested the use of **embolus** as the name for a loose clot that is "thrown in" the bloodstream, then becomes wedged in a smaller vessel, thereby impeding circulation.

embryo is a slight contraction of the Greek *embryon*, "the fruit of the womb," which, in turn, was derived from *en-*, "in," + *bryein*, "to swell or to cause to burst forth."

emergency is a circumstance attending a sudden and serious event requiring a prompt response. So frequent are these events in medical practice that hospitals maintain "emergency rooms" staffed by "emergency personnel." The word, in its origin, is not quite that exciting. It is related to **emerge**, which comes from the Latin *emergere*, "to raise, especially from the water," this being derived from *e[x]-*, "out of," + *mergere*, "to sink, to dip, to immerse." Literally, an emergency is whatever arises from submersion, or whatever "comes up." Confusion may arise when one seeks an adjective to describe whatever may pertain to an emergency. To refer to an "emergent operation" might be construed to mean a recently devised operation; a better choice would be "exigent operation."

emeritus is an honorific addition to the title of a person who has retired from the active ranks of his profession. The Latin *emeritus* is the past participle of *emereri*, "to earn by service." But I like the jocose explanation given by Dr. J. Edward Berk on the occasion of his own retirement as professor and chairman of the department of medicine at the University of California, Irvine. "Emeritus," he pointed out, "is derived from the Latin *ex-*, meaning 'out,' and *meritus*, 'deserves to be.'"

emesis comes from the Greek *emein*, "to vomit," which in Latin is *vomere*. To the Greeks *emetikos* meant "provoking sickness," and from this comes our word **emetic**, referring to an agent that induces **vomiting**.

emissary describes veins connecting the venous sinuses of the dura mater through foramina in the skull with external veins. The word is derived from the Latin *emissarium*, "drain or outlet," from a combination of *e[x]-*, "out," + *mittere*, "to send." The term was first applied in 1720 by Giovanni Domenico Santorini (1681-1737), the Italian anatomist, whose name is also associated with the accessory duct of the pancreas. The concept was that excessive pressure in the dural vessels could be alleviated by the escape of blood through these "drains."

emollient comes from the Latin *emollire*, "to soften or make mild." In pharmacy, an emollient is a substance, usually in the form of a cream or ointment, that softens or soothes the skin or an irritated mucosal surface.

empathy is derived from a combination of the Greek *en-*, "in," + *pathos*, "feeling." The concept is thought to have originated with the German psychologist Theodor Lipps in the word *Einfühlung*. The concept of "in feeling" connotes the emotional appreciation of another's feeling. But, in comparison with **sympathy**, which means "feeling along with" the sufferer, empathy implies an awareness of the observer's separateness from the observed. The distinction is nicely made by Dr. Charles D. Aring (*JAMA*. 1958;167:448), who points out, "Appreciation of another's feelings and problems is quite different from joining in them, and in so doing, complicating them beyond resolving." The conscientious medical practitioner, then, develops an empathetic understanding of the patient's feelings coupled with an expression of compassion, which implies an intent to relieve suffering.

emphysema is a borrowing of the Greek word meaning "an inflation," this coming from a combination of *en-*, "in," + *physan*, "to blow or puff." In the 17th century emphysema was any swelling of tissues caused by infiltration of air. "Surgical emphysema" sometimes followed trauma and produced the sign we now refer to as crepitus. René Théophile Hyancinthe Laënnec (1781-1826), the innovative French physician who also devised the first stethoscope, described pulmonary emphysema in the early 19th century. The term now is customarily reserved, for the most part, to the disease of the lungs characterized by increased air space.

empirical comes through the Latin *empiricus*, "self-trained physician," from the Greek *empeiros*, "skilled by experience." This, in turn, was derived from *en-*, "by," + *peira*, "trial." The "empiric school of medicine" arose in the 2nd century B.C., and its adherents were concerned only with what they perceived as the immediate cause of illness and its symptomatic expression. In their search for remedies, they were committed to acting on their own observations and scorned the more traditional and speculative approach of the "dogmatists." The dogmatists (or "methodists," as they were sometimes called) in turn looked upon the empiricists as charlatans. Fortunately, there is no longer such an acrimonious dispute. All capable physicians recognize and make use of empirical observations and beneficial treatments with the understanding that simply because these cannot yet be wholly or rationally explained does not render them invalid.

empyema is taken from the Greek word for "a suppuration." It is a combination of *en-*, "imbued with," + *pyon*, "pus or corrupt matter." Now the term usually is restricted to a suppurative collection in the pleural space or gallbladder.

encephalo- is a combining term derived from the Greek *enkephalon*, "the brain." This, in turn, comes from *en-*, "in," + *kephalē*, "the head." Indeed, the Greek word, slightly modified as **encephalon**, is still used to designate, collectively, the contents of the cranium, including the cerebrum, the cerebellum, the pons, and the medulla oblongata. **Encephalopathy** is a general term referring to almost any disorder of the brain; **encephalitis** is an inflammation of the brain.

enciente is the French way of referring to pregnancy. The term came into French from the Latin *in-*, "without," + *cingere*, "to gird." The allusion is to the fact that a woman well along in pregnancy cannot comfortably wear a girdle.

endarteritis is an inflammation of the innermost coat, the tunica intima, of an artery. The word has been derived from the Greek *endon*, "within," + *artēria*, which originally meant "windpipe," but later became a classical term for an artery. Endarteritis is not to be misconstrued as inflammation of an end artery, a small terminal branch that does not anastomose with another arterial channel. In this usage, "end" means "dead end."

endemic comes from the Greek *endēmos*, "native to the place," this being derived from *en-*, "in," + *dēmos*, "people." The Greek word appears in Hippocratic writings to refer to anything, particularly a disease, peculiar to

a people in a given area. In present usage, "endemic" denotes a disease that is not necessarily widely prevalent, but almost always to be found among the inhabitants of a particular place.

endo- is a combining prefix representing the Greek *endon*, "in, inner, or within," and serves a large number of medical terms.

endocardium (+ Greek *kardia*, "heart") is the membrane lining the inner chambers of the heart.

endocrine (+ Greek *krinein*, "to separate or put apart") is a term contrived to describe those glands that "put apart" and secrete substances which are then used within the body. This action is in contrast to that of **exocrine** glands, which excrete whatever they "put apart" into channels that communicate with the exterior of the body. The endocrine organs sometimes are called "glands of internal secretion."

endoderm (+ Greek *derma*, "skin") is an alternative spelling of **entoderm**, the innermost of the three germ layers of the embryo, the others being the **ectoderm** (outer) and the **mesoderm** (middle).

endometriosis is a condition wherein an endothelial tissue almost identical to that of the uterine mucosa proliferates in ectopic sites, usually in or near the pelvis.

endometrium (+ Greek *mētra*, "uterus") is the membrane lining the inner cavity of the uterus.

endorphin is a generic descriptor of certain opiate peptides recently found to be elaborated in the brain. Dr. Avram Goldstein, among the pioneer investigators in this field, credits his colleague Dr. E. J. Simon with having coined the term in 1975. Presumably, "endorphin" is a contraction of "*endogenous morphine*like substances." Dr. Goldstein explains that this is "analogous to 'corticotropin,' which denotes the biologic activity rather than a specific chemical structure" (*Science.* 1976;193:1081).

endoscopy (+ Greek *skopein*, "to look or inspect") is a technique whereby a diagnostician, using specially designed optical instruments, can peer into the innermost recesses of the body. Hardly any orifice or body cavity has remained virgin by resisting the probes of the endoscopist.

endothelium (+ Greek *thēlē*, "nipple") is an oddly derived word. Apparently, **epithelium** was first used to describe the outer covering of the nipple, then applied to the skin generally, and eventually used for any membrane communicating with the exterior of the body. In contrast, **endothelium** was contrived to denote the type of membrane that lines the cavities of the heart, the blood and lymph vessels, and the serous surfaces of the body. (*see* **epithelium**)

endotoxin (*see* **toxin**)

enema comes from the Greek *enienai*, derived from a combination of *en*, "in," + *ienai*, "to send." The procedure of injecting fluids into the anus was known and practiced by the ancients, probably originating with the Egyptians. In times not so long ago, the proper medical term was **clyster**, taken from the Greek *klyzein*, "to wash out." A Greek *klyster* was "a syringe." The intrarectal administration of fluid, either for cleansing or for the introduction of medicaments, was long held to be solely in the province of the doctor and, as such, was always called a clyster. When physicians tired of the practice and abandoned it to nurses, the procedure was the same but the name was changed to enema. The early Dutch were more straightforward and called it *aarsspuiting*.

ensiform comes from the Latin *ensis*, "a sword," + *forma*, "shape or appearance." Thus, the cartilage at the lower end of the sternum, having the appearance of a small sword, became known as "the ensiform process." Its other name is **xiphoid** and means the same but comes from the Greek *xiphos*, "sword," + *eidos*, "like."

entero- is a combining form derived from the Greek *enteron*, "the gut or intestine," this relating to the Greek *enteros*, "within." The same sense is expressed in the vulgar English term "innards."

enthesis means literally "whatever is introduced from without" and is related to the Greek *entithenai*, "to put in." An enthesis can be a disease propagated by inoculation, the site of attachment of a tendon or ligament to bone, or an artificial material used to repair a defect. "Enthesis" in the last sense has been largely replaced by **prosthesis**, which carries

the meaning not only of placement but also of substitution. (Incidentally, whatever is in **parenthesis** is "put in" beside something else.)

entoterm (*see* **endoderm**)

entropion (*see* **ectropion**)

enuresis is a New Latin adaptation of the Greek *enourin*, "to urinate in." The term is now applied to the uncontrolled or involuntary passage of urine, the prefix "en-" presumably referring to unrestrained urination in one's bed or in one's undergarments.

enzyme is contrived from the Greek *en*, as an intensive prefix, + *zymē*, "a leavening agent or ferment." The term was coined in 1858 by Moritz Traube (1826-1894), working in the laboratory of Ferdinand Cohn (1828-1898) in Breslau. Traube came up with the name for a substance he could only hypothesize to be responsible for the phenomenon of fermentation. Previously, fermentation of carbohydrates was thought to be dependent on the presence of living yeast cells. It was not until 1897 that the actual enzyme, then called **zymase**, was proved to exist by Eduard Buchner (1860-1917), a German biochemist.

eosin was given its name from the Greek *ēos*, "the dawn." The allusion was to the resemblance of the rosy color of the sky at daybreak to that of the dye, tetrabrom fluorescein, commonly used in tissue staining.

eosinophil is a cell that exhibits an attraction for eosin (hence the suffix "-phil," from the Greek *philos*, "an affinity") and refers specifically to those white blood cells that display prominent red cytoplasmic granules when stained with eosin.

ependyma was given as a name for the lining membrane of the cerebral ventricles by Rudolf Virchow (1821-1902), the celebrated German pathologist. How Virchow contrived this name is not clear. The Greek *ependytēs* was "an outer tunic," that is, a tunic worn on top of another (from *ep[i]-*, "over," + *en*, "on," + *dyein*, "to put on, to clothe"). The idea of clothing may be understood, but the allusion to an outer garment for an inner lining is confusing.

ephedrine is the name given to a sympathomimetic alkaloid originally obtained from *Ephedra equisetina*, commonly known as the "horsetail plant." The Greek *ephedraō* means

"I sit upon" (from *ep[i]*, "upon," + *hedra*, "seat or chair"), and a similar term was used in Hippocratic writings to refer to the buttocks. Apparently, there was something about the plant that suggested the tail end of a horse.

epi- is a classical prefix taken from the Greek preposition *epi*, which can mean "on, upon, at, by, near, over, on top of, toward, against, among."

epicondyle was contrived by adding the prefix "epi-" to a derivative of the Greek *kondylos*, "knob or knuckle," and became the term applied to an eminence above or on top of a condyle, the rounded projection at the end of a bone, usually where it articulates with another.

epicranius (*see* **galea**)

epicritic incorporates a derivative of the Greek *krinein*, "to separate or to decide," and has been applied to that sense of light touch which permits discrimination of fine variations in configuration or temperature. (*see* **protopathic**)

epidemic is a near borrowing of the Greek *epidēmios*, "among the people"; the Greek *dēmos* referred especially to "the common people or citizenry." Hippocrates used *epidēmios* when alluding to diseases rife among the populace.

epidermis is a current term also found in classical writings to refer to the outer layer of the skin (Greek *derma*, "skin").

epididymis is a direct borrowing of the Greek word, but to Galen, the famous 2nd century Greek physician, it meant the outer membrane of the testis. However, Herophilus, the Greek "father of anatomy," used the term as we do to mean the coiled portion of the spermatic ducts that cap the testes. The Greek *didymos* actually means "double, twofold, or twins," but also was used to refer to the paired testes and ovaries. "Epididymis" with its three "i's" and one "y" often poses a spelling problem for medical students, young and old. The puzzle of which goes where is solved by remembering the origin of the word, i.e., beginning with "epi-" followed by the "di-" of "two," and finally "dymis."

epigastrium is an almost direct borrowing of the Greek *epigastrion* (+ Greek *gastēr*, "belly"), which referred to the area of the anterior abdominal wall above the umbilicus. The area below the umbilicus was called the *hypogastrion* ("below the belly") or **hypogastrium**, as we know it now.

epiglottis is the term for the lidlike cap covering the entrance to the trachea. Apparently, the structure was once thought of as an appendage of the tongue, because its name combines "epi-" with the Greek *glotta*, a variant of *glossa*, "tongue."

epilepsy comes from the Greek *epilēpsis*, "a laying hold of." To the Greeks the word also meant "a seizure," the notion being that the victim of a seizure was "laid hold of" by some mysterious force or influence, presumably instigated by the gods. In fact, the Roman term for epilepsy was *morbus sacer*, "sacred disease."

epinephrine was so named from Greek sources in 1898 by J. J. Abel (1857-1938), the physiologist who isolated the sympathomimetic substance from the adrenal gland which happens to be situated above ("epi-") the kidney (Greek *nephros*). (*see* **adrenal**)

epiphysis is a direct borrowing of the Greek word for an outgrowth of bone that is separated in its development by a zone of cartilage from the end of the main portion of a long bone. Now, more particularly, the term refers to a secondary center of ossification commonly found at the ends of long bones. The Greek word for "growth" is *physis*.

epiploic is taken from the Greek *epiploon*, the name used for the **omentum** in Hippocratic writings. This, in turn, came from the Greek *epipleō*, "I sail upon or float upon." The allusion, presumably, is to the omentum "floating" on the abdominal viscera. The **appendices epiploicae** were so called because they appeared to be small, omentumlike appendages of the colon. The **epiploic foramen** is an opening into the lesser peritoneal space behind the lesser omentum. It is sometimes called "the foramen of Winslow" after Jacob Benignus Winslow (1669-1760), the Danish anatomist who described it.

episiotomy is a combination of the Greek *epision*, "the pubes or pudenda," + *tomē*, "a cutting." The term is said to have been proposed in 1857 by Karl von Braun (1822-1891), a Viennese obstetrician, for the procedure of incising the outlet of the birth canal to facilitate delivery.

episodic (*see* **periodic**)

epispadias refers to the congenital defect (Greek *spadōn*, "a tear or rent") wherein the urethra opens on the dorsum of the penis.

epistaxis is a direct borrowing of the Greek word meaning "a dripping," particularly of blood from the nose. The root verb is the Greek *stazein*, "to let fall, drop by drop." "Nosebleed" is more straightforward and should suffice.

epithelium originally was used to describe the membrane surfacing the nipple alone (Greek *thēlē*, "the nipple"). Later, Friedrich Gustav Jakob Henle (1809-1885), a German histologist, applied the term to all surface membranes, including the skin and other mucosal surfaces communicating with the exterior of the body. This is in contrast to **endothelium**, which has nothing to do with the nipple, but somehow was contrived from the same origin to refer to membranes lining closed, internal spaces, including blood and lymph vessels.

epizootic describes a disease rampant among animals (from the Greek *zōion*, "animal"), the bestial counterpart of "epidemic."

eponym is from the Greek *epōnymos*, "named after someone," this being derived from a combination of *epi-*, "upon," + *onyma*, "name." In medicine, a number of anatomic structures, diseases, diagnostic procedures, and methods of treatment have been named after the persons who discovered, described, or promoted them. A modern tendency has been to discourage or even disparage the use of eponyms. In part, this is understandable. "Bright's disease," named for Richard Bright (1789-1858), a notable physician who worked at Guy's Hospital in London, proved to be too nondescript a term for the various forms of nephritis. On the other hand, "Laënnec cirrhosis" clearly designates the micronodular consequence of alcoholic liver injury, and substitutes are either incomplete or unduly cumbersome. Moreover, eponyms often convey a nice sense of historical tribute.

Epsom salt once was the term for hydrated magnesium sulfate when this was commonly used as a laxative and also as a bath or soak to alleviate inflammation or swelling. An early source for the substance was the mineral springs at Epsom, England. The town is now better known as the site of Epsom Downs, a racetrack catering to the "horsey" set.

eradication (*see* **resection**)

ergasthenia is a state of impairment caused by overwork, at one time or another a complaint uttered by almost every medical student. The term combines derivatives of the Greek *ergon*, "work," + *asthenos*, "weakness."

ergot gets it name from the Old French *argot*, "a cock's spur." Rye plants infected by the fungus *Claviceps purpurea* yield grain that is purple and misshapen in a sickle-form that resembles a cock's spur. Such grains are carefully excluded from rye intended for consumption as a cereal, but are deliberately cultivated as a commercial source of various ergot alkaloids (e.g., D-lysergic acid, methysergide, ergotamine, and bromocriptine). The principal actions (but by no means the only effects) of ergot are contraction of uterine muscle and peripheral vasoconstriction. Ergot poisoning, from consumption of rye contaminated by the fungus, was rife in the Middle Ages. Abortion and gangrene were common consequences of ergot poisoning. The pain suffered by its victims was such that the condition was sometimes referred to as *ignis sacer* ("holy fire"), *ignis infernalis* ("hell's fire"), or Saint Anthony's fire (because it was at shrines dedicated to Saint Anthony that sufferers sought relief). "Saint Anthony's fire" also was a colloquial name for **erysipelas**.

erosion comes from the Latin *erodere*, "to eat away," which is a combination of *e[x]-*, "out or away," + *rodere*, "to gnaw." An erosion is a lesion wherein the affected skin or mucous membrane appears to have been "eaten away" or "gnawed." Incidentally, the Latin term explains why certain gnawing animals are called "rodents" and why mercury bichloride is sometimes called "corrosive sublimate."

eructation is a fussy substitute for "belch" or "burp." It comes from the Latin *eructare*, "to belch or vomit." **Belch** is the present-day spelling of the Old English *bealcian* and may be related to "boil" in the sense of generating gas. The Dutch *balken* means "to bray." **Burp**

is an imitative word; that is, it sounds like what it means, and that would seem to be a perfectly sound reason for using it.

erysipelas is a condition marked by redness and swelling of the skin and subcutaneous tissue resulting from infection by group-A streptococci. The name we use is the same as given by the ancient Greeks, although their application of the term may not have been as specific. Professor H. A. Skinner offers two origins of "erysipelas": (a) from the Greek *erythros*, "red," + *pella*, "skin"; or (b) from the Greek *eraō*, "I draw," + *pelas*, "near" (perhaps because of a tendency for the infection to spread to nearby parts). He points out that the sense of the first derivation is better, whereas the etymology of the second seems more correct. Erysipelas was also once known as "Saint Anthony's fire." Saint Anthony was a 3rd century Egyptian ascetic, a pillar of the early Christian church. His bones, discovered in 561 A.D., were enshrined at Vienne, France, where they reportedly performed miracles of healing during an epidemic of erysipelas in the 11th century.

erythema is a direct borrowing of the Greek word for "redness in the skin, or a blush." The Greek *erythros* means "red." Medically, the use of "erythema" has been extended to describe redness in any surface, external or internal, caused by dilatation and engorgement of the capillary bed.

erythrocyte is so called from a combination of the Greek *erythros*, "red," + *kytos*, "cell." As such, it could refer to any red cell but is reserved for those anucleate, disk-shaped, hemoglobin-laden cells that circulate in the blood.

eschar comes from the Greek *eschara*, which commonly meant "a hearth or fireplace" but also was used in Hippocratic writings to describe the scab that formed when a wound was healed by cautery. To call such a seal an eschar is nice usage, but to call every scab an eschar is a turgidity.

esophagus is a name for the **gullet** and was derived from the Greek *oise*, the future imperative of *pherein* "to bear or carry," + phago-, a learned combining form taken from the Greek *phagein*, "to eat or devour," and in this sense referring to "that which was eaten." Gullet comes through the Old French as a diminutive of the Latin *gula*, "throat," the idea presumably being that the narrower esophagus was a sort of "little throat." Until recent times not much attention was paid to what seemed a simple conduit connecting the pharynx with the stomach. Now we know that the esophagus is actually a quite sophisticated organ, subject to a variety of disturbances and disorders.

esoteric (*see* **exotic**)

esotropia (*see* **strabismus**)

essence has long been used to refer to the active principle of a drug, particularly one of botanical origin. The word comes from the Latin *essentia*, which in turn was derived from *esse*, "to be." Thereby, the "essence" is the "being" or fundamental quality of anything. For example, in a solution of a volatile oil in alcohol, where the alcohol is the vehicle, the volatile oil is the "essential oil." Aristotle added a "fifth element" that he called "essence" to his basic categories of matter: fire, air, earth, and water. This came to be called the **quintessence**, from the Latin *quintus*, "fifth." We now use this term for the most perfect embodiment of something.

essential acquired an odd meaning in medicine. It has been used to describe certain diseases presumed to be entities, but of unknown cause and obscure pathogenesis, and yet found to exhibit characteristic features. For example, essential hypertension was high blood pressure observed to occur with no evident cause, as compared with hypertension, the result of known adrenergic stimulation, such as that associated with pheochromocytoma. This was before the renal pathogenesis of most forms of hypertension was fully appreciated. "Essential" was sometimes used interchangeably with "idiopathic." To describe a disease as "essential" was to say, "There is something about it, a sort of 'essence,' but I don't know what it is." Fortunately, as medical knowledge expands, there is less need to describe diseases as "essential."

ester is a term said to have been coined by Leopold Gmelin (1788-1853), a German physiologist. His purpose was to generally designate compound ethers. The new term was made up of the first and last syllables, joined by a "t," of *Essigäther*, the German word for acetic ether.

estrogen is the generic term coined for hormonal substances that induce **estrus** in female mammals. It is a contrived combination of "estro-," denoting **estrus**, + "gen" (from the Greek *gennaō*, "I bring forth").

estrus refers to the regularly recurring periods of maximal sexual receptivity in female mammals, also known as periods of "heat" or "rut." "Estrus" (spelled "oestrus" by the British) comes from the Greek *oistros*, "the gadfly," an insect whose sting puts cattle in a frenzy. In gynecology, estrus relates to the cycle of changes in the female genital tract consequent to ovarian hormonal activity.

et al. is an abbreviation of the Latin *et alia*, literally "and others." It is regularly and correctly used after the initial author's name when referring to multiauthored papers, as in "Smith et al." A common error is to forget that et al. is an abbreviation and that a period belongs after the "al." even when it is not at the end of a sentence. Not knowing that, one is led to think that a fellow named "Al" is the most prolific writer in scientific history.

ether comes through the Latin *aethra* from the Greek *aithēr*, "the upper, purer air" (in contrast to *aēr*, "the lower or immediately surrounding atmosphere"). This explains why "ether" is used to refer to whatever is conceived to fill the vast upper regions of space and thus serves to transmit waves of the electromagnetic spectrum. The colorless, transparent, and highly volatile diethyl ether was known and named long before its use as an anesthetic agent was demonstrated. It was first called *spiritus aethereus*, "ethereal spirit," presumably because of its clarity and extreme volatility.

ethmoid comes from the Greek *ēthmos*, "a sieve," + *eidos*, "like." The name has been applied to the bone that forms a roof for the nasal fossae and part of the floor of the anterior fossa of the skull. The bone's numerous perforations give it the appearance of a sieve.

etiology is a combination of the Greek *aitia*, "a cause," + *logos*, "a discourse," and means a study or exposition of causes. "Etiology" often is mistakenly used as a synonym for "cause." For example, to say "the etiology is unknown" is not the same as saying "the cause is unknown"; a good deal may have been said about the etiology, though the actual cause remains obscure. Doctors of medicine have a penchant for using seemingly learned, polysyllabic terms in place of simple words. If one chooses the more pretentious of two words that mean the same thing, that is pedantic pomposity. If one uses the more highfalutin of two words that do not mean the same thing, that is ignorance. Other frequently encountered examples are the mistaken use of "methodology" when one means "method," and the almost ludicrous use of "symptomatology" when one means "symptoms." Tacking on a mistaken "-ology" should fool no one.

eu- is a combining form that represents the Greek adverb *eu*, "goodly or well," as opposed to the inseparable prefix *dys-*, "hard, bad, or ill."

eugenics has to do with improved breeding that aims toward enhancement of a species. The term was introduced into biology in 1883 by Sir Frances Galton (1822-1911), an English naturalist and cousin of Charles Darwin. The term is taken from the Greek *eugenēs*, "well born," itself a combination of *eu*, "good," + *genēs*, "that brought forth." The Greek word also brought forth the proper names "Eugene" and "Eugenia."

eunuch comes almost directly from the Greek *eunochos*, literally "a bed keeper," being a combination of *eunē*, "bed," + *echein*, "to hold or keep." In certain ancient courts it was customary that only men who had been deprived of their testicles could stand guard over the women's sleeping quarters. Such bed keepers, it must have been assumed, would have their minds more on vigilance than on venery; any transgression would be more venial than venal.

euphoria comes from the Greek *euphorus*, "well or patiently borne," being a combination of *eu* + *pherein*, "to bear." In present day usage, "euphoria" has been elevated in sense to mean elation or an abnormally exaggerated feeling of well-being.

euploidy (*see* -ploid)

euthanasia is a direct borrowing of the Greek

word (incorporating *thanatos*, "death") for a quiet and undisturbed exit from earthly existence, and this is what it meant, too, for 18th century English writers. Latterly, the term has come to mean a "mercy killing," death deliberately induced to end the suffering of a painful and incurable illness.

euthyroid has been coined to indicate a normal or "good" function of the thyroid gland.

evolution comes from the Latin *evolvere*, "to unroll," being a combination of *e[x]*, "out," + *volvere*, "to roll." The concept of a continuous and progressive emergence of varying forms of life from simpler antecedents is usually associated with the name of Charles Darwin (1809-1882), the celebrated English naturalist. Long before, it was Aristotle (384-322 B.C.) who broached the idea of organic evolution. The word "evolution" in its presently understood sense is said to have been introduced by Sir Charles Lyell (1797-1875), an English geologist, whose writings were intently studied by Darwin before and during his epochmaking voyage on HMS *Beagle*. In fact, it was Herbert Spencer (1820-1903), a radical English philosopher and contemporary of Darwin, who coined the phrase "survival of the fittest" in writings that preceded Darwin's painstaking treatises. Still, it is Charles Darwin who is rightly recognized as the scientific thinker who firmly established the theory of biologic evolution.

ex- is a combining form (sometimes shortened to just "e-") representing the Latin preposition meaning "out of, from" (in the sense of space); "from, after, since" (in the sense of time); "from, by, through, on account of" (in the sense of cause or origin); "after, according to" (in the sense of conformity); or "with, by means of" (in the sense of means).

exacerbation is taken from the Latin *exacerbare*, "to provoke or exasperate," this being a combination of *ex-* + *acerbare*, "to embitter, to aggravate." Thus, an acerbic remark is a bitter utterance that may provoke anger. In medicine, an exacerbation is a recurrence, usually with severity, of a disease or its symptoms.

exanthem is a near borrowing of the Greek *exanthēma*, "a breaking out," as in the blooming of flowers. In this Greek word, the

"x" represents the letters "xi" (not "chi"). *Anthos* is Greek for "flower," specifically its bloom or blossom. In medicine, an exanthem is an outbreak of lesions in the skin, particularly those associated with the familiar childhood diseases, such as measles. Formerly, a companion word "enanthem" was used to refer to lesions appearing in mucous membranes, but this is seldom heard nowadays.

excoriation comes from the Latin *excoriare*, "to flay," a combination of *ex-* + *corium*, "the skin." The sense here is that strips of skin are torn away by flaying. The violence implicit in the term has been toned down in medicine, where an excoriation can be merely a scratch.

excrescence comes from the Latin *excrescere*, "to grow out, to rise up," being a combination of *ex-* + *crescere*, "to come into being, to arise." In pathology, an excrescence is a lesion of any sort that "grows out" from a surface. Incidentally, the Latin *crescere* also gives us "crescent" as the name for the emerging moon.

excretion is derived from the Latin *excernere*, "to sift out, to separate," a combination of *ex-* + *cernere*, "to distinguish, to decide." Thus, the origin of this term makes an interesting and significant point. Whatever is excreted is not merely discarded or "put out" but rather has been purposely separated from something else. In physiology, excretion is the process whereby substances are separated for external discharge, as from the skin or mucous channels, while secretion is the process whereby substances, such as hormones, are separated for internal discharge.

exercise comes from the Latin verb *exercere*, "to keep someone busy or to keep something in motion, to train, or to drill." *Excercere*, in turn, was derived from *ex-* + *ercere*, the combining form of *arcere*, "to restrain or to keep pent up." Thus, exercise is not just moving about but also the release of tension and is often prescribed for this purpose.

exfoliate comes from a combination of *ex-* + the Latin *folium*, "leaf," and thus means "to shed," as happens to the leaves of growing plants. An exfoliative dermatitis is a severe form of inflammation wherein the necrotic skin peels away, as dead leaves fall from a tree.

exogenous is contrived from a combination of the Greek *exō-* (where the "x" represents the Greek "xi," not "chi") + *gennaō*, "I produce." Whatever is exogenous is produced or arises outside the body, whereas whatever is **endogenous** is produced or arises within.

exophthalmos describes a protruding eye or the condition of being "bug eyed," the term being a combination of the Greek *ex-* + *ophthalmos*, "eye." **Exophthalmic goiter** is a condition wherein a palpable swelling of the thyroid gland is associated with a hypermetabolic state, a sign of which is protrusion of the eyeballs. Formerly, this was called "Graves' disease" in tribute to Robert James Graves (1796-1853), the brilliant Irish physician who lived and taught in Dublin and who published a perceptive account of the disease in 1835. Graves was a reformer of clinical teaching and an innovator often given to irreverent humor. Whereas in his time the dictum was "Feed a cold and starve a fever," Graves requested that his epitaph should read, "He fed fevers."

exostosis is an outgrowth of bone (Greek *osteon*, "bone") beyond its normal contour.

exotic is derived from the Greek *exotikos*, meaning "foreign or alien." Originally, it was used to describe anything strange that came from a foreign land. An exotic disease is one usually observed in faraway places and rarely, if ever, occurs in one's own habitat. "Exotic" is not to be confused with **esoteric**, which means "known only to a select few." That the two words often are mixed up suggests the distinction is esoteric. "Esoteric" comes from the Greek *esōterō*, the comparative of *esō*, "within."

exotoxin (*see* **toxin**)

exotropia (*see* **strabismus**)

expectorant comes from the Latin *expectorare*, "to expel from the chest," being derived from a combination of *ex-* + *pectus*, "the chest." An expectorant, then, is a medicament that enables the patient to expel phlegm from the bronchial tubes and trachea. To expectorate is not exactly the same as to spit, though often the polysyllabic term is used as a delicate substitute. One spits from the mouth; whatever is spit may or may not come from the chest. **Spit** comes from the Old English *spatl*, "saliva," whence "spittle": all of these English words are of echoic origin.

experiment is a slight contraction of the Latin *experimentum*, "a test." This relates to *experiri*, "to try out," which in turn combines *ex-* + *periculum*, "a trial," implying risk or danger. In this sense, to perform an experiment is to run the risk of success or failure, a hazard well known to research workers.

exsanguinate is to make or become bloodless (Latin *sanguis*, "blood").

extensor comes from the Latin *extendere*, "to stretch out." An extensor muscle is one that "stretches out" a joint as opposed to a **flexor** muscle, which bends a joint.

extirpate means to remove completely or "to root out," as a surgeon might wholly resect a tumor (*see* **resection**). The word comes from the Latin *ex-* + *stirps*, "stalk, stem, or root."

extrinsic (*see* **intrinsic**)

extrovert is made up of a combination of the Latin *exterius*, "on the outside," + *vertere*, "to turn." In psychology, "extrovert" describes a person whose attitudes "turn out" toward other persons or things rather than being "turned in" to himself, in which case he would be described as an **introvert**.

exude is a contraction of the Latin *exsudare*, "to sweat out." The Latin word for sweat is *sudor*. In pathology, an **exudate** is the substance that seeps or oozes from an inflamed surface (*see* **transudate**). **Ooze** is a perfectly good word, coming from the Anglo-Saxon *wōs*, "juice or moisture."

eye comes through the Anglo-Saxon *ēage* from the Teutonic *auge*, all of which refer to the organ of vision. Incidentally, the Old Norse *vindauga*, "wind-eye," became our "window." In years past, the upper canine tooth was called the "eyetooth" in the mistaken belief that it was connected to a branch of the same nerve that supplies the eye.

Facet comes through the French *facette* as a diminutive derivative of the Latin *facies*, "face," thus "a little face." In anatomy, a facet is any small, smooth surface of a bone, particularly at a site of articulation.

facies is a direct borrowing of the Latin word for "face." To the Romans it also meant "visage or appearance," in the sense of what was externally apparent. We also use "face" figuratively when we say, "On the face of it...." In medicine, the **facies Hippocratica** is the visage of a moribund patient. In the *Prognostic of Hippocrates*, this was described as "a sharp nose, hollow eyes, collapsed temples; the ears cold, contracted, and their lobes turned out; the skin about the forehead being rough, distended, and parched; the color of the whole face being green, black, livid, or lead-colored." "Cassius facies" is an expression that comes from Shakespeare's *Julius Caesar* (Act I, .scene ii), where Caesar observes, "Yon Cassius has a lean and hungry look." Caesar was prescient when he followed this by remarking, "He thinks too much; such men are dangerous."

factitious is taken from the Latin *facticius*, which is related to the verb *facere*, "to make, fashion, or build," and hence refers to whatever is made to occur, as opposed to that which occurs naturally or spontaneously. Thus, a **factitious fever** is one that is induced, and **factitious diarrhea** is the consequence of a deliberate or inadvertent use of cathartics. "Artificial" and "factitious" are nearly synonymous but, in medicine, "factitious" tends to bear the connotation of surreptitious, with intent to deceive.

Fahrenheit (*see* **centigrade**)

falciform is contrived by a combination of the Latin *falx, falcis*, "scythe or sickle," + *forma*, "shape." The **falciform ligament** is a sickle-shaped peritoneal fold by which the anterior and superior surface of the liver is attached to the abdominal wall and the diaphragm.

fart is disdained by many as a vulgar word, perhaps because it contains only four letters. The word has a venerable origin in the Old Teutonic *fertan*, "to break wind." Why "to pass gas" is more respectable than "to fart" escapes me. I find euphonious Chaucer's phrase "...to flee a fart" found in *The Miller's Tale*.

fascia is the singular of the Latin feminine noun meaning "a band or bandage." To the Romans, the word also meant "a wisp of cloud." Both senses are evident in the anatomic use of the term. In ancient writings, "fascia" meant only a narrow fibrous band, whereas a broad sheet of connective tissue was called "an aponeurosis." **Fasciculus**, being a diminutive related to fascia, is "a little bundle." In anatomy, the term is applied to various small bundles or clusters of nerve or muscle fibers.

fasciculation refers to focal, clonic contractions of a small bundle of muscle fibers resulting from irritability in a single neuromuscular component. In literature, a **fascicle** is a part of a book or journal that is published and bound separately.

fat comes from the Old English *faētt*, the past participle of *faētan*, "to cram or adorn." Fat tends to invest certain tissues. A related word is "vat," which comes from the Old English *faet*, "a vessel." In olden days, for a man or beast to be "well upholstered" was looked upon with favor.

fatal is derived from the Latin *fatalis*, "destined by fate," which is related to *fatum*, the past participle of *fari*, "to speak," referring to the pronouncement of oracles. Apparently, because such pronouncements often were ominous, even in ancient times *fatum* was taken as calamitous or portending of death. (*see* **mortal**)

fauces is a direct borrowing of the Latin word for "a small passage," particularly that into the throat or gullet. In anatomy, the **faucial tonsils** (also called "palatine tonsils") are the glandlike aggregates of lymphoid tissue situated in the throat.

favism refers to an acute hemolytic anemia that occurs in persons who have a genetic deficiency of glucose 6-phosphate dehydrogenase in their erythrocytes and who thereby suffer a hemolytic reaction when they eat fava beans. *Fava* is the Italian word for "bean," particularly the "broad bean." The Latin word for bean is *faba*. This serves as an example of the frequent interchange of "b" and "v" in Romance languages.

favus is a kind of tinea capitis, resulting from infection by the fungus *Trichophyton schoenleini* and characterized by the formation of yellow, cup-shaped crusts. *Favus* is the Latin word for "honeycomb," which the crusts resemble.

febrifuge (*see* **fever**)

febrile (*see* **fever**)

feces comes from the Latin *faex, faecis*, "dregs or sediment." In the 15th century and for at least 200 years thereafter, English writers used the Latin word, variously spelled, to refer to the dregs of any fermenting substance. Beginning in the 17th century, "faeces" (later Americanized as "feces") became restricted in reference to the dregs or excrement of the bowel. There is no singular of the term in English, British or American. **Defecate** is taken from the Latin *defaecatio*, "a cleansing," that is, a removal of the dregs.

fecund is a contraction of the Latin *fecundus*, "to be fruitful." In the biology of reproduction, **fecundity** denotes the capacity to bear offspring. (*see* **female**)

feldsher as used to describe a physician's assistant comes from the German *Feldscherer*. An old German word for "barber" was *Scherer*, which reminds us of our word "shearer," one who shears sheep or human heads. Taking to the field, as with an army, the *Scherer* became a *Feldscherer* (German *Feld*, "field"), among whose duties was also that of pulling teeth and otherwise assisting the military surgeon. Today, "feldsher" designates a minimally trained medical practitioner, particularly one who serves in rural Russia. The Chinese counterpart is a "barefoot doctor."

fellow is used in medical or scientific circles to designate one who is a full member in good standing of a professional group. To be a Fellow of the American College of Physicians or similar specialty society is a distinction. "Fellow" comes through the Old English *fёolaga* from the Old Norse *fёlagi*, "business partner." These forerunners relate, in turn, to a combination of *fё*, "chattel or money," + *lag*, "a person who lays something down." One who pledges his valued effort to a common cause is thus "a good fellow."

felon (*see* **whitlow**)

female comes from the Latin *femina*, "woman," related to the verb *felare*, "to suckle," and the Greek *phēlē*, "breast." The adjective should be spelled "femal," but a terminal "e" was added at some point, probably to correspond with **male**. Related words based on the root *fe-* include **fecund**, **fertile**, and **fetal**. What is neither male nor female is **neuter**, which looks like a single word but really is a collision of the Latin *ne*, "not," + *uter*, "the other," i.e., "neither." (*see* **male**)

femto- is the prefix used in the metric system to denote powers of 15. It is from the Danish *femten*, "fifteen." The units by which the mean corpuscular volume (MCV) of erythrocytes are expressed are femtoliters, i.e., 1×10^{-15} liter, an exceedingly small volume.

femur is the Latin word for "thigh." In anatomy, it is used as the name for the thigh bone. The derived adjective **femoral** is used to designate structures, such as blood vessels and nerves, that bear a relation to the femur.

fenestra is the Latin word for "window," being related to the Greek *phainein*, "to show, to bring to light, to disclose." "Fenestra" is used as an anatomic term to describe certain windowlike openings, especially in the ear, such as the fenestra ovalis (in the middle ear) and fenestra rotunda (in the cochlea). **Fenestration** is the operation of creating an artificial opening (as from the external auditory canal to the labyrinth of the inner ear to improve hearing) or the condition of being perforated (as in aortopulmonary fenestration, an anomaly wherein the aorta and the pulmonary artery communicate just above the semilunar valves). In another context, to defenestrate means to throw something, or someone, out of a window.

ferment is a contraction of the Latin *fermentum* that to the Romans meant "yeast" and was recognized as the ingredient necessary to promote conversion of sugar or starch-containing substances to alcoholic beverages. The word was derived from the Latin verb *fervere*, "to seethe or to boil," doubtless because gas (carbon dioxide), generated in the process, gives an appearance of boiling. Fermentation occurs both normally and abnormally in the human digestive tract.

fertile is an almost direct borrowing of the Latin *fertilis*, "fruitful or productive," including the sense of bearing offspring. The adjective was derived from the Latin verb *ferre*, "to bear." (*see* **female**)

fester is descended from the Latin *fistula*, "a pipe or tube," by way of the Old French *festre*, also spelled *fistle*, "a draining or rankling sore." It was not unusual in Old French for a terminal "-le" to change to "-re" (another example being the change from *epistle* to *épître*). In early medical usage, a fester was a fistula, but later the word came to be used as an intransitive verb to describe the behavior of any exuding sore. Incidentally, we use "rancor" to describe mental irritation or resentment, and this word comes from the Middle French *rancier*, the "d" having been dropped from the Old French *draoncier*, "to fester." This, in turn, came from the Late Latin *dracunculus*, the diminutive of the Latin *draco*, "serpent," from which also sprang "dragon." The bite of a serpent was known to be venomous and productive of a sore. What might be called a draconian remedy is so called not from *draco* the serpent but from Draco (or Dracon), the 6th century B.C. Athenian politician remembered for having levied harsh laws.

fetal (*see* **fetus**)

fetish is used by psychiatrists and psychologists to refer to any object to which a disturbed patient has an irrational attachment. To anthropologists, a fetish is an object to which primitive people attribute supernatural powers. The word comes, by way of the French *fetiche*, from the Portuguese *feitiço*, "charm or sorcery," which is related to the Latin *facticius*, "made by art."

fetor can be spelled **foetor**, and either is a direct borrowing of the Latin *fetor*, or *foetor*, "stench," which also gives the adjective **fetid**. **Fetor hepaticus** is a peculiarly musty odor detected in the breath of patients with advanced liver disease, often when such patients are in a state of hepatic encephalopathy. The odor can be traced to excess mercaptans of metabolic origin.

fettle is a word for "condition or trim" that is now only occasionally heard and then in combination as "in fine fettle," meaning physically and mentally fit. In Old English, a *fettle* was a girdle of sorts, and to be in fine fettle was to be well girded. This brings to mind a verse composed by German students in 1817 at Wartburg in celebration of the burning of the male corset:

> A corset girds with great élan
> The waist of every proud Uhlan,
> So that when he in battle stands
> His heart won't fall into his pants!

fetus is a direct borrowing of the Latin masculine noun, which had numerous meanings, such as "breeding, producing, offspring, fruit," all in the sense of successful reproduction. Probably the term is related to the Latin *ferre*, "to carry, to bear, to bring forth, to produce." Now the word is restricted to designate the unborn offspring, more mature than an embryo, of any mammal. Curiously, the word is sometimes misspelled, especially in Britain, as "foetus," perhaps because that looks more learned, as if related to Greek. It is not. This is one instance in which American spelling is correct.

fever comes through the Old French *fevre* from the Latin *febris*, all of which mean the same. The word is thought to be of Sabine origin, related to the Latin *fervere*, "to seethe or to steam" (from which, incidentally, comes our word "fervent"). In Hippocratic practice, fever was regarded as beneficial in the sense of being a symptom of the body's natural antagonism to disease. Indeed, more recent investigation indicates this might be the case. The Latin *febris*, then, may also relate to the verb *februare*, "to cleanse or purify." **February** is so named as the month for cleansing and purification in anticipation of the coming spring. Only a few generations ago it was customary early in the year for people to dose themselves with cathartics, as a "spring tonic." **Febrile**, a Latinized way of saying "with fever," is favored by doctors and nurses. **Feverish** would be a more English way of saying the same thing, but this is a word used by patients and is not quite learned enough for professionals. A **febrifuge** (incorporating a derivative of the Latin *fugare*, "to drive away") is a remedy intended to "make a fever flee." To describe a fever as "hectic" is redundant; the Latin *hecticus* means "feverish."

fiber is an almost direct borrowing of the Latin *fibra*, which means the same thing, that is, "a tough filament or thread." A **fibril**, as the diminutive, is "a fine thread."

fibrillation in cardiology refers to an incoordinate twitching of individual muscle fibers in the atria or ventricles.

fibrin is the product of plasma that forms the proteinaceous fibers that constitute the matrix of a blood clot.

fibroid is a hybrid term combining the Latin *fibra* + the Greek *eidos*, "like," and can refer to anything that appears to be composed of fibers. More specifically, "fibroid" was long used mistakenly as the name for a benign, smooth muscle neoplasm arising in the myometrium. This, of course, is a **leiomyoma** of the uterus and is now, correctly, so called.

fibula is the Latin word for "clasp or broach (or brooch)," particularly the needle of a brooch or the tongue of a buckle. Probably, this was derived from the Latin verb *figere*, "to fasten." The relation of the two bones of the lower leg was likened to that of the bar and clasp of a brooch, the fibula being the clasp.

filariasis is the disease caused by *Filaria*, a genus of nematodes or "thread worms," which, in some areas, are common parasites of man and beast. The name comes from the Latin *filum*, "a thread." One manifestation of filariasis can be grotesque swelling of the affected leg consequent to lymphatic obstruction; the name **elephantiasis** also has been given to the affliction. A **filiform** structure is threadlike.

filter began with the German *Filz*, "felt," nonwoven fabric made from the hair or fur of animals by the application of heat, moisture, and pressure. It was of a thin layer of this fabric that the first efficient fine strainers were made, and *Filz* became Latinized in medieval times as *filtrum*. This term later was applied to any porous material through which a fluid mixture could be passed to remove its particulate matter.

fimbria is the Latin word for "fringe" and the name given to any fringelike border, such as that of the distal end of the oviduct.

finger as the name for a **digit** of the hand is of Teutonic origin and possibly goes back to *pengros*, related to *penge*, "five." The Romans named rather than numbered the fingers: pollex (thumb), index (the pointing finger), medius (the middle finger), annularis (the ring finger), and minimus (the smallest finger). The fifth finger is sometimes called **pinkie**; this comes from the Indo-European *penk^we*, "five" or "fifth."

fissure is taken from the Latin *fissura*, "a cleft," which was derived from the Latin verb *findere*, "to cleave." The postulated Indo-European root is said to have been *bheid*, "to split" (from which, incidentally, we get the words "bit," "bite," "bitter," "beetle," and "boat"). "Fissure" has been applied to the names of various cleft structures, particularly those of the surface of the brain. An anal fissure is a painful split in the mucosa or skin of that keenly sensitive area.

fistula is the Latin word for "pipe or tube." To the Romans, this usually meant a water pipe, but could also mean the opening of an ulcer. It is in this latter sense that, in medicine, a fistula is any drainage tract whereby an abnormal or artificial communication, internal or external, has occurred.

fit has two medical implications and, not surprisingly, they are of different origins. "Fit" in the sense of ready, prepared, "all together" is derived from the Middle English *fitten*, "to array," coming from the Old Norse *fitja*, "to knit together." "Fit" as a paroxysm or dangerous crisis comes from the Old English *fitt*, "strife or conflict," akin to "a fight," and originated in the Old English verb *feohtan*, "to fight."

fix as a goal to which all medical effort is aimed is a contraction of the Latin *fixus*, the past participle of *figere*, "to fasten or to make firm." This is the precise sense in which a fracture is "fixed." The common meaning of the word has been broadened to include repair or restoration to a normal, functioning state. By extrapolation, a drug addict, in a state of deprived disrepair, demands a fix.

flagella is the plural of the Latin *flagellum*, "a whip." The whiplike appendages providing motility to various microorganisms are called flagella. The word is a diminutive of the Latin *flagrum*, "a scourge," which in turn can be traced to the Indo-European root *bhlag,* "to strike." The English "flog" has been said to be a schoolboy's (though perhaps it was a sailor's) abbreviation of flagellate.

flail describes a joint of unusual or abnormal mobility. This is an allusion to "flail" as the name of a tool for threshing grain, which consists of a freely swinging bar at the end of a staff or handle. The term comes from the Old French *flaiel* that in turn relates to the Latin *flagellum.*

flatus is the Latin word for "blowing," as a breeze or a snort. Formerly, **flatulence** meant the disagreeable presence of gas in the gut generally, but latterly "flatus" has come to be restricted to gas expelled through the anus. The Greek word for "breaking wind" was *perdomai,* and from this word came *perdix,* the Greek name for the gallinaceous game bird we call the "partridge." Anyone who has flushed a partridge in the field can recognize the Greeks' allusion to the whirring sound as the partridge takes flight. (*see* **fart**)

flavivirus (*see* **yellow fever**)

fletcherism is a term now almost forgotten but one that had wide play in the early 1900s. It referred to the nutritional fad promoted by Horace Fletcher (1849-1919), a retired San Francisco businessman, whose book *The ABC of Nutrition* was published in 1903 and promptly caught the public fancy. A key principle, Fletcher insisted, was that each mouthful of food be chewed 32 times—once for each tooth. William James, the famous psychologist and philosopher, gave "fletcherism" an honest try but after 3 months was quoted as saying, "I had to give it up. It nearly killed me."

flex comes from the Latin verb *flectere,* "to bend or to turn." Muscles that bend a joint are **flexors** as opposed to **extensors,** which straighten a joint. Sometimes the action of joints and muscles are confused. One can flex a joint but not a muscle, common parlance notwithstanding.

flocculation is derived from the diminutive of the Latin *floccus,* "a tuft of wool." Particulate matter coming out of solution as a result of chemical or physical action may resemble little tufts of wool.

fluke in the descriptive sense of "flat" is related to the German *flach* and probably to the Latin *plaga,* "a flat surface." The name "fluke" is given to a flatfish (also called a flounder). Parasitic flatworms also are commonly called "flukes," according to their habitat, be it blood, the intestine, the lung, or the liver (*see* **trematode**). The origin of "fluke" as an unexpected or accidental stroke of good luck is obscure. It seems to have come from the game of billiards where an accidentally successful shot, especially by a novice, was called "a fluke shot," perhaps because the common flatfish is easily caught by even an unskilled angler, or perhaps because a fish caught by its fluke is a lucky, if misdirected, catch.

fluorescence is a word coined in 1852 by Sir George Stokes (1819-1903), a British physicist, to denote glowing of the mineral fluorite, or fluorspar, when exposed to certain rays of the electromagnetic spectrum. In conceiving "fluorescence," Sir George chose to follow the custom of incorporating the names of other minerals in similar terms, such as "opalescence" and "phosphorescence." **Fluorite** was known as "a fluxing stone," i.e., when heated it melted into a sort of enamel, hence its name from the Latin *fluere,* "to flow."

fluorine was so named because it was first recognized in fumes produced when the mineral fluorspar was heated in combination with sulfuric acid. (*see* **fluorescence**)

fluoroscopy is a means of viewing an image generated by X-rays acting on a fluorescent screen. Actually, the **fluorescent** screen used to capture the image generated by X-rays was coated with calcium tungstate, not calcium fluoride or fluorite. What is now called fluoroscopy in a modern radiology department employs a television screen.

flux in its medical applications and derivatives relates to its origin in the Latin *fluere,* "to flow." A "bloody flux" is a flow of relatively fresh blood, usually from the bowel. An **effluent** (or *effluvium* if the Latin word is used) is "anything that flows out." (To be **affluent** is to be in the fortunate position of having wealth "flow toward" one.) **Reflux** is a "backward flow," i.e., in a direction contrary to the normal course. **Reflux esophagitis** is the consequence of a backward flow of corrosive gastric juice into the distal esophagus.

focus is a direct borrowing of the Latin word that to the Romans meant "hearth, fireplace, or altar." The hearth, in a Roman home, was the place where most of the essential household activities converged. Now, we use the word to refer to any point of convergence or center of attention. A focal pain, for example, is clearly where the patient's attention is centered.

folates are compounds related to folic acid, so called because the parent substance was first isolated from vegetable leaves. *Folium* is the Latin word for a leaf. Folic acid, a member of the vitamin B group, also is found in certain fruits, liver, and yeast. A deficiency of folic acid can result in a megaloblastic anemia.

folie à deux is a term used in psychiatry for the sharing of delusions simultaneously by two closely associated persons. It is obviously French and combines *folie*, "madness," + *à*, "in," + *deux*, "two." The French *folie*, incidentally, also can mean "playful, frisky, or extravagant" and in this sense gives us the show business term "the follies."

follicle comes from the Latin *folliculus*, the diminutive of *follis*, "a leather bag or bellows." A follicle, then, is "a little bag" and an apt name for a host of saccular or encapsulated structures, usually occurring as aggregates, in biology and medicine.

fomentation is a quaint term for the application of hot packs. "Foment" as a verb, now usually used in a figurative way to mean "heat up," was derived as a contraction of the Latin *fovimentum*, "a warm application," from the Latin verb *fovere*, "to warm."

fomite is taken from the Latin *fomitis*, the genitive of *fomes*, "tinder." In medicine, a fomite is an inanimate object that can be a source of infection, such as a doorknob or toilet seat might be suspected. The idea is that such an object might "light the fire" of infection. Unduly fastidious persons tend to exaggerate the risk of infection from such a source.

fontanelle is from the diminutive, through the Italian, of the Latin *fontana*, "spring or fountain." The term refers to the incompletely ossified junctions of the bones in a baby's skull, also known as "soft spots." The allusion to "a little fountain" may have arisen because of pulsations felt at the fontanelles.

food is a word of obscure Old Teutonic origin of which cognates are known in most Germanic languages. It is possible there is a tenuous connection between the words "food" and "fat." In the obese patient, the connection is more obvious. A related word is "fodder," meaning food for animals. Incidentally, the German *Drachenfutter*, literally "dragon fodder," is the expression used for a gift brought home by a timorous, errant husband to allay the ire of his wife.

foot comes from the Anglo-Saxon *fot*, which can be traced to the Indo-European root *ped, pod*. The Greeks used the word *pous*, and the Romans used *pes*. All of these mean "foot." Related words include **fetch**, **fetlock**, and **fetter**.

foramen is the Latin word for "a hole or an opening." In anatomy, holes or openings in all sorts of structures have been called "foramina," which is the Latin plural.

forceps is a direct borrowing of the Latin name for an instrument used to grasp, pluck, or lift. Probably, the term was derived from a combination of the stems of the Latin *formus*, "hot," + *capere*, "to grasp," thereby designating an appliance designed to pick up whatever is too hot to handle, as one would use a pair of tongs. Incidentally, "forceps" is grammatically the singular (the Latin plural is *forcipis*), but it is almost always treated as plural. At home, a similar instrument is called a **tweezers**, but this too can be a medical term. As noted by the Reverend Skeat (in *A Concise Etymological Dictionary of the English Language*, 1882), a surgeon's box of instruments was formerly called a **tweese**, and the delicate tools therein were called tweezes and, later, tweezers. "Tweese" can be traced as an apheretic derivative of the French *étui*, "a sheath or case for storing needles."

forensic is an adaptation of the Latin *forensis*, meaning whatever pertains to a forum. To the Romans, the Latin *forum* originally designated the marketplace where people gathered to conduct all sorts of transactions, including the business of public affairs. Later, the word became more restricted in reference to courts of law. Now, forensic medicine relates to medical jurisprudence.

formaldehyde is the aldehyde (HCHO) of **formic acid**, which was so called because it was first obtained, in the 17th century, by distilling, of all things, a batch of red ants. *Formica* is the Latin word for "ant."

formalin is a 40% solution of gaseous **formaldehyde** and is used widely as a fixative for tissue specimens and as an embalming fluid. In years past diluted (1:200 to 1:2000) solutions of formalin were commonly used as disinfectant, and their pungency accounted for the peculiar odor that pervaded hospitals of a bygone era.

forme fruste describes an incomplete or atypical expression of a disease. These are French words which together mean "a defaced, rough, or unpolished form." The Latin *frustra esse* means "to be mistaken," especially in the sense of "confused." In medicine, for example, a patient may exhibit sudden, intense, epigastric pain and a rigid abdomen. He is thought to have a perforated peptic ulcer. But at operation only a penetrating ulcer is found, sealed off by adhesion to the omentum or anterior abdominal wall. Such a patient is said to have a forme fruste of acute free perforation as a complication of his peptic ulcer disease. A *forme pleine*, also French but seldom used by English-speaking clinicians, is a term for the complete or full-blown form of a disease.

formication is a neuropathic symptom wherein the sensation is that of small insects crawling over the skin. The term is contrived from the Latin *formica*, "ant."

fornix is the Latin word for "arch or vault." In anatomy, the fornix of the cerebrum is an arched fiber tract having two lateral halves that are united under the corpus callosum. The fornix of the vagina is the vaultlike recess between the vaginal wall and the protruding uterine cervix. **Fornication**, as a term for sexual intercourse between a couple unblessed by holy wedlock, has a similar classical origin. In ancient Rome prostitutes customarily loitered under the arches of certain public buildings, and an illicit dalliance therewith came to be known euphemistically as "going under the arches."

fossa is the Latin word for "ditch or trench." This, in turn, relates to the Latin verb *fodere*, "to dig." In anatomy, a variety of concavities that resemble excavations are referred to as **fossae**.

fourchette is the diminutive of the French *fourche*, "fork," hence "a little fork." In anatomy, the fourchette is the posterior union of the labia minora of the female **pudendum**.

fovea is the Latin word for "a small pit" and is used in anatomy to designate small depressions in various structures. The fovea of the eye is a tiny pit in the center of the retinal macula where registration of vision is most precise.

fracture is derived from the Latin verb *frangere*, "to shatter or to break in pieces." The term is applied to the common injury to which bones are subject.

frambesia tropica (*see* **yaws**)

fremitus is the Latin word for "grumbling or growling." In physical diagnosis, the word denotes the vibration perceived by **palpation**, particularly over the chest as the patient makes a vocal sound. Fremitus is increased when there is consolidation of the underlying lung and is absent in pneumothorax.

frenulum is the diminutive of the Latin *frenum*, "a bridle." In anatomy, various ligamentous or membranous folds that have a restraining function and hence resemble a bridle are known by this term. An example is the frenulum of the tongue, a vertical fold of mucous membrane under the tongue that attaches the tongue to the floor of the mouth. A person in whom this "bridle" is unduly short is said to be "tongue-tied."

friable is derived from the Latin *friare*, "to crumble into small pieces." Thus, Marcus Terentius Varro (116-26 B.C.), the Roman scholar and encyclopedist, wrote of *terra quae facile frietur*, "earth that crumbles easily." "Friable" appeared in English as early as the 16th century but was applied mainly to mineral substances. The ancient meaning serves well in pathology to describe tissues that are readily fragmented. A related word is "frayed."

frontal comes from the Latin *frons, frontis*, "forehead or brow," and hence describes whatever pertains to the forehead, such as the frontal nerve or the frontal sinus. The Latin meaning also encompassed "countenance or facade" in the sense of whatever was seen first, and thus "front" and "frontal" commonly are used in a figurative sense.

fructose (*see* **glucose**)

fuchsin is a brilliant red dye formerly used as a topical antiseptic agent, but now more widely employed as a stain for bacteria and tissue in the preparation of slides for microscopic examination. The dye was discovered as a product of coal tar in the mid-19th century and was so named because its color resembles that of fuchsia blossoms. The plant, in turn, was named for Leonhard Fuchs (1501-1566), a famous German botanist. Fuchsin is not to be confused with **fuscin**, a brown pigment occurring in the retinal epithelium, or with **lipofuscin**, a fatty pigment observed as the intracellular product of certain degenerative processes.

fulguration refers to the use of electrical energy in the form of sparks to desiccate and destroy unwanted tissue, such as that comprising small tumors. The term is derived from the Latin *fulgar*, "a flash of lightning." Although it is perfectly proper to refer to a doctor who fulgurates a lesion as a "fulgurator," to the Romans a *fulgurator* was a person who interpreted the mystical significance of lightning.

fumigate is taken from the Latin verb *fumigare*, "to expose to the fumes of smoke." In turn, this was derived from *fumus*, "smoke," + *agere*, "to drive." The ancients knew that fire and smoke could have a disinfectant action. Homer's Odysseus called for burning sulfur to fumigate the palace at Ithaca. Our word "perfume" is related, being a combination of *per-*, "through," + *fumus*. In the Middle Ages dwellings were "perfumed" to prevent or counteract the plague. Out of this evolved the idea that anything fetid would be cleansed if it was made fragrant. Thus, a substance that conferred fragrance came to be known as perfume.

function is derived from the Latin *functio*, "a performance," which in turn comes from the Latin deponent verb *fungor*, "to perform or accomplish." Thus, physiology as a major arm of biomedical study concerns itself with how organs and organisms perform. In medical practice, so-called "functional disorders" are those in which there is a defect of performance or behavior in the absence of any known or recognized defect in structure.

fundus is the Latin word meaning "bottom." In anatomy, the term indicates that portion of a hollow structure that is farthest from its opening. Thus, the fundus of the gallbladder is the very bottom of the bag, and the fundus of the uterus is that part farthest from the cervix. The fundus of the stomach, being that portion superior to the entrance of the esophagus, is a little harder to explain, except that it is the most dependent part when the body is recumbent. Perhaps the meaning is that it is the farthest part of the stomach from the pylorus.

fungus is a Latin word that means the same as in English, i.e., a class of vegetable organisms that includes mushrooms, toadstools, and various molds. The Latin word is said to have been derived from the Greek *spho[n]ggos*, "a sponge" (the initial "s" having been expunged in transition). The allusion, of course, is to the spongy texture of the various forms that the Romans came to call *fungi*.

funiculus (taken from the diminutive of *funis*, i.e., "a little cord") is used especially to designate certain nerve tracts in the spinal cord. *Funis argenteus* (Latin *argentum*, "silver") was a classical term for the spinal cord.

funis is the Latin word for "rope or cord," and has been applied in anatomy to indicate any cordlike structure, especially the umbilical cord. **Funisitis** is an inflammation of the umbilical cord, as seen in newborns, and possibly related to congenital herpes virus infection.

funny bone is an expression used by an occasional patient to refer to his elbow or, more specifically, to the olecranon process of his ulna. Punsters have tried to explain this by pointing out that the ulna articulates with the humerus. The real explanation for "funny bone" is that the ulnar nerve lies in the exposed ulnar groove of the olecranon, which, when bumped, causes a strangely "electric" sensation in the forearm and hand.

furuncle is from the Latin *furunculus*, "a petty thief," being the diminutive of the Latin *fur*, "a thief," presumably of standard dimension. Roman writers on agriculture used the term to mean a knob on a vine. A word of related origin is "furtive," meaning sly and stealthy, like a thief. What all this has to do with a small focus of suppuration in a hair follicle has baffled most medical linguists. A guess might be that extensive furunculosis can result in a loss or "theft" of hair. Another possibility is that because boils were once thought of as a form of corruption, little boils might be considered evidence of only petty corruption.

fuscin is a dark brown pigment found in the retinal epithelium. The term is taken from the Latin *fuscus*, "dark or indistinct." This Latin word also gives us "obfuscation," rumored to be a major course of study in law schools. (*see* **fuchsin**)

fusiform means spindle-shaped, and this is appropriate because the Latin word *fusus* means "spindle" or, as the past participle of the verb *fundere*, "spread out." Fusiform aneurysms are spindle-shaped dilatations of arteries or veins.

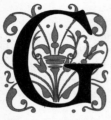 **alactose** (*see* **glucose**)

galea is the Latin word for "helmet," particularly one made of leather or skin. The **galea aponeurotica** (the latter term indicating an early confusion of connective tissue and nerves) is the tough, tendinous connection between the anterior and posterior bellies of the occipitofrontalis muscle, now called the **epicranius**. It covers the scalp as a cap.

galenical denotes a medicinal preparation composed mainly of herbal or vegetative ingredients. The term is taken from the name of Galen (129-200 A.D.), a Greek physician born in Pergamum, Asia Minor, who gained prominence as court physician to Marcus Aurelius, a contemporary Roman philosopher and emperor. Galen adhered to the principles of Hippocrates, Plato, and Aristotle, while advancing his own pronouncements in an astonishing array of treatises on philosophy, philology, and medicine. His appeal lasted for well over a millennium, when many of his concepts were superseded by those of Andreas Vesalius (1514-1564) in anatomy and William Harvey (1578-1657) in physiology.

gall as a name for **bile** is descended from the Old English *gealla*, which meant the same, being probably related to *geolo*, "yellow." Thus, the English word for bile seems to refer to its color. In all likelihood there was a primordial root, probably the Indo-European *ghel*, also indicating "yellow," that led to the Greek *cholē* as a word for bile. There happens to be another "gall," quite unrelated to bile, which comes from the Latin *galla*, meaning a nutlike deformity found on plants infected by the larva of certain insects. **Gallic acid**, an astringent substance, was first found in a decoction of gallnuts. In Late Latin, *galla* became a word for "tumor," particularly that

which seemed to result from focal irritation. This also yielded the verb "to gall," meaning to rub harshly or repetitively so as to produce a sore. A saddlesore on either a horse or its rider can be said to result from galling. One occasionally hears the word used figuratively, as in "His rude behavior galls me."

galvanometer designates an instrument for determining the strength and direction of an electric current. The name comes from that of Luigi Galvani (1737-1798), a professor of anatomy at Bologna, who was fascinated by the wondrous properties of the newly discovered electricity. The story is told that one day in 1786 Galvani was working with a machine that produced static electricity, while on a nearby table lay some skinned frog legs. Through a scalpel held by an assistant, an impulse of electricity was transmitted to the frog muscle, which thereupon jerked. Galvani seized on this curious observation and expanded it into a rather fanciful theory of "animal electricity," which later was discredited. Nevertheless, Galvani went on to invent a chemical battery to release a flow of electric current, and on this his fame rests secure. By an interesting turnabout, in 1902 Willem Einthoven (1860-1927), a Dutch physiologist, invented a string galvanometer so sensitive as to detect the electric impulse generated in the heart, and this became the basis for modern electrocardiography.

gamete designates a germ cell, either an ovum or a spermatocyte, essential to sexual reproduction. The term comes from the Greek *gametēs*, "husband," or *gametē*, "wife." These nouns, in turn, relate to the Greek verb *gamein*, "to marry." The biologic usage of "gamete" was advanced by Johann Gregor Mendel (1822-1884), an Austrian monk who gained fame as the naturalist who discovered the fundamental principles of genetics.

ganglion is a slight transliteration of the Greek *ga[n]gglion*. The Greek letter gamma is pronounced as "n" in "ng" when it appears before certain consonants, such as gamma, kappa, chi, and xi; this explains the change of Greek "gg" to "ng" in derivatives as they appear in Latin and modern languages. In

Hippocratic writings *ga[n]gglion* was used for any small subcutaneous nodule, and this sense has persisted in the use of "ganglion" to refer to a tendinous cyst, such as is commonly found at the wrist. Galen, the 2nd century Roman physician, used the term to refer to nerve complexes, which often appear as small nodes, and it is in this usage that "ganglion" has been most widely applied in anatomy.

gangrene comes from the Greek *ga[n]ggraina*, "an eating sore ending in mortification." The Greek root verb may have been *grainein*, "to gnaw." The Greeks referred to the degeneration and necrosis of tissue in stages. That which led to mortification was *ga[n]ggraina*; the final stage of tissue death was *sphakelos*, an archaic term for the eventual slough of a gangrenous mass.

gargle is an imitative word that sounds like what it means, just as does the French *gargouiller* and the Greek *gargarizein*, "to wash the throat." A somewhat related word is "jargon," referring to an obfuscating language, such as doctors of medicine and other experts are sometimes said to speak. The word is taken from the French *jargon*, which originally meant "the chattering of birds," indicating a sound, typically unintelligible, arising in the throat.

gargoylism is a rare familial condition characterized by a grotesque facies, stunted and deformed body and limbs, an enlarged liver and spleen, and mental impairment. The term comes from "gargoyle," which is a type of rainspout affixed to the gutters of buildings of medieval architecture. Often the end of the spout was decorated with a caricature of a human or animal face. "Gargoyle" refers to the function of the spout, not the face. The word comes from the French *gargouille*, "waterspout," which relates to the Latin *gurgulio*, "gullet." Incidentally, "gargantuan," the adjective describing anything of immense size, is taken from the name Gargantua given to a fictional giant by the French author François Rabelais (1494?-1553), a doctor of medicine turned novelist. The giant was so called because he had an enormous throat (Spanish *garganta*) to accommodate his huge meals.

gas is such a short, simple word, one might take it for a primordial utterance. It is not. It was invented by Johannes Baptista van Helmont (1577-1644), a Flemish physician and naturalist, who felt called upon to distinguish between carbon dioxide in its usual state and the ultrafine disposition of water that became a vapor when exposed to cold. Later, van Helmont explained that his invention of the word was prompted by the Greek *chaos*, meaning "space," particularly in the sense of a rude, unformed mass. To the ancients, *chaos* was the disordered mass of elemental substances that existed before creation. Hesiod, the Greek poet of the 8th century B.C., wrote:

> Light, uncollected, through the chaos urged its
> infant way,
> Nor order yet had drawn his lovely train from
> out of the dubious gloom.

This concept is echoed in the first chapter of the Book of Genesis:

> In the beginning God created the heaven and
> the earth. And
> the earth was without form, and void; and
> darkness was upon
> face of the deep....And God said, Let there be
> light: and there was light....

gastric comes from the Greek *gastēr*, "the paunch or belly." To the ancients, this could refer to anything roundly protruding. In modern medical terminology, "gastric" is used only as an adjective to qualify whatever pertains to the stomach as an organ, e.g., a gastric ulcer. Also, it provides the combining form **gastr-**, as in **gastrectomy** or **gastroscopy**.

gastrocnemius is the name of the large muscle forming the calf of the leg. Originally, the Greek *gastroknēmia* (from *gastēr*, "belly," + *knēmē*, "leg") referred generally to the calf, or "belly," of the lower leg.

gauze as the word for a light, loosely woven fabric, is said to have originated in the name of Gaza, a town near the eastern Mediterranean shore in what is now the oft-disputed strip of land between Egypt and Israel. The Old French term was *gaze*, and supposedly the fabric was imported from Gaza, but this may be only a fabrication.

gel comes from the Latin *gelare*, "to freeze." The

Latin *gelidus* refers to whatever is cold or frosty. Anything liquid that "sets" into a solid when cooled is a gel.

-gen is a suffix that appears at the end of a number of biomedical terms to indicate either a producer (e.g., **androgen**) or a product (e.g., **nitrogen**, a gaseous element that can be obtained from nitre). The combining form is taken from the Greek *gennaō,* "I produce"; *gennan,* "to produce"; or *genos,* "a descendent."

gene is the biologic unit of heredity through which certain characteristics are passed from generation to generation. The name was taken from the Greek *gennaō,* "I produce, I beget (of the father), or I bring forth (of the mother)."

generic means "relating to or descriptive of an entire group or class." The word is taken from the Latin *genus,* "a kind, sort, or type." Generic names for drugs, in distinction to proprietary names, are composed and assigned by the U.S. Adopted Names Council, formed in 1964 and sponsored by the American Medical Association, the American Pharmaceutical Association, and the U.S. Pharmacopoeial Convention. Generic drugs are now usually thought of as those whose manufacture and purveyance are in the public domain, that is, not restricted by patent or purveyed under a tradename.

geniculate (*see* **genu**)

genio- is a combining form used to designate that which pertains to the chin or, specifically, to the mandible. Thus, the **geniohyoid** muscle connects the mandible and the hyoid bone. "Genio-" is derived from the Greek *geneias,* "a beard"; in its plural the word means "the cheeks."

genital as an adjective designates whatever may pertain to biologic reproduction and is a slight contraction of the Latin *genitalis,* "productive," which in turn is related to the Greek *gennan,* "to produce or bring forth." In the plural it can be a noun indicating, collectively, the organs of reproduction. However, even in this modern day, one usually hears of "the genitals" being called by their classical name **genitalia.**

genotype (*see* **mutation**)

gentian sounds like an adjective but really is a noun and the name of a plant with showy blue blossoms. An extract of the root of *Gentiana lutea* was long used as a tonic and an antidote to poisons. The plant is said to have been named after King Gentius, who ruled over Illyria in the 2nd century B.C. and supposedly discovered the plant's useful properties. Gentian violet is an aniline dye that has nothing to do with the plant other than reproducing the color of its flowers. The dye formerly was used as an antiseptic solution but now is used mainly as a stain for cytology, especially of bacteria.

genu is the Latin word for "the knee," being related to the Greek *gonu,* which has the same meaning. In the brain, the genu of the internal capsule is the point where the fiber tracts bend. **Geniculate**, being the diminutive, refers to whatever resembles a little knee and has been applied to knotty or nodal structures, especially when they are shaped in a kneelike bend, as is the geniculate ganglion of the facial nerve. A related word is **genuflect**, meaning to bend the knee or to bow down.

geriatrics is the treatment of disorders or diseases characteristic of elderly people. The term was coined by combining the Greek *gerōn,* "an old man," + *iatreia,* "the treatment of disease." **Gerontology** is a study of aging in all its aspects. The primitive Indo-European root may have been *gar,* "to wear away," or *ger,* "to mature, to grow old." From this came the Latin *granum,* "grain," in the sense of grain being the ripe fruit of the mature plant. The classical Latin *grandis,* "full-grown, great, aged," became favored in popular or Vulgar Latin over *magnus* and led to the French *grande* and the English "grand." In the sense of advanced age, this led to "grandfather" and "grandmother."

germ is a derivative of the Latin *germen,* "a sprout, bud, or offshoot." Thus, a **germinal** cell is so called because it is capable of proliferating into a more mature tissue, organ, or organism. The use of "germ" in the sense of bacteria carries the idea that these minute bodies are the origin of certain diseases, a concept now firmly established but at one time disputed as "the germ theory of disease." The word also is aptly used in a figurative sense when one says, "Now that is the germ of an idea."

gerontology (*see* **geriatrics**)

gestation is derived from the Latin verb *gestare*, "to carry or bear," and thus has been applied to pregnancy. Curiously, the Latin *gestare* could also mean "to carry a tale, to blab," and there are few in the bloom of pregnancy who are not anxious to converse on their condition.

-geusia is a combining form taken from the Greek *geuma*, "the taste of a thing." Thus, **ageusia** is an absence of the sense of taste, **hypogeusia** is a diminished sense of taste, **hypergeusia** is a heightened sense of taste, and **dysgeusia** is an altered or perverted sense of taste.

giddy describes a common form of dizziness also known as lightheadedness, but distinct from a true rotary hallucination (*see* **vertigo**). "Giddy" in Old English was *gidig*, which meant "insane." This, in turn, can be traced to the Teutonic *gudo* or "god." Thus, to be giddy once meant to be possessed by a god. Incidentally, our word "enthusiasm" once meant much the same thing, from the Greek *enthousiasmos*, which was formed from *en*, "in," + *theos*, "god."

gingiva is a direct borrowing of the Latin word for the gum of the mouth. It has been suggested that "gingiva" is a transposed derivative of the Latin *gignere*, "to bear or to produce," the allusion being to the observation that teeth spring from the gums.

glabella refers to the smooth area of the frontal bone between the superciliary arches or to the overlying smooth area of skin between the eyebrows. The term is taken from the Latin *glaber*, "hairless or bald." The Romans also used *glaber* as a fond nickname for a prepubescent slave. A related word is **glabrous**, meaning devoid of hair or signs of pubescence.

gladiolus is a diminutive derivation of the Latin *gladus*, "a sword," and is a term sometimes used for the pointed sternum or breastbone, the allusion being the same that led to "ensiform" and "xiphoid." The *gladus* was a short Roman sword such as that wielded by gladiators. "Gladiolus" is, and was in ancient times, also the name of a flowering plant, so called because of the shape of its leaves.

gland is a derivative of *glandulus*, being the diminutive of the Latin *glans*, "a nut or acorn," a term also used to mean the end of the male organ, as glans penis, because of its shape. The Greeks referred to lymph glands as *adenos*, which apparently was derived from *adēn*, a word for "acorn." **Adeno-** has become the combining form to designate whatever pertains to gland or glandlike structures, as in **adenoid**, **adenopathy**, **adenoma**, and **adenocarcinoma**, among other medical terms.

glanders is mainly a disease of horses but is communicable to man. In horses the disease is featured by an eruption of subcutaneous or submucosal nodules (hence the relation to the Latin *glandulus*, "a little nut") which then coalesce, ulcerate, and discharge pus. In man the disease affects both skin and lungs and, in its acute form, can result in often fatal septicemia. The causative microorganism is *Pseudomonas mallei*, formerly called *Malleomyces mallei*. Here we enter an etymologic thicket. *Malleomyces* was the name given to what was supposed to be a genus of schizomycetes; the organisms are rods with rounded ends, hence the name incorporated the Latin *malleus*, "hammer or mallet," + the Greek *mykēs*, "fungus." The organism is now classified as a bacterium. *Mallei* presumably relates to the disease that was known by the ancients as a devastating affliction of horses and was called, by the Romans, *malleus*. This particular use of malleus can be thought to relate either to *male habitus*, "a bad condition," or to *malleus* as the term for a pole-ax used by the Romans to destroy animals.

glaucoma is an almost direct borrowing of the Greek *glaukōma*, "a silvery swelling," being a combination of *glaukos*, "gleaming or silvery, especially of the sea," + *-ōma*, "a swelling or tumor." The early Greeks used *glaukōma* to refer to any condition of degeneration wherein the eyeball appeared silvery-green, such as occurred with a dense opacity of the crystalline lens. Later, a distinction was made between lenticular opacities and deeper degeneration consequent to increased intraocular pressure. "Glaucoma" came to be applied to the latter condition.

glenoid refers to the shallow concavity in the scapula which serves for articulation with the humerus. "Glenoid" (with the "oid" taken from the Greek *eidos*, "like"), however, originated with the Greek *glēnēs*, by which the ancients meant the eyeball. Perhaps the shiny cartilaginous concavity in the humerus suggested an appearance similar to that of the socket of the eyeball.

glia is a near borrowing of the Greek *gloia*, "glue." Presumably, the supporting and connective tissue was looked on as a sort of glue that held together the functional elements of the nervous system. A **glioma** is a tumor originating in glial cells.

globulin is the diminutive of the Latin *globus*, "sphere," wherein the suffix "-in" denotes a derivative. Hence, the term "globulin" was applied in the early 19th century to the substance thought to originate in the "globules," i.e., the particulate cellular elements of blood. Later, with a better appreciation of blood chemistry, "globulin" was reserved for certain plasma proteins of high molecular weight.

glomerulus is the diminutive of the Latin *glomus*, "a ball of yarn," related to the Latin verb *glomerare*, "to form into a ball." The glomerulus of the kidney, a minute ball-shaped capillary tuft, was so named by Mercello Malpighi (1628-1694), the great Italian anatomist, and formerly called a "malpighian corpuscle."

glomus is directly borrowed from the Latin (*see* **glomerulus**) as an anatomic term for an agglomeration of small arteries, veins, and neural elements that serves as a chemoreceptor responding to changes in blood content. The best known are the paired **carotid bodies** that lie in the bifurcation of the right and left common carotid arteries and respond to changes in blood pH levels and variations in concentration of blood gases.

glosso- is a combining form descended from the Greek *glōssa*, "the tongue." The **glossopharyngeal** (or ninth cranial) nerve serves the tongue and the pharynx. Incidentally, by the relation of "tongue" to language, we have "glossary," a listing of specialized terms. **Glossitis** is an inflammation or erythema of the tongue often seen in various states of nutritional deficiency.

glottis comes from *glōtta*, the Attic variant of the Greek *glōssa*, "the tongue." The Greeks also used their word for "tongue," as we do,

to mean "a voiced language," and it is this sense that "glottis," in anatomy, has been applied to the vocal apparatus. Incidentally, the related word "polyglot" means a mixture, and sometimes a confusion, of several languages.

glucagon is a pancreatic hormone that increases blood glucose levels, thus opposing the action of insulin. The name is contrived by combining the Greek *glukus*, "sweet," + *agōn*, "leading or driving."

glucose is a word contrived by a committee of the French *Académie des Sciences* in a report dated 16 July 1838. The purpose was to name the principal constituent sugar of the grape, of starch, and of diabetic urine. The committee settled on glucose as a Gallicized transformation of the Greek *glukus*, "sweet to the taste," + a derivative of the Latin *-osus*. "Glucose" was the prototype term, and its last three letters, -ose, became a biochemical suffix indicating a carbohydrate. Such a suffix, of course, already was used in a quite different way in English, where adding "-ose" (derived from the Latin *-osus*, equivalent to the Greek *-os*, "condition") is a way of converting substantives to adjectives, with the sense of "full of or abounding in," as in "bellicose" and "verbose." Glucose, as the term usually is applied, is a dextrorotary monosaccharide ($C_6H_{12}O_6 \cdot H_2O$) and as such should be specifically designated as D-glucose or **dextrose**. The levorotary counterpart is **levulose**, also called **fructose** ("the sugar of fruit," from the Latin *fructus*). There then followed **galactose**, or milk sugar (from the Greek *gala*, "milk"), **maltose** (from the Anglo-Saxon *mealt*, "grain," usually barley, steeped in water, this relating to the Latin *mollis*, "soft"), et cetera. Monosaccharides are further designated according to the number of carbon atoms in their respective molecules: diose (2), triose (3), tetrose (4), pentose (5), hexose (6), septose (7). Glucose, then, is a hexose.

gluten (*see* **agglutination**)

glycine (*see* **amino acids**)

glycosuria is a neologism made up from the Greek *glukus*, or *glykus*, "sweet," + *ouron*, "urine." Medieval physicians prided themselves on their divination of all sorts of things by their scrutiny of urine, including its taste, and a small flask for the collection of urine was an accouterment of every up-to-date doctor of "physick" in the Middle Ages. But it remained for Thomas Willis (1621-1675), an English physician, to relate the sweet taste of diabetic urine to the disease. It was not until the early 19th century that François Magendie (1783-1855), a pioneer French physiologist, demonstrated sugar in the blood as glycemia, and it was Magendie's pupil, Claude Bernard (1813-1878), who went on to conduct basic investigations of the biochemistry of sugars.

gluteal comes from the Greek *gloutos*, "the buttock," and refers specifically to that area of the anatomy.

gluten is the substance in wheat and other cereal flours that imparts a sticky consistency when moistened. The word is the same as the Latin *gluten*, "glue." Of more concern in medicine is that gluten is responsible for impaired absorption of nutriments in patients with celiac disease.

glycogen is a polysaccharide serving as the principal carbohydrate storage material in animals, being formed and largely stored in the liver and, to a lesser extent, in muscle. The substance was recognized as a constituent of the liver in the mid-19th century, when it was found that sugar could be obtained by hydrolysis of liver tissue. The term is a derivative of the Greek *glukus* or *glykus*, "sweet," + *-gen*, from *gennaō*, "I produce," and it was introduced by Claude Bernard (1813-1878), the renowned French physiologist.

gnash (*see* **bruxism**)

goiter comes, through French, from the Latin *guttur*, "gullet, throat, or neck." However, the Romans referred to a swelling of the neck as a "bronchocele." According to Professor H. A. Skinner, *gutterosi* was used in reference to persons with visibly swollen thyroid glands by Gerolama Fabrizio (1533-1619), better known as Fabricius ab Aquapendente, a famous Italian anatomist and surgeon. At that time, and for at least two centuries thereafter, the condition usually was called by the Latin **struma**, a generic term for "swelling in the neck," not being distinguished from scrofula. In the late 18th and early 19th centuries, the relationship between thyroid enlargement and hypermetabolism was recognized and variously known as Parry's disease, after the Englishman Caleb Parry (1755-1822); Graves' disease, after the Irishman Robert Graves (1797-1853); or Basedow's disease, after the German Karl von Basedow (1799-1854).

GOK is a flippant acronym for "God only knows." Neophyte doctors have been known to list GOK as their "diagnosis" when stumped by a perplexing and incomprehensible case. A seemingly more learned acronym, useful in the same way, would be "ygiagam," which sounds as though it might come from the Greek but, of course, it does not. It stands for "Your guess is as good as mine."

golgi apparatus should be spelled with an initial capital "G" but seldom is, even though it is an eponym commemorating the investigations of Camillo Golgi (1843-1926), an Italian anatomist. The term refers to an intracellular complex of fine membranes and vesicles, the exact function of which remains a subject of inquiry. Golgi's name also is associated with certain types of nerve cells and neural end-organs in muscle.

gomer (*see* **crazy**)

gonad comes from the Greek *gonē*, which means, variously, "the offspring, the seed, childbirth, the womb, or a generation," all having to do with reproduction. In zoology the gonads are the organs of sexual procreation, both in the male (the testes) and in the female (the ovaries).

gonio- is a combining form taken from the Greek *gōnia*, "a corner or an angle." The Indo-European root was *genu*, "knee," the predecessor of the Greek *gonu* and the Latin *genu*, both terms designating that joint which is the "angle" of the leg. In medicine, "gonio-" refers to that angle in the anterior chamber of the eye between the iris and the cornea. Thus **gonioscopy** (+ Greek *skopein*, "to observe") is the direct visual examination of that angle, and **goniotomy** (+ Greek *tomē*, "a cutting") is the operation performed in the anterior chamber of the eye to facilitate drainage as a remedy for the open-angle type of glaucoma. However, a **goniometer** is an instrument used to measure the range of motion in a joint.

gonococcus (*see* coccus; *also* **gonorrhea**)

gonorrhea is a word contrived by the ancient Greeks by combining *gōne*, "a seed," + *rheos*, "a flowing," their idea being that the urethral discharge characteristic of the disease was a leakage of semen. Though this notion was early learned to be erroneous, the disease was so ancient and ubiquitous that the name stuck. Even the causative organism, when discovered in 1879, was named **gonococcus**. Meanwhile, other people of other cultures have called the disease by a variety of names. Of particular interest is **clap** and the French *chaude pisse* ("hot piss"), which is vividly descriptive of the chief symptom.

gout is attributed to the French *goutte* and the antecedent Latin *gutta*, "a drop of fluid." The term apparently grew out of the medieval belief that the concretions that characterize the malady were the result of distillation, "drop by drop," of "bad humors" in the diseased part. A classic account of gout for the general reader, but also fascinating for doctors, was written by Berton Roueché and published in the 13 November 1948 issue of *The New Yorker* magazine. (*see* **saturnine**)

gracilis is the Latin word for "slender," and became, in anatomy, the name of a long, thin muscle originating at the inferior ramus of the pubis and inserting along the upper medial aspect of the tibia.

graft sounds as if it might be related to "graph," and it is, though the uses of the words are quite different. The origin of both is the Greek *graphein*, "to write." The relation of this to graph as a recording is obvious. But what about "graft" as an artificially implanted tissue? The explanation is that the Romans, in the propagation of trees, used a thin, sharpened shoot to affix to the root stock, and this was called a *graphium*, from the Latin word for "a stylus." The principal of grafting in botany was later applied to medicine, as in skin or bone grafting. Incidentally, "graft" as a word for an illicit, underhanded reward relates to the botanical graft in the sense of "something added on."

Graham crackers are so named after the Reverend Sylvester Graham (1794-1851), a self-styled reformer and nutritionist who attracted a surprisingly large following in his crusade against refined white flour and in favor of brisk cold showers. He espoused the belief that eating natural cereal foods suppressed the baser passions. Graham advocated the use of only whole, coarse grain flour for baking, and his name became attached to "Graham bread" and "Graham crackers," then known as "digestive biscuits." Doubtless Graham's ghost revels in the recent revival of the high fiber diet.

grain (*see* **gram**)

gram as a basic unit of mass and weight in the metric system is taken, by way of the French *gramme*, from the Late Latin *gramma*, "a small weight." The Greek *gramma* means "a marking," such as an inscribed letter or symbol and, by extension, an account given of weight. With the establishment of the French metric system of weights and measures, *gramme* was assigned as the weight of 1 cubic centimeter (or 1 milliliter) of distilled water at 4°C (*see* **metric**). Also from the Greek *gramma* comes our combining form **-gram**, as in electrocardiogram (the abbreviated reference, "EKG," is taken from the German *Elektrokardiogram*). Another small unit of weight, now outmoded in pharmacy, is the **grain**, from the Latin *granum*, "a grain or seed of a cereal plant." Doses of medication were once measured in grains, 1 grain as an apothecary weight being 0.065 gram. There is another **gram**, unrelated in its origin, and this is the name of a stain widely used in bacteriology. This "gram," which formerly was spelled with a capital "G," is taken from the name of Hans Christian Joachim Gram (1853-1938), a Danish physician who devised the method wherein microorganisms are first stained with crystal violet, treated with a 1:15 dilution of Lugol's iodine, washed with ethanol or ethanol-acetone, then counterstained with a contrasting dye, usually safranin. Those microorganisms that retain the crystal violet are said to be "gram positive," and those that lose the violet stain but take the counterstain are said to be "gram negative." This is a helpful means of distinguishing species of microorganisms that are otherwise morphologically similar.

grand mal (*see* **petit mal**)

granuloma is a swelling or tumorlike aggregation of granulation tissue, a form of inflammatory reaction. Its texture is like that of small grains. The term is derived from the diminutive of the Latin *granum*, "grain or seed," + the Greek *-ōma*, "swelling."

graph is a word in itself as well as a combining form directly descended from the Greek *graphein*, "to write." **Agraphia** is an inability, due to a cerebral lesion, to express thoughts in writing.

gravid describes a pregnant uterus or a pregnant woman and comes from the Latin *gravitus*, "pregnancy." This, in turn, was derived from the Latin adjective *gravis*, "heavy or burdensome," which has numerous descendants, including **grave** (in the sense of weighty or serious when applied to an illness), **gravity** (as an earthly force), and **aggravate** (only distantly related to the Latin *gravidare*, "to make heavy, to impregnate").

gray (*see* **radiology**)

grenz rays are "soft" X-rays, sometimes used therapeutically, whose wavelength is on the border of the electromagnetic spectrum between X-rays and ultraviolet rays. The term is from the German *Grenz*, "boundary."

grippe is French and more properly called *la grippe*, "a seizure or attack," particularly by an acute febrile illness. Influenza, in bygone days, was commonly called *la grippe* or, in English, "the grip." The English verb "to grip" and the noun (and sometimes verb) "gripe" are related, being descended from the Anglo-Saxon *gripan*, "to clutch or grasp."

groin is of uncertain origin but may have been taken from the Old English *grynde*, "a trench of abyss." That the groin is a depression or cleft between the lower abdominal wall and the thigh, especially when the thigh is flexed, would support this supposition.

gtt. formerly appeared commonly in prescriptions as an abbreviation of the Latin *gutta*, "a drop of fluid." Thus, "℞: gtt. v" meant "take 5 drops." *Gutta serena* is an old term for ocular opacity, such as might be caused by cataract. In guttate psoriasis, the spots on the skin may resemble drops.

guaiac comes from the Spanish *guayaco*, derived from the Taino Indian name *waiacan* for a tree originally found in the West Indies and South America. The tree was prized for its resin and became known as *lignum vitae*, "the wood of life." A preparation of the resin was once used as a tonic medicine and also was applied topically as a remedy for rheumatism and skin rashes. Now, a tincture of the resin is used as a reagent to detect blood in stains or feces, as in the "guaiac test." A widely used form of this test is known as Hemoccult, a tradename contrived by hybridizing the Greek *haima*, "blood," + the Latin *occultus*, "concealed."

gubernaculum is the name of two structures involved in developmental anatomy. One is the gubernaculum testis, a fibrous cord connecting the lower portion of the epididymis to the fold of skin that becomes the fundic portion of the scrotum. The other is the gubernaculum dentin, a band of connective tissue attaching the dental sac of an unerupted permanent tooth to the gingiva. In both cases, the gubernaculum (the Latin word for "rudder or helm") is thought to serve as a guide or "governor" to the testicle as it descends into the scrotum or to the tooth as it erupts from the gum.

gullet is now almost a colloquial name applied to the throat or esophagus. The word is descended from the Middle English *golet*, taken from the Old French diminutive of *gole*, "throat," which is related to the Latin *gula*, meaning the same.

gum as the name for the membrane covering the alveolar process of the jaws began with the Anglo-Saxon *goma*, "jaw." In Middle English this was *gome*, pronounced "goom." One may still hear an elderly, provincial person complain, "Ay, an' me gooms hurt!"

gumma is a term for a circumscribed lesion of chronic granulation tissue, particularly that of tertiary syphilis. It comes from the Latin *gummi*, "gum," in the sense of a rubbery resin. A gumma is so called because its center has a gummy consistency.

gurney is the name given to a wheeled stretcher on which patients are transported. One can suppose it might have originated with the surname of an early maker of the vehicle. According to Dr. Richard Gordon in his *Alarming History of Medicine* (New York, St. Martin's Press, 1993), Sir Goldsworthy Gurney (1793-1875) was an ingenious Cornish surgeon who invented limelight, an oxyhydrogen blowpipe, a piano that played on musical glasses, a jet-propelled steamboat, a steam carriage, a fire extinguisher to be used in coal mines, a signaling lamp, a means by which seamen could identify lighthouses, and the Gurney stove to warm up the House of Commons. With all of these accomplishments, who is to say he did not also come up with the idea of a wheeled stretcher?

gustatory in referring to the sense of oral taste comes from the Latin *gustatus*, "taste or flavor," and is related to the Greek *geuma*, "the taste of a thing" (*see* **-geusia**). The Spanish and Italian *gusto* means both "a pleasing and appetizing flavor" as well as "pleasure" in a general sense. Taken into English, "gusto" means an even more exuberant relish. Incidentally, "relish" is derived from the Old French *relais*, "that which is left behind," which came to be used in the sense of an aftertaste.

gut is an old English word for "the entrails," as the contents of the abdominal cavity. Probably the term originated in the Anglo-Saxon *gēotan*, "to pour," as an allusion to the entrails having the appearance of being poured into the abdominal cavity as molten metal is poured into a cast. The plural "guts" is a slang word for courage or nerve, sometimes euphemized as "intestinal fortitude." The *Oxford English Dictionary* states that gut "formerly, but not now, [was] in dignified use with reference to man." The *OED* notwithstanding, *Gut* is the current name of the official journal of the prestigious British Association of Gastroenterology.

gynecology comes from the Greek *gynē, gynaikelos*, "woman, womanly," + *logia*, "a study." According to a strict etymologic definition, then, a gynecologist would be one steeped in the study of women. Those doctors who actually practice gynecology would rightly disclaim such a bold and sweeping purview. Their concern is limited to disorders of the female reproductive apparatus. One hears varying pronunciations of "gynecology," either with a hard "g" coupled with the sound of a long "i," or with a soft "g" coupled with the sound of a short "i." In classical Greek, the letter gamma was always pronounced as a hard "g." In Latinized Greek, "g" is softened to sound like "j" before "e," "i," and "y" (as in "geriatrics") but keeps the hard "g" before "a," "o," and "u" (as in "gastric"). This brief explanation is not intended to dictate a proper pronunciation of "gynecology"; one can do as one prefers.

gyrus is Latin for "ring, circle, or orbit," being related to the Greek *gyros*, meaning the same. In anatomy, the term is applied to the intricate rugal configuration of the cerebral cortex and incorporated in the names of its particular areas, such as the "hippocampal gyrus." An alternative term is **convolution**, from the Latin *convolvere*, "to roll together, as a scroll," which also describes the infoldings of the intestinal mucosa.

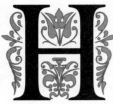

Habitus (*see* -sthenia)

haggard describes a person of gaunt, worn, and anxious appearance. It was also once used in falconery to designate a wild female hawk caught only after it had attained adult plumage, presumably having already undergone the rigors of the hunt on its own. The pejorative "hag," meaning an ugly, malicious, old woman, may have been the original term, coming from the Old English *haegtes[se]*, "witch."

hair is of Teutonic origin, through the Anglo-Saxon *hǽr*. Latin provides a variety of words denoting different kinds of hair, and some of them have been carried over into medical terms. **Capillus** means hair generally, but in particular the fine hair of the head. The Latin term is a contraction of *capitis pilus*. From this, much later, was derived **capillary** as the name for the fine, hairlike blood vessels that connect arteries and veins. The ancients had no idea these vessels existed. **Pilus**, related to the Greek *pilos*, "carded wool," referred to hair generally, and from this we have **pilonidal** (+ Latin *nidus*, "nest"), a hairy dermoid cyst that occurs as a developmental defect at the base of the spine; **pilomotor**, a minute muscle that moves a hair to stand on end; and **depilatory**, an agent that removes unwanted hair. **Cirrus**, a Latin word related to the Greek *skirros*, means "curly hair" and describes a type of wispy cloud formation; also it is used as a term for various flexible, filamentous appendages of certain protozoa and other primitive creatures. *Cilium* is Latin for "eyelid," especially its margins and lashes, hence use of the plural **cilia** for vibratile, hairlike projections from the surface of certain cells such as those that make up the respiratory epithelium. Above the *cilium* is the *supercilium* or "eyebrow." The Latin *vellus* and *villus* both mean "fleece" (*villus* more specifically is "a tuft of hair") and also referred to

the fine body hair or "down," especially that of children and women (also known by the Latin **lanugo**); thus, we have the French *velours,* the English "velvet," and **villus** (plural, **villi**) as the anatomic term for the slender mucosal projections lining the lumen of the small intestine. **Vibrissa**, from the verb *vibrare*, "to quiver," refers to hair in the nostrils or the whiskers of a cat. The Greek *mystax* refers to hair on the upper lip and led to **mustache**. *Barba* is Latin for "beard," hence "barber" (but not "barbarian," which can be traced to the root *bar-bar*, an echoic term imitating the supposed stammering of outlanders unfamiliar with classical languages). **Seta** is a New Latin term for "bristle" such as found on pigs. From this comes *Setaria*, the name of a genus of filarial nematodes, and **seton**, a strip of nonabsorbable material drawn through a wound to facilitate drainage.

haircut at one time was heard as a dialect word for the primary lesion of syphilis. The allusion was to the former medical custom of shaving the pubic hair when applying topical therapy for venereal disease.

hale as in "hale and hearty," referring to a state of ebullient wellness, is descended from the Old English *hāl*, meaning "whole" in the sense of all parts intact and functioning in good order. (*see* **heal**; *also* **healthy**)

halitosis comes from the Latin *halitus*, "breath or vapor," and this relates to "inhale" and "exhale." Strictly speaking, halitosis means "a condition of the breath." But, thanks to the gratuitous efforts of the advertising industry, everyone knows that halitosis is a euphemism for "bad breath." One could hardly expect the denizens of Madison Avenue to handle the full and proper Latin term: *halitus oris fetidus*, "breath of a stinking mouth."

hallucination comes from the Latin *hallucinari*, "to dream or to talk wildly." An earlier Latin deponent verb was *alucinari*, "to engage in small talk or to ramble." This, in turn, related to the Greek *aluein*, "to wander, as in mind, or to be distraught."

hallux is the Latin word for the big toe and is so

used in terms referring to deformities such as hallux valgus. Hallux came from the earlier form *allex*, which is thought to have been derived from the Greek *allomai*, a deponent verb meaning "to leap." The Latin adjective for bowlegged is *valgus*, obviously referring to the knee, as in genu valgus. But the metatarsophalangeal joint of the big toe could become bowed, too, and came to be known as hallux valgus. A better term is simply **bunion**, from the Old French *buigne*, "a swelling or bump due to a blow."

halogen is derived from the Greek *als*, "salt," + -gen from *genesis*, "origin or source." Thus, a halogen is a "source of salts." To designate chlorine, bromine, and iodine as halogens seemed appropriate to early chemists because these elements were commonly found in seawater, and the Greek *als* particularly referred to the salt of the sea. Fluorine was later added to the group of halogens.

hamartoma is derived from a combination of the Greek *hamartanein*, "to fail of purpose, to go wrong," + *ōma*, "a swelling." The idea is that a hamartoma is a tumor resulting from something gone awry in development. The term is said to have been introduced by Karl Albrecht (1851-1894), a German anatomist, to denote a tumorlike nodule of superfluous tissue. The essential feature of a hamartoma is that it contains elements or variants thereof that are indigenous to the part involved, and that these have proliferated because of an ontogenetic defect. Hamartomas are thus distinguished from neoplasms that arise later in life and may or may not contain elements normally found in the part affected.

hamate is the name of one of the carpal bones that has a hooklike process extending from its volar surface, and its name is taken from the Latin *hamatus*, "hookshaped." **Hamulus** is the diminutive, and the pterygoid hamulus, a process of the sphenoid bone, is shaped like a little hook at the end of the medial pterygoid plate.

hamstring as a noun refers to the prominent tendons of the flexor muscle at the back of the knee; as a verb it means to cut these tendons, a sure way of crippling an animal or a human adversary in battle. The relation of "string" to tendon is obvious. The "ham-" part is taken from the Old Teutonic *ham*, "crooked," that was applied to the crooked part of the leg at the knee. "Ham" also came to mean the thigh of an animal prepared as food, later being restricted to that of the pig, then extended to include most of the meat of that particular animal. All of this has nothing to do with "ham" as an overly zealous performer; this use of "ham" is an aspersion cast on the inept actor who vainly attempts to play the protagonist of Shakespeare's *Hamlet*.

hamulus (*see* **hamate**)

handbook (*see* **manual**)

handicap is a disadvantage or burden that diminishes the chance of success and, when applied to a person, refers to a physical impairment. The term originated in sport in the 18th century, and the term is still used specifically for the added weight placed on the back of an otherwise favored entry in a horse race. The custom was to place the wager money in the cap of an impartial umpire who decreed the extent of burden to be borne by the superior horse so as to ensure a fair race. The challenged and the challenger each put his hand in the cap. If either withdrew his money, the race was off. If both pulled back an empty hand, the terms were accepted, and the race was on. The gesture of the "hand in the cap" came to be called simply "handicap."

hangnail is the term for a tender, split cuticle at the edge of the fingernail or toenail, but it has nothing to do with hanging. It is derived from the Anglo-Saxon *ang*, "painful," + *naegl*, "nail." How or why "h" became the initial letter is a mystery. Perhaps "hangnail" seemed easier to pronounce, at least to cockneys.

haploid describes one of a pair or a single set, usually in reference to chromosomes. The term is from the Greek *haplous*, "single," + *eidos*, "like." (*see* **-ploid**)

haptin is derived from the Greek *haptein*, "to fasten or bind." The term, sometimes spelled **haptene**, was introduced by Paul Ehrlich (1854-1915), the renowned German bacteriologist and immunologist. Ehrlich's "side-chain theory" postulated the presence of receptors in cell membranes that served as binding sites for various antibodies, a remarkably prescient idea. A haptin is not a whole antigen, but rather is that part of the antigenic molecule or complex that determines its immunologic specificity.

harelip is a congenital defect in the upper lip consequent to failure of the median nasal and maxillary processes to unite in the course of embryonic development. It is so called because the hare, a close relative of the rabbit, normally has a divided upper lip.

haruspication is hardly an everyday word, but it should be of interest to diagnosticians. A *haruspex* was a priest of ancient Rome who sought to foretell the future by inspection of the entrails of sacrificed animals. The name comes from a combination of the Latin *haru, hira,* "the empty gut," + *specere,* "to look at." This sounds bizarre, but there was a precedent. Ancient Persian soothsayers claimed to predict the outcome of battles by examining sections of animal livers. Knowing this can open a renewed purview for hepatologists.

hashish is the dried, flowering tip of the hemp plant, which is smoked, chewed, or brewed as a potent source of the intoxicant drug cannabis. *Hashish* is the Arabic word for dried vegetation, such as hay. Thus, "hashish" is analogous to "grass," a common street word for marijuana in the United States. **Cannabis**, incidentally, is a direct borrowing of the Latin word for hemp, being related to the Greek *kannabis.* The ancients were acquainted with the psychotropic property of hemp. Smoking for pleasure is by no means a recent discovery.

haustrum is the Latin word for "a scoop or bucket" and, as the neuter plural *haustra,* has been applied to the bucketlike pouches that characterize the wall of the colon.

hay fever was first described in 1819 by John Bostock (1773-1846), an English physician who himself suffered from the condition that he called "summer catarrh" because it recurred perennially in the late summer season. Shortly thereafter, it was correctly surmised that the cause was the inhalation of pollen, but the source was mistakenly thought to be the ripening grasses mown for hay. Only later was pollen from the ragweed plant properly indicted. And, of course, the allergy is not marked by fever. So, "hay fever" is a misnomer all around, but its common use persists.

heal comes from the Old English *haelen,* "to make sound or whole," and thus has its similar counterparts in most Teutonic languages.

health is derived from Old English (*see* **heal**) and can be defined as a state of soundness or wholeness or, as might be said today, "to have it all together." Related words are **hail**, "a greeting," and **hale**, "a poetic or dialect word for health."

heart is descended from the Anglo-Saxon *heorte.* Through the ages, despite an ignorance of the circulation of blood, the heart was somehow associated with the essence of life and vigor and was looked upon as the seat of courage, hence the figurative use of "hearty" and "to hearten" or "to dishearten."

hebephrenia is a form of schizophrenia observed in adolescents and takes its name from a combination of the Greek *hebe,* "puberty," + *phrēn,* "the mind." Hebe, the wife of Hercules, was the mythologic goddess of youth who purportedly had the power to make the aged young again. "Hebiatrics," sometimes called "ephebiatrics," is a perfectly good name for the practice of medicine limited to pubescent youngsters, but most practitioners of this specialty prefer "adolescent medicine."

hectic owes its present meaning to a medical association. Galen, the renowned 2nd century A.D. physician, described recurring flushing and fever with the Greek *hektikos,* "habitual." In the 15th century "hectic fever" was associated with tuberculosis which, in advanced stages, was not only persistent but marked by flushed cheeks, nervous excitability, and confused agitation. Thereupon, the meaning of "hectic" changed from "habitual or repetitive" to "feverish, reckless activity."

HeLa cells are used in biomedical research at the cellular level and are the product of a perpetual culture of malignant cells originally isolated in 1951 by Dr. George O. Gey at the Johns Hopkins Hospital in Baltimore. The source was a cervical carcinoma harbored by a patient named Henrietta Lacks. The term is taken from the first two letters of her first and last names. This is yet another example of unexpected immortality, of a sort.

helix is borrowed from the Greek *helix,* "a coil," and is related to the verb *helissein,* "to twist or roll." The helix of the ear is the rolled superior and posterior margin of the pinna of the ear. In modern biology the "double helix" is the paired, coiled structure of DNA (deoxyribonucleic acid) that enables reproduction of genetic information in living cells.

helminth is an almost direct borrowing of the Greek *helmins*, "a worm," and is used in medicine, either alone or as a combining form, to refer to any wormlike parasite.

hema-, hemato-, hemo- are combining forms indicating a relationship to blood and are derived from the Greek *haima*, "blood."

hemangioma is an abnormal proliferation of blood vessels, often as a **hamartoma**. The term incorporates "hema-" + *a[n]ggeion*, "vessel," + *-ōma*, "tumor."

hematemesis is the vomiting of blood, adding to "hema-" a derivative of the Greek *emein*, "to vomit."

hematochezia is the passage of recognizable, usually fresh red blood at stool. A derivative of the Greek *chezein*, "to defecate," is added to the prefix "hemato-." This is in contrast to **melena**, the passage of tarry black stools, though in some cases the blood in stools is mixed, both red and black.

hematocrit is the percentage of cellular elements in blood when plasma, the fluid component, is separated by centrifugation. The term combines "hemato-" + a derivative of *krinein*, "to separate."

hematopoiesis is the process whereby the cellular elements of blood are formed. The Greek *poiēsis*, "creation," is borrowed for the second portion of the term. Originally, the liver and spleen were thought to be the principal blood-forming organs. It was not until the mid-19th century that the hematopoietic role of the bone marrow was recognized.

hematoxylin is a common tissue stain, often used in combination with eosin, as in the familiar "H&E" preparation of histologic sections. The heavy, reddish-brown heartwood of a West Indian and Central American tree called "logwood" is used as a source of the dye. The generic name for the tree is *Haematoxylon* (+ Greek *xylon*, "wood"). The name presumably was suggested by the bloodlike color of the wood. The dye, extracted from the wood by ether, became known as "hematoxylin" and has been applied to tissue sections since the mid-19th century.

hemochromatosis is a condition characterized by an accumulation of excess iron pigment in the liver, pancreas, heart, skin, and other organs. At one time the disease was occasionally called "bronze (or bronzed) diabetes." The name "hemochromatosis," incorporating the Greek *chrōma*, "color or complexion," was proposed by Friedrich Daniel von Recklinghausen (1833-1910), a German pathologist. Presumably, the original idea was that the affected organs were discolored by iron from blood; it is now known that the iron accumulates from exogenous sources.

hemodynamic describes the physical principles governing blood pressure and flow. The term incorporates the Greek *dynamis*, "power, force."

hemoglobin is a word that can fool the armchair etymologist. Professor Alexander Gode points out (*JAMA.* 1965;192:1066) that, when dissected, "hemoglobin" seems to be a combination of "hemo-" + glob, "ball," + "-in," indicating a substance; this would add up to "blood-ball stuff," which sounds silly, yet this is an almost literal translation of the German *Blutkügelchenstoff*. Actually, the original form of the word probably was "haematoglobulin," which for convenience was shortened to "hemoglobin." Only later, when the chemical composition of hemoglobin was better understood, did the word make sense as indicating a composition of "heme," the pigment component, and "globin," the protein moiety.

hemolysis refers to the consequence of a disruption of red blood cells and the dispersion of their contents into whatever medium they were suspended. The second portion of the term is a borrowing of the Greek *lysis*, "a breaking up."

hemophilia is a disease that has been recognized since biblical times, being mentioned in the Talmud. In this collection of Judaic law, the condition was cited as exempting the sufferer from the rite of circumcision because of the hazard of hemorrhage. The term combines "hemo-" with the Greek *philos*, "loved or dear." The idea is not that blood is held dear or that a condition of the blood affects loved ones; rather, "-philia" here means "tendency," in this case to bleeding.

hemoptysis incorporates the Greek *ptysis*, "a spitting" (an onomatopoeic word if ever there was one). The ancients used "hemoptysis" to refer to the spitting of blood from any source. Only later was it restricted to the coughing up of blood from the respiratory tract.

hemorrhage means a free and forceful escape of blood. The tail of the term is taken from the Greek *r[h]ēgnumai*, "to break forth."

hemorrhoid comes from the Greek *hemorrhoia*, "a flow of blood," a term combining *haima* + *rheein*, "to flow." In this case the ending "-oid" does not originate in the Greek *eidos*, "like." Rather, our word came through the French *emoroyde*. Apparently, the flow of blood from distended, prolapsed, anal veins was familiar to the ancients. Because the condition was frequent, the source of the bleeding was referred to, anatomically, as "the hemorrhoidal veins." In other words, the bleeding was named first and then the name was transferred to the source. The British, of course, spell it "haemorrhoid," more in keeping with the original Greek. Some years ago, a highly regarded English proctologist was invited to address the American Gastroenterological Association on the subject. He began by pointing out, "No wonder you Yanks have trouble dealing with this condition—you can't even spell the word!"

hemi- is a combining form derived from the Greek *hēmisus*, "half," and is equivalent to the Latin *semi-*. As a rule, which is not always followed, "hemi-" is attached as a modifier to words of Greek origin and "semi-" is attached to those of Latin origin.

heparin was the name given by William Henry Howell (1860-1945), an eminent American physiologist, to an anticoagulant phospholipid substance extracted from canine liver. The name was concocted from the Greek *hēpar*, "the liver," + the suffix "*-in*," meaning "a substance of." Howell thought this substance was equivalent to what he had postulated as the "anti-prothrombin principle" that prevented circulating blood from clotting. The "anti-prothrombin" notion figured in a mistaken theory of blood coagulation that was propounded in Howell's *Textbook of Physiology* through several editions from 1911 to 1921. It was in the 1930s that a quite dif-ferent substance having potent anticoagulant activity was extracted from beef lung by A. F. Charles and D. A. Scott in Toronto. But the original name "heparin" stuck. The refined substance used in clinical practice today is a mucopolysaccharide prepared from beef lung or from beef and hog intestinal mucosa; it has nothing to do with the liver.

hepatic can describe anything related to the liver, being a near borrowing of the Greek *hēpatikos*, "of the liver." Not so many years ago there was a once popular, over-the-counter, proprietary medicinal known as Sal Hepatica, literally "the salt of the liver." According to the rules of Latin syntax it should have been "Sal Hepaticum." It was a saline laxative containing magnesium sulfate and purportedly stimulated the flow of bile, which doubtless it did to some extent. Touted as a tonic, it was supposed "to get the juices going." The Greek name for the liver is *hēpar*, now modified and used only as a combining form, as in **hepatitis**, an inflammation of the liver. Strangely, the Latin word for liver, *jecur*, never appears in medical usage, with the possible exception of **jecorize**, an arcane term for imparting to food, by any means, the therapeutic qualities of cod liver oil.

hermaphrodite is a person or animal whose body exhibits anatomic features of both sexes. The word comes from Hermaphroditus, so named in Greek mythology because he was the son of Hermes and Aphrodite. Hermaphroditus was beloved by a nymph Salmacis, who shamelessly pursued and embraced him, imploring the gods to unite them "so the twain might become one flesh." Her fervent prayer was not only heard but granted, one might think to the dismay of Hermaphroditus. Sailors know a "hermaphrodite brig" as a two-masted vessel that is square-rigged forward and schooner-rigged aft.

hernia probably comes from the Greek *hernos*, "a sprout," as it referred to the protruding bud of a plant. The allusion originally was to any unsightly bulge from the body. Only later was the essential definition established as a protrusion through an abnormal opening.

heroin was first described in 1874 as a semisynthetic derivative of morphine, but it gained attention in 1898 when commercially introduced by the Bayer company of Germany. The name "heroin" reportedly was bestowed on the drug by Dr. Heinrich Dreser, then head of Bayer's research department, who adapted the name from the German *heroisch*, "heroic, strong." The claim was that heroin was both strong (true: the drug has more than twice the potency of morphine) and benign (false: the malignant addicting property of the drug was soon apparent but slow to be believed). Curiously, heroin was at first touted as a cure for morphine addiction. Whoever believed that must have forgotten that morphine was once touted as a cure for opium addiction. Some lessons are difficult to learn.

herpes is a borrowing of the Greek word that appears in Hippocratic writings as a term for a spreading cutaneous eruption. The root word is the Greek *herpein*, "to creep." The Latin equivalent is *serpere*, "to crawl, to move or spread slowly." To the Romans a *serpens* was a creeping thing, a snake. The Greek *zōstēr* denotes a girdle. Hence, **herpes zoster** is an eruption that tends to creep around the torso. But it is only "half a girdle" because the eruption of herpes zoster (or **shingles**, as it is popularly known, this term being hobson-jobsoned from the Latin *cingulum*, "a girdle") almost never crosses the midline from one side to the other. **Herpes simplex** (Latin *simplex*, "simple or plain") is the name given to a virus that occurs in two types. Type I causes ordinary "cold sores," such as those that erupt around the mouth, sometimes in response to fever, but Type II causes recalcitrant genital sores that are anything but simple for the sufferer.

hetero- is a combining form taken from the Greek *heteros*, "different," or "the other of two." This is in contrast to the Greek *homoios*, "like or resembling," from which is derived the combining form **homo-**. Whatever is **heterogeneous** is made up of different things, particularly of things from different sources; whatever is homogeneous is from the same source, hence "all the same." Whatever is **heterotopic** (+ Greek *topos*, "place") is in a location other than where it should normally be.

hiatus is the Latin word for "an opening, a gaping mouth, or a chasm." The Latin verb *hiare* means "to yawn or gape." The word has been incorporated in various medical terms, such as "hiatus semilunaris," which is the crescentic groove anterior and inferior to the bulla of the ethmoid bone into which the paranasal sinuses drain. What is commonly called "hiatal hernia" is a protrusion of the cardial portion of the stomach superiorly into the opening in the diaphragm that is normally occupied by the esophagus.

hiccup is an imitative word that when pronounced sounds like what it means. Similar sounding words of the same meaning occur in most European languages, as, for example, the Spanish *hipo* and the French *hoquet* (the German *Schlucken* has a juicier sound). Occasionally, there comes along a pseudosophisticated pedant to whom "hiccup" looks inelegant. He then insists on spelling it "hiccough," which is nonsense. **Singultus** is highfalutin "medicalese" for hiccup. It is a Latin word meaning "a gasp or a sob," especially those that occur repetitively. "Singultus," in turn, is related to the Latin adjective *singuli*, "one at a time."

hidro- is a combining form taken from the Greek *hidros*, "sweat." Hence, **anhidrosis** is an absence of sweating, and **hidradenitis** is an inflammation of the sweat glands. "Hidro-" is not to be confused with "hydro-," a pitfall for the unwary speller.

hilum is the Latin word for "a little something, a trifle." The Romans used the word to refer to the small spot on a seed or bean that marked its point of attachment to a stalk. Hence, in anatomy, the hilum of the lung or kidney is the point of attachment by the serving vessels. Hilum is a neuter singular noun; to use "hilus" would be imputing an incorrect gender, and the proper plural of hilum is **hila**. The Romans are said to have had an expression *ne hilum*, meaning "not even a trifle," often shortened to *nihil*, and even to *nil*. From this comes our "nihilism," "nil" (as an expression for zero), and "annihilate" (utterly destroyed, reduced to nothing). It would seem the Old English expression "not worth a hill of beans" is a miscarriage. At today's prices a hill of almost any kind of beans would be valuable. The phrase probably should be "not worth the hilum on a bean."

hip is a word of Anglo-Saxon origin that in its earliest form may have meant "a bump or a lump," the humps on either side of the pelvis being sufficient to hang one's pants on. The same word appears in rose hips, meaning the lumplike fruit of the rose plant, now purveyed in so-called natural food stores as a source of vitamin C.

hippocampus is a curved gyrus in the medial part of the floor of the inferior horn of the lateral ventricle of the brain. Functionally, it is part of the olfactory cortex. Its shape suggests that of the seahorse, which exists both in mythology as a sea monster with the head of a horse and the tail of a fish, and as an actual small sea creature, a member of the pipefish family. The name comes from the Greek *hippos*, "horse," + *kampos*, "a sea monster."

hirsute is a Latin way of saying "hairy" and is an almost direct borrowing of the Latin adjective *hirsutus*, which to the Romans meant "bristly" or even "rude." *Hirsutus* probably is related to the Latin verb *horrere*, "to bristle," i.e., to make one's hair stand on end. Descended from *horrere* are the English words horror, horrid, and horrendous.

histo- is a combining form that refers to any biologic tissue or composite of cells. The Greek *histos* means "a ship's mast," but it also came to be used for the upright pole supporting the web of a loom (the warp of ancient looms was stretched horizontally rather than suspended vertically). Later, the term was applied to the web as well and, by extension, to the fabric, then further still to organic tissues. Building on "histo-," we have **histology** (+ Greek *logos*, "a treatise"), **histamine** (an amine occurring in various tissues), and **histolytic** (+ Greek *lysis*, "a loosening"). **Histio-** is a variant of "histo-" and used in the same sense of pertaining to tissues, as in **histiocyte**, a macrophage found in a variety of tissues. The Greek *histion* means "anything woven, particularly a sail."

hive as a localized swelling of the skin (and, because multiple, usually called "hives") traditionally related to the verb "to heave," in the sense of raising up. However, it would seem more likely that the bump in the skin suggested the shape of a beehive, a conical or domed structure. This kind of "hive" is descended from the Icelandic *hufr*, "a ship's hull."

holistic (*see* **eclectic**)

homeopathy is a concept of medical therapy promoted by Christian Friedrich Samuel Hahnemann (1755-1843), a German physician. The concept did not originate with Hahnemann but was embodied in the ancient aphorism *Similia similibus curantur* ("Like things are cured by like things"). According to this notion, symptoms are best treated by agents believed to induce the same reaction. An example would be an attempt to combat fever by administering a pyrogenic agent, thus to "fight fire with fire." In this sense, "homeopathy" was derived from the Greek *homo-*, "the same," + *pathos*, "suffering or disease." Hahnemann himself suggested the contrasting term **allopathy** (concocted from the Greek *allo-*, "other," + *pathos*) to refer to the use of medications having effects antagonistic to symptoms, then and still now a prevalent view. To Hahnemann's credit, he advocated the use of minute doses of drugs synergistic to symptoms, and thus his prescriptions were generally innocuous. Some wag derisively suggested that Hahnemann would make coffee by plugging the cloaca of a duck with a coffee bean, then chasing the duck across a lake. Ambrose Bierce, in his *Devil's Dictionary*, defined homeopathy as "a school of medicine midway between allopathy and Christian Science. To the last, both of the others are distinctly inferior, for Christian Science will cure imaginary diseases, and they cannot."

homo- is a combining form taken from the Greek *homos*, "like or similar." The Greek *homologos* (+ *logos*, "a statement") means "an agreement or being in accord with." (*see* **hetero-**)

homogeneous incorporates the Greek *genos*, "race or tribe" and denotes whatever is made up of the same elements or is of the same quality throughout.

homologue in biology is often shortened to **homolog** and denotes a part having the same structure and origin in different organisms, whereas an **analog** (Greek *ana*, "again") is a part having the same function but of different origin in different organisms. Analog is not to be confused with **anlage**, borrowed from the German word meaning "a laying on," which, in biology, refers to a primordial structure or rudiment.

Homo sapiens (*see* **sapid**)

homozygote is an individual organism possessing an identical part of alleles in regard to a given phenotype. The latter portion of the term is taken from the Greek *zygōtos*, "yoked together."

homunculus is a direct borrowing of the Latin word for "a little man," the diminutive of *homo*, "a human being." In neuroanatomy, homunculus is the proportional representation of the human figure superimposed on the motor and sensory areas of the cerebral cortex as a device to depict localization of neural control.

hordeolum is a polysyllabic term for a stye, an inflamed meibomian gland in the eyelid. It comes from the diminutive of the Latin *hordeum*, "barley"; the lesion was fancied to resemble a little barleycorn. Meibomian is taken from the name of Heinrich Meibom (1638-1700), a German anatomist who described the tarsal glands of the eyelid in 1666. (*see* **acne**; *also* **stye**)

hormone is derived from the Greek *hormē*, "impulse." The Greek word appears in Hippocratic writings to denote the action of supposed "vital principles," the notion of "getting the juices going" being an ancient one. The term was revived in 1902 by W. M. Bayliss and E. H. Starling when they described the stimulus to pancreatic secretion (*J Physiol.* 1902;28:325) as mediated by a humoral agent they called **secretin**, taken from the Latin *secretus*, "that which is separated." This marked the discovery and recognition of the first true hormone.

hospital is from the Latin *hospitalia*, "apartments for strangers or guests." This, in turn, was derived from the Latin *hospes*, which could mean either a visitor or one who entertained a visitor. Related words are **hospital**, **hospice**, **host**, **hostel**, and **hotel**, all in the sense of contributing to the congenial accommodation of guests. A time-honored French proper name for a hospital is *Hôtel-Dieu*, "God's hospice." But, as Professor Alexander Gode pointed out (*JAMA.* 1965;194:1230), all

visitors are not friendly, hence the use of the word "host," from the Latin *hostis*, "enemy," to mean a confronting army, and the word "hostile."

human is said to have originated in the postulated Indo-European root *ghdhem*, which referred to earth or soil. From this comes the Latin *humus*, "earth or land"; *humilis*, "common or colloquial," whence "humble"; *homo*, "a person" (*Homo sapien* is "a wise, knowing, or sensible person"); and *humanus*, "kind or compassionate," whence "humane." Also, presumably from this root came the Anglo-Saxon *guma*, "man," which in Old English was incorporated into *brydguma*, "a bride's man," and later became "bridegroom."

humdudgeon is an imaginary illness or a woeful hypochondriac's complaint. Probably the word is a contracted combination of "humbug" and "dudgeon," meaning "sullen." In Grose's *Dictionary of the Vulgar Tongue* is the quotation, "He has got the humdudgeon; nothing ails him except low spirits."

humerus is derived from the Latin *umerus*, related to the Greek *ōmus*, both meaning "shoulder." To ancient anatomists, the scapula, the clavicle, and the humerus were known collectively as the *ossa humeri*, "bones of the shoulder." Later, humerus came to denote the bone of the upper arm alone. Exhaustive research yields no evidence supporting the notion that the humerus is so called because it is connected to the **funny bone**.

humoral comes from the Latin *umere*, "to be moist," which seems close to the modern sense of "humoral" as denoting those regulatory effects transmitted by internal (endocrine) secretions. This is in contrast to neural regulatory effects transmitted by nerve pathways. The action of insulin, secreted by the islet cells of the pancreas, on tissues involved in carbohydrate metabolism is an example of a humoral effect. Of course, "humoral" was used historically to characterize a concept of physiology and pathology that entailed four "humors" contained in the body: blood, phlegm, yellow bile, and black bile. Health was a state in which the four were in proper balance. Disease resulted from an imbalance, and treatment required the purging or strengthening of such "humors" as were considered excessive or deficient. Even today we speak of people being "good humored" or "bad humored."

hyaline comes from the Greek *hyalos*, "a transparent stone (as a crystal) or glass." The word used by the Greeks is said to have originated in ancient Egypt where the making of glass began. Hyaline cartilage is so called because of its glassy appearance.

hybrid apparently did not originate directly with the Greek *hybris*, "wanton violence, insolence, or arrogance"; this, rather, has given us **hubris**, of which modern day doctors of medicine are sometimes accused. "Hybrid," in biologic usage, probably began with the Latin *hibrida*, the term for an untamable offspring of a domestic sow and a wild boar. Later, the term was applied to any mongrel, especially to a child born of a Roman father and a barbarian mother.

hybridoma is a newly contrived term to designate the product of an amazing technologic feat wherein certain components of antigen-bearing cells and antibody-producing cells are genetically combined. (Here the suffix "-oma" presumably is used in the sense of "body" rather than "swelling.") The combination can result in a **monoclonal** (Greek *mono-*, "single," + *klōn*, "twig") antibody of incredible specificity. Such hybridomas give promise of more precise diagnosis and treatment of disease than heretofore possible.

hydatid is a near borrowing of the Greek *hydatoeis*, "watery," being related to *hydor*, "water," and refers to a watery cyst or vesicle. Hydatid cysts, often of large size, can occur in the liver, lungs, or other organs as a consequence of infection by the *Echinococcus* genus of tapeworm. **Echino-** is from the Greek word for "a prickly husk," and "-coccus" suggests its berrylike appearance.

hydro- is a combining form derived from the Greek *hydor*, "water."

hydrocele is a collection of serous fluid in the tunica vaginalis of the testicle. The tail of the term was taken from the Greek *kēlē*, "hernia," because the collection was originally mistaken as a serous sac from the peritoneum protruding into the scrotum. (*see* -cel-)

hydrocephalus is literally "watery head" (Greek *kephalē*, "head"), but more specifically denotes an excessive accumulation of cerebrospinal fluid in the ventricles of the brain.

hydrogen is so named because the gas was observed to generate water when burned in the presence of oxygen.

hydrolysis is the splitting of a compound by the addition of water, wherein the hydroxyl group (OH) attaches to one fragment and the hydrogen atom (H) attaches to the other. Use of the Greek *lysis*, "a dissolution," refers particularly to the change induced in the substrate rather than the breakup of H_2O.

hydrophobia is a name by which the disease rabies became popularly known and can be explained by the intensely painful spasm of the throat muscles felt by the victim of the disease when he attempts to drink, suggesting a dread of water (Greek *phobos*, "fear"). Incidentally, the Greek *hydropotēs* was literally "a water drinker" but actually meant "a drinker of thin potations," in contrast to a drinker of more robust beverages; hence to the Greeks it meant "a thin-blooded fellow." This notion survives in the present-day description of a lean, asthenic person as "a long drink of water." Note again that "hydro-" is not to be confused with **hidro-**, a distinct combining term borrowed from the Greek word for sweat. (*see* **rabies**)

hydrops is derived from the Greek *hyderos* or *hydrōps* as used by ancient writers to refer to any abnormal accumulation of watery fluid in the tissues or in a body cavity. A colloquial rendering of "hydrops" became **dropsy**, a now archaic term for serous swelling of a part. The edema of congestive heart failure was once called dropsy. Presently, hydrops is restricted to mean an accumulation of serous fluid, particularly in a chronically obstructed yet distensible gallbladder.

hygiene is the science of preventive medicine and the practice of healthy habits. It is so called from Hygeia, the name of one of the two daughters of Asklēpios (in Latin, Aesculapius), the Greek god of medicine. The other daughter, Panaceia, became the goddess of healing. Hygeia, as the goddess of health, was credited with supplying a wholesome environment, thus promoting sound growth and the ability to ward off diseases. It is perhaps understandable that a somewhat acrimonious competition arose between the two legendary sisters. After all, if Hygeia had her way Panaceia would have little to do.

hygroma is an endothelial-lined cyst filled with serous fluid. The word is derived from the Greek *hygros*, "moist," +*ōma*, "a swelling." In modern medicine, a hygroma is a lymphatic cyst, usually found in the neck of infants or children.

hygroscopic describes a substance that attracts moisture; here the "scopic" relates to the Greek *skopos*, "target," rather than to the verb *skopein*, "to observe."

hymen is a direct borrowing of the Greek *hymēn*, "a skin or membrane." The Greek word was used for all sorts of membranes, including the pericardium and peritoneum, in addition to the membranous fold occluding the external vaginal orifice. Later, Hymen became the name of the god of marriage, a sort of overgrown Cupid. It was not until the 16th century that "hymen" was restricted to denote the vaginal, or virginal, membrane. *Hymenoptera* (+ Greek *ptōron*, "wing") is an order of insects bearing two pairs of membranous wings, including bees and wasps.

hyoid is a classical way of saying "u-shaped." The "hy-" is derived from the Greek equivalent of "h" (the aspirate sound of which was written in Greek not as a letter but as a mark ['], called "a rough-breathing") followed by the Greek letter upsilon (Υ). The suffix is from the Greek *eidos*, "like." The hyoid bone is shaped like a "U."

hyoscine (*see* **scopolamine**)

hyoscyamine is an anticholinergic alkaloid originally obtained from the henbane plant, so called because its poisonous substance was the bane of domestic fowl. The hairy beans of the plant were known to the ancient Greeks as *hyskyamos*, "hog bean," either because swine ate it or its bristly surface appeared to resemble the hide of swine.

hyper- is a combining form signifying "over, above, beyond, or exceeding." It is said to have originated in the postulated Indo-European root *uper*, "over." This became the Greek *hyper*, the Latin *super* or *supra*, and the Anglo-Saxon *ofer*, predecessor of the English "over." The list of biomedical terms in which "hyper-" has been incorporated as a prefix is almost endless. In vernacular speech, "hyper" has become almost a word in itself

when used to mean an excessively animated state. The exaggerated and extravagant manner in which some patients describe their symptoms is called "hyperbole," a direct borrowing of the Greek word meaning "a throwing beyond." This word meant the same to ancient Greeks as our modern expression "to lay it on thick" or "to pile it on."

hyperalimentation (*see* **alimentary**)

hyperbaric (*see* **baro-**)

hypercapnia (*see* **acapnia**)

hyperesthesia (*see* **anesthesia**)

hypergeusia (*see* **geusia**)

hypersthenic (*see* **asthenia**)

hypesthesia (*see* **anesthesia**)

hypnosis comes from the Greek *hypnos*, "sleep," and was introduced in 1843 by James Braid (1795-1860), a Scottish surgeon, to refer to an induced, "nervous" sleep. At one time this was known as "braidism." "Hypnosis" later became the preferred term for the state induced supposedly by a mysterious force called "animal magnetism" by Anton Mesmer (1734-1815), a Swiss physician. More is told of Mesmer under **mesmerism**.

hypo- is a combining form signifying "below, under, or deficient" and is the same as the Greek *hypo*. The prefix has been attached to a host of chemical and biomedical terms. **Hypochlorite**, for example, was so named because it contains less, or is deficient in, oxygen when compared with the chlorate.

hypochondrium locates the anatomic area beneath the cartilagenous costal margins (Greek *chondros*, "cartilage"). The ancients looked upon the spleen as the seat of melancholy, and even today a "splenetic" person is thought of as irritable, peevish, or spiteful. The spleen being located in the hypochondrium, **hypochondriac** came to be applied to patients whose complaints seemed to have no organic basis. We now know that in many cases this is because of the "splenic flexure syndrome," a common expression of functional bowel disorder often seen in nervous persons.

hypogastrium (*see* **epigastrium**)

hypogeusia (*see* **geusia**)

hypophysis is a name for the endocrine appendage that is now better known as the pituitary gland, which appears to "grow below" the brain (hypo- + Greek *physis*, "growth"). (*see* **pituitary**)

hypospadius is a condition wherein the urethral orifice appears to be "drawn under" the penis (hypo- + Greek *spaein*, "to draw").

hypothesis is a supposition "placed under" (hypo- + Greek *thesis*, "a placing") an idea as its foundation (which may or may not be sound), just as "supposition" is derived from the Latin *sub*, "under," + *positus*, "a placing."

hysterectomy is derived from a combination of the Greek *hystera*, "the womb or uterus," + *ektomē*, "a cutting out." To the Greeks, *hysterikos* meant "a suffering in the womb." Professor H. A. Skinner tells us, "Plato and his followers described the uterus as an animal endowed with spontaneous sensation and motion, lodged in a woman, and ardently desiring to bear children. If it remained sterile long after puberty, it became indignant, dissatisfied, and ill-tempered and caused a general disturbance of the body until it became pregnant, when it became normal again." This is in keeping with the age-old proclivity to attribute various abnormal manifestations to specific organs of the body. Emotional instability, thought to be more characteristic of women than men, was attributed to the uterus. A safe assumption is that this notion was proclaimed and promoted, in the main, by men. From this anatomic designation comes the term **hysteria**, a term doubtless conceived by a confirmed male chauvinist.

Iatr-, -iatric, iatro- are combining forms taken from *iatros*, the Greek word for "healer," and these words are related to the verb *iasthai*, "to cure." The suffix is incorporated into the names for specialized branches of healing, such as **pediatrics**, more properly **paediatrics** (+ Greek *pais, paidos*, "child") or geriatrics (+ Greek *gerōn*, "an old man"). Of the Greek *iatros* the Roman counterpart was *medicus*, derived from the Latin verb *medeor*, again "to heal." Modern Romance languages have followed suit; witness the Spanish *medico*. The Swedish *läkare* is derived from *läka*, "to heal." The German *Artz* is said to have descended from the Greek as a contraction of *archiatros*, "the master healer." The concept that one who ministers to his fellows' illness or injury is a healer is heartening and inspiring. The pity is that in English we do not say "healer." For some reason we prefer **doctor**, which, strictly speaking, is the title of a teacher, or **physician**, one who is steeped in "physic," that is, one who knows "the nature of things."

iatrapistic is a somewhat arcane word that refers to a lack of faith in doctors (iatr- + *a-*, "lacking," + Greek *pisteuō*, "I trust in.")

iatrogenic refers to the consequence of treatment (iatro- + Greek *gennan*, "to bring forth, as a product of"). Often, "iatrogenic" is used to refer to a secondary or adverse effect rather than to the primary and favorable effect.

iatromelia indicates ineffective or negligent medical treatment (iatro- + Greek *meleos*, "fruitless or vain").

iatromisia is an intense dislike of doctors (iatro- + Greek *miseō*, "I hate").

ichthyosis comes from the Greek *ichthys*, "a fish," and refers to a rough, scaly skin resulting from overgrowth or excessive retention of the keratin layer. A "fishlike" skin can be an inherited affliction or an acquired metabolic disorder.

ictal is a near borrowing of the Latin *ictus*, the past participle of *icere*, "to strike." Hence, whatever is ictal pertains to a stroke or an epileptic seizure. **Interictal** refers to the period between such repeated events. "Ictal" from the Latin is not to be confused with **icterus** from the Greek.

icterus is a Latinized form of the Greek *ikteros*, that to the ancients meant both "jaundice" and "a yellow bird," probably the oriole, a familiar small bird with golden-yellow plumage. "Oriole," incidentally, comes from the Latin *aureum*, "golden." According to Professor Alexander Gode (*JAMA.* 1963; 184:615), the connection between the bird and the disease is explained in Pliny. The disease purportedly could be cured by having the patient gaze upon the bird. Through a mysterious transmigration, the disease was supposed to pass from the patient to the hapless bird.

idio- is a frequently applied prefix that comes from the Greek *idios*, meaning that which is "personal, private, or one's own." In the sense of being opposite of public or popular, *idios* might also mean "peculiar."

idiolalia is the use of an invented language peculiar to the prattler himself (idio- + Greek *lalein*, "to chatter or babble").

idiopathic has come to be a word sometimes used to describe a condition of which one is uncertain or ignorant of the cause, yet to which one wishes to apply a high-sounding word intended to mask the fact. In this sense, "idiopathic" (idio- + Greek *pathos*, "disease") is equivalent to "essential" or "cryptogenic." Originally, an idiopathic condition was thought of as arising in the patient himself rather than occurring as a consequence of any recognized outside cause. Later, the sense shifted slightly to that of a condition peculiar to a given individual, in contrast to that being representative of a widely recognized disease.

idiosyncrasy in common parlance is an expression of a temperament peculiar to a given individual (idio- + Greek *sy[n]gkrasis*, "a mixing together or blending"). Medically, it is an abnormal susceptibility or allergy peculiar to an individual, a drug, or a chemical agent.

idiot is derived from the Greek *idiotōs*, which originally was the word for a man engaged in private pursuits, as contrasted to a man who holds public office. From the implication that such a man was ignorant of public affairs, the term became restricted in a deprecatory sense and was applied to persons judged to be of less than normal intelligence. To the laity, an idiot is any utterly foolish or senseless person. To psychologists, an idiot is an adult whose intellect has become arrested at a mental age of less than 3 years. A mongolian idiot is a mentally retarded person with mongoloid facies, now known to be the result of a chromosomal aberration. The term was suggested by Landon Down (1828-1896), an English physician. What was once called **mongolism** is now more properly known as **Down's syndrome**.

idiotropic refers, in psychology, to a type of personality satisfied with its own inner intellectual or emotional experiences (idio- + Greek *tropos*, "a turning").

idioventricular describes an impulse, conduction, or rhythm originating within the cardiac ventricle alone (idio- + Latin *ventriculus*, "little belly [of the heart]").

-igo (*see* **lentigo**)

ileum is derived from the Greek *eileos*, "twisted." When the abdomen is opened at operation or at necropsy, all of the small intestine appears twisted. So why should only the distal portion be called "ileum"? One explanation is that insofar as the distal small intestine is more often the seat of obstruction, the ancients may have used *eileos* also as a pathologic term. This also could account for the use of "ileus" as a reference to an apparent obstruction due to paralysis of the gut. The British, classical scholars that they are, pronounce "ileum" as "eye-leum."

ilium is the Medieval Latin term for the hip bone, and it is so used today. But to the Romans, the *ilia* (the neuter plural noun) referred generally to the belly, groin, and guts. Possibly the later connection was that the hip bones were looked upon as delimiting and protecting the flanks of the belly. "Ilium," of course, is not to be confused in spelling or meaning with **ileum**.

imbecile comes from the Latin *imbecillus*, "weak or feeble." It has been suggested that this might have been derived from a combination of the Latin *in-*, used in the sense of "on," + *baculum*, "a rod or staff," thus referring to one who was obliged to lean on a crutch. Before long the meaning was transferred from weakness in body to weakness in mind. The ranking of imbecile in the Binet-Simon scale of mental retardation is cited in the entry **moron**.

immunity is an almost direct borrowing of the Latin *immunitas*, which to the Romans meant "an exemption from taxes or from public or military service." The Latin word comes from a combination of *in*, "not," + *munus*, "tribute or service." The legal sense, both lay and judicial, became the principal meaning of the word in English, too. In the late 19th century, when knowledge of toxins and infection evolved, the meaning was extended in reference to persons "exempt from" or protected against the onslaught of foreign substances, thus were said to be "immune."

impetigo comes from the Latin *impetus*, "a vehement attack or assault," which also is the origin of "impetuous." Originally, "impetigo" was given as a name for a variety of inflammatory skin afflictions. Currently, the term usually refers to an infectious, pustular dermatitis. (*see* **petechia**)

inanition comes from the Latin verb *inanire*, "to empty," which is akin to the Latin *inanis*, "empty." "Inanition" is used especially with reference to that which has been rendered void or hollow by depletion. In medicine, "inanition" describes the condition of a patient who has been depleted by lack of nourishment. From the Latin *inanis* also comes "inane," meaning whatever is empty, void, or worthless.

incarcerated describes a hernia wherein the protruding tissues are stuck or held fast and hence cannot be restored to their normal location. To the Romans, *incarceratus* meant "imprisoned," the word being a combination of the Latin in-, "in," + carcer, "a prison."

incidence relates to the Latin verb incidere, "to happen, occur, or befall," this being derived from a combination of the Latin in-, "in or on," + cadere, "to fall." In citing statistics, many medical authors tend to use "incidence" and "frequency" interchangeably. This is not quite proper. Incidence expresses the rate at which a certain event occurs within a given period of time, particularly as that rate may rise or fall; it is the time frame that is important. Frequency, in the medical sense, expresses the number of occurrences of whatever is being described in a given population.

incise comes from the Latin incidere, "to carve or cut into." An **incisura** is "a notch or cleft," as if the result of cutting into, and an **incisor** tooth is one capable of cutting into anything that is bitten, as compared to a molar or grinding tooth.

incontinent meant "immediately" in Shakespearean English, as it does in modern French. Desdemona remarks that Othello will "return incontinent." She does not mean that Othello will come back with a loss of bladder or bowel control, which would be the sense of "incontinent" in medical usage. It happens the medical usage conforms to the word's origin in the Latin in-, "not," + continens, "restrained."

incubate is taken from the Latin incubare, "to lie in or on; to brood," this being a combination of in-, "in," + cubare, "to lie down or to recline." An incubator is usually warm, but it is the idea of "lying in" rather than heating that is essential. The incubation period of any infectious disease is the time during which the causative organism "lies in" before the disease is "hatched." A related term is **incubus**, a demon descending to lie in with and oppress a sleeper, as in a nightmare. The meaning of "incubus" has been extended to designate any nightmarish mental burden.

incus is the name of one of three little bones in the middle ear. The name is the Latin word for an anvil, related to the verb incudere, "to strike upon." Thus, to transmit sound in the ear, the **malleus** (Latin for "hammer"), a tiny bone attached to the eardrum, strikes the incus, which conveys the impulse to the **cochlea** by way of the third little stirrup-shaped bone, hence its name **stapes**, the Latin word for "stirrup."

index is the Latin word for "a sign or mark of something." It is related to the verb indicare, "to point out or disclose." Thus, the index of a book is supposed to be a guide to its contents, and the index finger is used to point out whatever merits attention.

indolent has changed its meaning in common usage but retains its original sense when used as a medical adjective. The Latin indolentia means "freedom from pain," being a combination of in-, "not," + dolens, "painful or distressing." The Latin dolor is preserved intact in the Spanish word for pain. Hence, an indolent ulcer is a painless ulcer. Although most such ulcers also are long standing, the true meaning of the term emphasizes a lack of pain, not chronicity. In common usage, "indolent" has come to mean "lazy or slothful." Presumably, a person so disposed feels little or no pain.

induration comes from the Latin indurare, "to harden," and refers to tissues that have become stiff and firm as a consequence of inflammation, hyperplasia, or neoplasia.

inexorable sometimes is used to describe the unalterable progress of a disease. The word is an almost direct borrowing of the Latin inexorabilis, which, to the Romans, meant "not to be removed by prayers." This, in turn, is a combination of in-, "not," + ex, "out of," + orare, "to pray or beg." Whatever is inexorable, be it disease or taxation, is beyond getting out of by prayer.

infant comes from the Latin infans, "speechless," which is derived from in-, "not," + fari, "to speak." Because an ability to speak usually becomes evident at the age of 2 years, all those younger are generally considered to be infants. By an odd twist, some adults betray their infantile attitudes only when they open their mouths to speak. Incidentally, bambino, the Italian word for "baby," is related to the Greek bambainō, "I stammer."

infarct is derived from the Latin infarcire, "to plug up or cram." The original use of the term in ancient pathology referred to consolidation or cramming of "humors" in the affected part. We now recognize an infarct as a necrotic lesion that results from acute deprivation of circulating blood. The swelling is due to transudation of fluid and inflammatory infiltration. The process of infarction is in the affected tissue. The emphasis was originally, and should be now, on the reaction and not its cause. To refer to a myocardial infarct is to designate the pathologic changes occurring in the heart muscle; the cause of these changes is another matter. Linguistically, "infarct" is not quite correct. The past participle of *infarcire* should be *infart*, but perhaps some prudish person insisted on inserting an extraneous "c" to avoid the sound of a socially unacceptable word. The Italian *infarto* and the Spanish *infartacion* are classically more correct, but then they do not contend with the Anglo-Saxon "fart."

infection comes from the Latin *inficere*, "to dye or stain" but also "to corrupt or spoil." The ancients conceived that disease could result from the entrance of invisible agents in the body, hence a sort of "tainting." But it was not until the latter part of the 19th century that the germ theory of disease gained currency and the true nature of infection was appreciated.

inferior is a comparative form of the Latin *inferus*, "low or beneath." In anatomy, the meaning is confined to a spatial relation, as in the statement that the liver is inferior to the heart. This implies no value judgment in comparing the merit of the liver with that of the heart.

infestation means the invasion of the body by arthropods, such as insects, mites, and ticks. The word comes from the Latin *infestare*, "to annoy," as is the wont of bugs. Invasion of the body by parasites is often referred to as infestation. This is not quite correct. Invasion by amebas or any other animalcules that do not have jointed legs is an **infection**, not an infestation.

infiltrate is taken from the French *infiltrer*, "to soak in," as through the pores or interstices of a filter. In pathology, an infiltrate is a substance, composed of either fluid or formed cellular elements, that has percolated into a tissue, usually in response to an injurious stimulus.

infirmary comes from the Latin adjective *infirmus*, "weak, feeble, or sick," in the sense of "not firm," and hence an infirmary is a place

where persons so afflicted are cared for. In former times, the term designated places of treatment for the destitute poor, in contrast to private hospitals for the more well-to-do.

inflammation is derived from the Latin *inflammare*, "to set on fire, to kindle." It was Celsus, in the 1st century A.D., who set down in his celebrated *De Medicina* the four cardinal features of inflammation: *rubor* (redness), *tumor* (swelling), *calor* (heat), and *dolor* (pain). These features suggested those of a smoldering fire.

influenza is an Italian word meaning, "influence," but it includes the further sense of "a visitation," as by an epidemic disease. It was in this way that "influenza" came to be used in the 14th century. Possibly the thought was that episodic and devastating illness was due to the influence of an ominous configuration of the planets and stars. Only in recent times, when infectious diseases have been more properly sorted out, has "influenza" been restricted to a viral disease of notorious contagion. Curiously, through the years, epidemics occurring in one place have been blamed on some other place. In Russia influenza was called "the Chinese disease"; in Germany, "the Russian pestilence"; in Italy, "the German disease"; and so on. Even today in the United States we claim to suffer from "the Hong Kong flu." What the people in Hong Kong suffer from is not recorded. Perhaps it is the "Malay malaise."

infra is the Latin preposition meaning "below or beneath" and, by extension, "less than." **Infrared** rays or waves that generate heat are so called because their wavelength falls below that of the red end of the visible spectrum (*see* **ultraviolet**). An infradiaphragmatic abscess is situated below the diaphragm.

infundibulum is the Latin word for "funnel" and comes from the verb *infundere*, "to pour into." "Infundibulum" has long been used to describe any funnel-shaped structure or passage. The infundibulum of the Fallopian tube refers to its funnel-shaped distal end.

infusion is derived from the Latin *infundere*, "to pour into." The term currently is used for the administration of fluids through a catheter, as in a vein, usually by means of gravity. There is an older meaning of "infusion" that accounts for the name Infusoria as the class of protozoa characterized by the presence of cilia. The older meaning was "to soak or steep" in water for the purpose of extracting some constituent, as in the steeping of tea from a bag of crushed tea leaves. Anton van Leeuwenhoek (1632-1723), the Dutch pioneer microscopist, observed tiny organisms in stagnant water and applied the term **infusoria** to these organisms.

inguinal is taken from the Latin *inguen*, "the groin," and hence the adjective applies to ligaments, lymph nodes, or hernias situated in the groin. To the Romans the plural *inguinis* meant "the private parts."

inject comes from the Latin *injicere*, "to throw into," being a combination of *in-* + *jactare*, "to toss, throw, or hurl." In the scientific sense "to inject" means to put something in under pressure, as compared to the gentler "infuse" or "instill." To **ejaculate** means "to hurl out."

innominate is a near borrowing of the Latin *innominatus*, literally "without a name." The innominate artery, a major branch of the aorta that serves the right side of the head and the right arm, was described by Galen, but he gave it no name. Later, Vesalius simply called it the "unnamed artery." It is now more properly known as the brachiocephalic trunk. The pelvis is made up of three bones: the ilium, the ischium, and the pubis. Each of these components was named, but the whole structure was not, so Galen referred to it as the innominate or "unnamed" bone. Actually, Celsus did call it the *os coxae*, "the bone of the hips."

inoculate comes from the Latin *inoculare*, "to ingraft," being derived from *in-* + *oculus*, "the eye." That seems a strange connection until one recalls how the ancients accomplished grafting. An emerging sprout or bud, which resembled an eye, was taken from one plant and inserted in a niche cut into another plant. Thus, the process was "putting in the eye." When the idea evolved of inducing immunity by grafting vaccine onto or into a person's body, the procedure was called **inoculation**. Even closer to the ancient meaning is the inoculation of a culture medium for the purpose of inducing the growth of whatever is inoculated.

inquest in forensic medicine is a preliminary inquiry as to the cause and circumstance of an unexpected death. The term comes from the Latin *inquisitio*, "a questioning into or investigation."

insanity is a near borrowing of the Latin *insania*, "madness or mania" beyond the bounds of normal mental composure. The term combines *in-*, "not," + *sanus*, "sound or rational." "Insanity" is a legal term. It has never been given the status of a medical diagnosis.

insemination is contrived by combining *in-* + the Latin *semen*, "seed," and refers to the deposition of the male sperm into the reproductive tract of the female, usually by what comes naturally but sometimes, if needed, by artificial means. **Sperm** is derived from the Greek *sperma*, "seed."

insidious as a feature of a disease means one that lurks inconspicuously, being deceptively quiescent. The word is borrowed from the Latin *insidiae*, "deceitful" in the sense of "ambush." *Incidiae* relates to a combination of *in-* + *sedere*, "to sit." So, an insidious disease is one that is "sitting in," waiting to wreak havoc. "Ambush," incidentally, comes through the Old French from the Late Latin *imboscare*, "in the woods or among the bushes."

insipidus (*see* **diabetes**)

in situ is a Latin term combining *in-* + the ablative of *situs*, "position or place." The anatomic reference is to something "in place" and not wandering around.

insomnia (*see* **somnus**)

inspissate is a near borrowing of the Latin *inspissatus*, being a combination of *in-* (here used as an intensive) + *spissatus*, "condensed, concentrated, or thickened." A liquid becomes inspissated by the loss of water or other fluid by evaporation or by selective absorption. Dehydrated and hardened fecal fragments lying in the bowel are said to be inspissated.

instill (*see* **distill**)

insufflation comes from the Latin *insufflare*, "to blow into or inflate." The word provides still another example of polysyllabic inflation encountered in the language known as "medicalese." A doctor would insufflate a balloon, whereas an ordinary mortal would simply blow up a balloon.

insula is Latin for "island." A triangular area of the cerebral cortex forming the floor of the lateral cerebral fossa was described by the German anatomist Johann Christian Reil (1759-1813) and is known as the insula of Reil.

insulin is the hormone essential to glucose metabolism, so named because it was found as a product of the pancreatic **islets of Langerhans**, described in 1869 by Paul Langerhans (1847-1888), a German pathologist and histologist, in his inaugural thesis. It was not until 1893 that these islets were associated with internal secretion.

integument is an almost direct borrowing of the Latin *integumentum*, "a covering," this being derived in turn from the verb *tegere*, "to cover" (*see* **tectum**; *also* **tegmen**). The skin is our integument. *Tegere* originated in the Indo-European *teg*, "to hide or cover," which through the Dutch gives us "deck" and through the Hindi "thug," a furtive criminal whose identity might be uncovered by a "detective."

inter is the Latin preposition meaning "between or among" and serves as a combining prefix to a host of medical terms, such as **intercostal**, between the ribs, and **interosseous**, between the bones.

intercalated means "inserted between" and is derived from the Latin *intercalaris*, a combination of *inter-* + *calare*, "to proclaim." Originally, the Latin term referred to an extra day that was inserted in the calendar by proclamation. ("Calendar" comes from the Latin *calends*, the first day of the Roman month and the day on which proclamations customarily were made.) **Intercalated discs** are the stripes extending across fibers of heart muscle, and **intercalated neurons** are those situated between primary afferent and efferent nerve cells.

interdigitate refers to a configuration such as that produced by the fingers of two hands when brought in alternate apposition to each other (*inter-* + Latin *digitus*, "finger").

interferon designates a class of cellular glycoproteins endogenously produced in response to viral infection, which then act to inhibit replication in a broad spectrum of viral agents. The substance was named by Jean Lindenmann, a Swiss microbiologist, working in the laboratory of Alick Isaacs at the National Institute for Medical Research, Mill Hill, London. The name, which appeared in a seminal 1957 publication (*Proc Royal Soc London.* 1957;147(B):258), was obviously modeled on the English verb "to interfere." This, in turn, comes through the Old French *entreferer*, "to meddle," from the Latin *interficere*, "to destroy." The Latin word combines *inter-*, "between," + *ficere*, "to strike."

interictal (*see* **ictal**)

intermediate means literally "in the middle" (*inter-* + Latin *medius*, "middle").

intermittent refers to a sequence wherein a pause, whether long or short, is inserted between repeated occurrences. The Latin *intermittere* means "to send between." (*see* **periodic**)

intern is now an obsolete term because the internship, by that name, no longer exists; the first year of postgraduate training for new MDs is now known as "PGY-1" (postgraduate year 1). In years gone by the word was spelled interne, befitting its French origin, and literally referred to one who was confined within a certain geographic limit. To put it another way, the neophyte physician was stuck in the hospital. The custom, while restrictive, was instructive.

internal medicine is a term of somewhat disputed origin. It refers to the practice of those specially trained physicians who deal with the diagnosis and nonsurgical treatment of diseases affecting the internal organs. One explanation is that its use arose in 19th century Germany as *innere Medizin* to distinguish internists from the large number of doctors whose specialty was dermatology and the external manifestations of various diseases, especially those of venereal origin.

internuncial describes certain neurons that serve to connect other neurons, thereby conveying an impulse (*inter-* + Latin *nuntius*, "messenger").

interstitial means whatever is placed between (*inter-* + Latin *sistere*, "to put or to place"). An example is interstitial fibrosis.

intertrigo is the result of chafing that occurs between opposing skin folds that rub on each other (*inter-* + Latin *terere*, "to rub"), such as under a pendulous breast.

intestine is a near borrowing of the Latin *intestinus*, which as the adjective generally means "internal" and as the plural noun "the guts." The latter usage is analogous to **innards** as a colloquial term for the **viscera**.

intima is the Latin word for "innermost." In anatomy, the term refers to the innermost lining of blood vessels, composed of a cylindrical sheet of endothelial cells surrounded by elastic and collagen fibers.

intoxication is derived from the Latin *intoxicare*, "to smear with poison." The Latin *toxicum*, "poison," is related to the Greek *toxon*, "a bow" as used by an archer. The connection between the Greek and Latin words is that the arrow shot from a bow might be tipped with poison. This is unfair to the Greeks, whose principal weapon was the spear, whereas bows and arrows were favored by the Persians. Be that as it may, intoxication was, and still is, viewed as a form of poisoning, most commonly by alcohol.

intra is the Latin preposition meaning "within or inside" and serves as a combining prefix for numerous medical terms. For example, **intramural** refers in anatomy to whatever may be contained within the walls of an organ, such as the intestine or heart (intra- + Latin *murus*, "wall"). In common parlance, the reference to wall is in the plural sense. Intramural sports are those enjoyed within the walls of a given institution.

intractable means difficult to manage or govern; in medicine an intractable symptom or disease is one that is difficult to alleviate or remedy. The word is descended from the Latin *intractabilis*, "unmanageable or formidable," this being a combination of *in-*, as a negative, + *tractare*, "to handle or to deal with." "Intractable" is sometimes used interchangeably with **refractory** or even **recalcitrant**, although their meanings while similar in reference are not exactly the same. A **refractory** period or disease is one that has reverted to a state of unresponsiveness; a **recalcitrant** patient is one who blatantly or surreptitiously disobeys instruction.

intrinsic is a near borrowing of the Latin *intrinsecus*, "on the inside," being derived from a combination of *intra-* + *sequi*, "to follow or accompany." Thus, the reference is to whatever "goes on inside." **Extrinsic**, from the Latin *extrinsecus*, by the opposite token, is whatever goes on outside.

introvert is derived from a combination of the Latin *intro-*, "inward," + *vertere*, "to turn." In psychiatry an introvert is a self-centered person who is more interested in his own emotions than in other people or external events. (*see* **extrovert**)

intussusception was made up by combining the Latin *intus-*, "within," + *suscipere*, "to pick up, to take up, or to receive." John Hunter (1728-1793), the renowned English anatomist and surgeon, gave the name to a condition wherein a proximal segment of intestine is telescoped or "taken up" into a succeeding segment, thus causing an obstruction.

investigation (*see* **vestige**)

in vitro (*see* **vital**)

in vivo (*see* **vital**)

involution comes from the Latin *involvere*, "to roll up or to wrap up," particularly in the sense of concluding something. The Latin *volvere*, among its various meanings, could refer to the rolling along of a river. Thus, *involvere* could refer to a river not rolling along or to one drying up. It is in this sense that "involution" is used in pathology as a word for the process whereby an organ withers in old age. An example is the involuted ovary of the postmenopausal woman.

iodine is derived from the Greek *ioeides*, "violet-colored, as the sea." The element was first discovered in 1812 by a French chemist, Bernard Courtois, who observed that the ash of kelp imparted an unusual violet color when held in a flame. Another Frenchman, Joseph Louis Gay-Lussac, proposed the name "iode" which his English contemporary Sir Humphry Davy changed to "iodine" to be more analogous to the other halogens, chlorine and fluorine. It was not until the late 19th century that the antiseptic properties of iodine were appreciated.

ion was so named from the Greek *iōn*, the present participle of *ienai*, "to go." Michael Faraday (1791-1867), the celebrated English physicist, named the particle set free by electrolysis "to go" to either the positive or negative pole of an electrically charged system (though some say it was Faraday's contemporary William Whewell who originated the neologism). Faraday proposed the term **anion** (Greek *ana*, "up") for the negatively charged particle that is attracted to or "goes up" to the positively charged **anode** (Greek *odos*, "track or course"); bicarbonate (HCO_3^-), chloride (Cl^-), and sulfate (SO_4^-) are examples of biologically important anions. Incidentally, the Greeks had the word *anodos*, meaning "the upward way," and they used it to refer to the path of the rising sun. The name **cation** (Greek *kata*, "down") was given to the positively charged particle that is attracted to or "goes down" to the negatively charged **cathode** (Greek *kata* + *odos*); hydrogen (H^+), potassium (K^+), and sodium (Na^+) are examples of biologically important cations.

ipecac is a shortened form of a native Brazilian word *ipecacuanha*. In the Guanari language this is said to be a combination of *pe*, "flat," + *kaa*, "an herb," + *quana*, "to vomit," hence "a small creeping plant that makes one throw up." The ending *-nha* indicates the passage of the word through the Portuguese. In the 17th century, ipecac was touted as a remedy for dysentery.

iris is a direct borrowing of the Greek word for "rainbow" and is derived from *eirō*, "I announce." To the ancient Greeks, a rainbow was a sign from the gods and was personified as Iris, their messenger. Much later, the name was given to a genus of flowers. Because of the association with different colors, Jacob Benignus Winslow (1669-1760), a Dane who served as a professor of anatomy in Paris, applied the same name to the varicolored circular membrane that surrounds the aperture of the eye.

ischemia is derived from the Greek *ischanein*, "to hold in check" (a related verb *ischainō* means "I make dry"), + *aima*, "blood." The Greek *ischaimos* means "quenching the flow of blood," as a styptic substance would do. Rudolf Virchow (1821-1902), the famed German pathologist, used the term in reference to focal deprivation of blood.

ischium is from the Greek *ischion*, a word that appears in Homer and means "the socket in which the thigh bone turns." Ancient Greek

anatomists extended the meaning to include the bone in which the socket sits (and on which we sit). The Greek source of the term (and **ischio-**, its combining form) dictates its pronunciation as "isk-," not "ish."

islets of Langerhans (*see* **insulin**)

iso- is a combining form derived from the Greek *isos*, "equal to, the same as, or like."

isomer designates one of two distinct compounds having the same atomic composition (iso- + Greek *meros*, "part or share") but different molecular configuration and exhibiting different properties.

isotonic describes solutions of equal osmotic pressure (iso- + Greek *tonos*, "tension"), the standard of reference in physiology usually being serum.

isotope is the term used for one of two or more forms of an element, all occupying the same place in the atomic table (iso- + Greek *topos*, "place").

isthmus is a near borrowing of the Greek *isthmos*, "a neck or narrow passage, particularly as a neck of lands between the seas." The term has been applied in anatomy to various necklike structures. The **thyroid isthmus** is that narrow, midline segment of the gland that connects the larger lateral lobes.

itch (*see* **pruritus**)

-itis is a Greek suffix that converts a noun into an adjective. When used as such, the Greek *nosos*, "disease," is understood as following the adjective but is not stated. In other words, by adding "-itis" to the name of any anatomic structure, it is understood that reference is being made to a disease affecting that structure. For example, *nephro-*, "kidney," + "-itis" means a condition affecting the kidney; if completely spelled out, this would have to be *nephritis nosos*, "disease of the kidney." Thus, "-itis" saves a lot of effort and space. Originally, "-itis" meant any sort of disease, but later it became restricted to denoting inflammation in the structure to whose name it was added.

Jade is a highly esteemed ornamental stone, so called because it once was thought to be a remedy for colic or flank pain. The ancient Spaniards called it *piedra de ijada*, "stone of the side." The French shortened this to *jade*. The adjective jaded, as in "jaded appetite," comes from a quite different source. In Old Norse *jalda* meant "a mare." In English, "jade" became a contemptuous term for a horse, particularly one of inferior breed or one that was old and decrepit. Hence, a jaded appetite is one that is weakened by fatigue, perhaps by overwork.

jaundice is considered to be ultimately derived from the Latin *galbinus*, an adjective describing a light greenish-yellow. In French this became *jaune* and in German *gelb*. In its trip across the channel, the Old French *jaunisse*, "yellowness," became the English "jaundice." (Dr. John H. Dirckx explains that "the 'd' is a phonetic parasite like the one that often creeps into the middle of 'drowning.' ") Nonmedical persons use the word in an interesting way when they refer to regarding something with "a jaundiced eye." In this sense the allusion is to an attitude of distaste or satiety tinged by prejudice. This use is understood by the clinician who knows that a person ill with a disease characterized by jaundice typically has lost his appetite, is often disturbed by nausea, and is generally torpid. At one time jaundice was known as *morbus regius*, "the regal disease," from the belief that only a king's touch could cure it.

jaw originated in the Anglo-Saxon *ceowan*, "to chew," which led to *chawe* or *jawe* (the conversion of "ch" to "j" being not unusual). Chaucer spelled the word "jowe," and this suggests the current "jowl." The old form is preserved in the colloquial "chaw," as in "a chaw of tobacco."

jecorize (*see* **hepatic**)

jecur is the Latin name for the organ we call "the liver." The Romans used *jecur* especially for their concept of the liver as the seat of emotions, such as anger and lust. The Latin *jecur* is mentioned here because of a curious incident, the curious incident being that neither "jecur" nor any derivative has found a place in the current medical lexicon (with the possible exception of "to jecorize," an obscure term meaning to impart to a food the therapeutic quality of cod liver oil). One is reminded of the repartee in Sir Arthur Conan Doyle's tale of *Silver Blaze*:

> Inspector: "Is there any other point to which you wish to draw to my attention?"
> Sherlock Holmes: "To the curious incident of the dog in the night-time."
> Inspector: "The dog did nothing in the night-time."
> Holmes: "That was the curious incident."

jejunum is a near borrowing of the Latin adjective *jejunus*, "fasting or hungry," in the sense of being empty and devoid of food. The ancient Greeks, impressed by their observation at necropsy that the lumen of the proximal small intestine was always empty, used the descriptive term *nēstis*, "fasting," and this was translated into Latin as *jejunus*. In his treatise on the function of different parts of the body, Galen says that this part of the intestine is always found to be empty. In lay language, a jejune argument is empty, devoid of substance.

joint comes through the Old French *joinct* from the Latin *junctura*, "a joining or connection." Anatomically, a joint is a juncture between two articulating bones.

journal comes from the Old French word meaning "daily." This, in turn, was taken from the Latin *diurnus*, "of the day," the adjectival derivative of *dies*, "day." Obviously, our word **diurnal** is closer to the origin. Before A.D. 1500, "journal" was used itself as an adjective, as in "journal account." Then the modified noun was dropped, and the account that was kept daily was called simply "a journal." Strictly speaking, every medical "journal" should be a daily publication.

jugular comes from the Latin *jugulum*, "the throat," which is related to *jugum*, "a yoke or collar." Thus, the jugular vein is "the vein of the neck." Galen referred to this structure as *phleps sphagitis*, "the sacrificial vein," an ominous allusion.

jupe is an old dialect word for tuberculosis. "Jupe" was once commonly used among poor black Americans as a name for the dread "consumption." Its origin is not known, but a source in an African tribal language would be a good guess.

juxta- is a prefix taken from the Latin preposition meaning "nearby." Thus, **juxtapyloric** refers to the vicinity of the junction between the stomach and the duodenum, and **juxtaglomerular** means adjacent to the renal glomerulus.

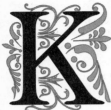**K**ala-azar is the Hindi name for "black fever," so called by the people of the Assam province in northeast India where the disease is endemic. The common name was given because of the dusky hue of the skin assumed by victims in the later phase of the disease. The cause is infection by a protozoon now called *Leishmania donovani*, and the visceral form of the disease is known as **leishmaniasis** (the "ei" is pronounced "ee"). It was Sir William Leishman (1865-1926), of Her Britannic Majesty's Indian Medical Service, who first discovered the parasite in a spleen at necropsy in 1900, a finding later confirmed by his colleague, Dr. Charles Donovan (1863-1951), an Irish physician in the Indian Sanitary Service.

kallikrein was the name given by H. Kraut, E. K. Frey, and E. Werle (*Hoppe Seyler's Z physiol Chem.* 1930;189:97) to a hypotensive substance of which they found the pancreas to be a major source. The name is contrived from a Greek word for the pancreas. It is possible that the Greeks may have referred to the pancreas (which they usually called *pa[n]gkreas*) as *kallikreas*, this being a combination of *kalli*, "beautiful, delectable," + *kreas*, "a piece of meat."

kaolin is taken from a French version of the Mandarin Chinese *kao-ling*, "high hill," which describes the place where the claylike silicate of aluminum was first found in an area of Jiangxi province. Originally, it was used by the Chinese in the manufacture of porcelain, then exported to Europe for the same purpose. Later, a pulverized form was used in pharmacy as a coating for pills and then emulsified as a medicine itself in the treatment of diarrhea because of its adsorptive properties.

karyo- is a combining form taken from the Greek *karyon*, "a nut," and used in reference to the nucleus of a cell. A **karyocyte** is a nucleated cell.

karyolysis is a degenerative process wherein the nucleus of a cell swells, then loses its chromatin (karyo- + Greek *lysis*, "a dissolution").

keloid is usually attributed to the Greek *kēlē*, "a rupture, as a hernia," though it could also come from the Greek *kēlis*, "a blemish." Professor H. A. Skinner has suggested yet another origin: the Greek *chēlē*, "a hoof, claw, or talon." Any or all of these could describe the tough, tumorlike scar that occurs after the healing of skin wounds in certain susceptible persons. Such a scar was called "keloid" by Jean Louis Albert (1768-1837), a French dermatologist, in 1835.

keratin is the name for the protein constituent of skin, hair, nails, and horny excrescences. It is attributed to the Indo-European *ker*, "horn," which led to the Greek *keras*. The rhinoceros gets his name from his nose horn.

keratosis is an abnormal horny excrescence of the skin or squamous mucosa.

kernicterus is a potentially dangerous form of jaundice observed in hemolytic disease of newborns. Babies are unable to conjugate the burden of bilirubin catabolized from heme that is released by dissolution of red blood cells; the unconjugated bilirubin then spills over the blood-brain barrier and lodges destructively in various vital centers of the brain, including bulbar, cerebellar, and cerebral nuclei. The term is a hybrid of the German *Kern*, "kernel," or, in anatomy, "nuclei," + the Greek *ikteros*, "jaundice."

keto- is a prefix denoting the presence of a carbonyl group (:C:O) in an organic compound. (*see* **ketones**)

ketones are organic compounds containing a carbonyl group (*see* **keto-**). The prototype was **acetone** (dimethyl ketone), named from the Latin *acetum*, "vinegar," + the Greek *-ōne*, "a female descendent," in the sense of a weaker derivative. One might conclude that acetone was first thought to be a "weak sister" of acetic acid. The German word for acetone is *aketon,* and the generic term "ketone" emerged by simply dropping the initial "a" and adding a terminal "e."

kidney as a name for the paired, retroperitoneal organs of urinary excretion is hard to track down. In Middle English, says the Reverend Skeat, the spelling was variously *kidneer, kidnere,* or *kidenei.* The second syllable of the first two forms would seem to be related to a common Indo-European root from which the Greek *nephros,* the Old Icelandic *nyra,* and the German *Niere* are derived; all mean "kidney." *Kidenei* has been postulated as a combination of the Anglo-Saxon *cyd,* "pod or husk," + *[n]ei,* "egg." Apparently, there was confusion in ancient times as to whether the testis or the kidney was the source of sperm. The Romans gave up and called the kidneys *renes,* from which we take our adjective **renal.** The Latin *rigare* means "to convey water." "Kidney" also has been used as a figure of speech to refer to a sort of temperament or nature. This is in keeping with the old proclivity to ascribe temperamental characteristics to certain organs of the body. Two fellows who take much the same view of things might be described as "men of the same kidney." The ancient Hebrews believed the kidneys were the seat of affections or passions. Solomon proclaimed, "Yea, my reins [kidneys] shall rejoice when thy lips speak right things" (Proverbs 23:16).

kilo- is the prefix denoting 1000 or 10^3 of anything. It comes from the Greek *khilioi,* "a thousand." (*see* **numbers**)

kindred in both lay language and in genetics means "a family relationship." "Kin" can be traced to the Old English *cynn,* "one's own people or race," and is analogous to the Greek *genos* and the Latin *genus.* The sense is that of persons or things related by a common origin or stock. Similarly derived is our word "kind," with the meanings both "of similar type" and "of acting in a nice way." Thus, to be kindly is to treat one as a member of the family. Would that all members of a kindred always treat each other kindly!

kine-, kinesio- are prefixes denoting movement and come from the Greek *kinēsis,* "motion." Another derivative is "cinema," a highfalutin name for the movies.

kinesthesia is the sense by which movement of a part is perceived (kine- + Greek *aisthesis,* "feeling").

king's evil was a medieval term for scrofula or cervical lymphadenopathy, which probably in most cases was tuberculous adenitis. The original Late Latin term was *morbus regius* (also applied to **jaundice**), the reference being not to a king afflicted but rather to the belief that a "laying on" of the royal hand was a sure cure. England's Edward the Confessor in the 11th century was a foremost practitioner of the royal touch, and Charles II is said to have "laid hands" on 100,000 of his subjects, doubtless in a effort to bolster his shaky reign (1660-1685). The ancient practice of "laying on of hands" persists today. One of my wise professors of medicine advised, "Always put your hand where the patient says it hurts."

kinins are endogenous peptides having an effect on the movement of smooth muscle. The term is derived from the Greek *kinēsis,* "motion." **Bradykinins** (Greek *brady,* "slow") cause slow movement or contraction of gut muscle.

knee originated in the Indo-European *gneu* or *genu,* the latter being taken directly into Latin and into Greek as *gonu.* In Anglo-Saxon this became *cneow,* from which "knee" eventually emerged. The names of geometric figures are derived from the Greek *gonu.* A pentagon has five angles or "knees."

knock-kneed (*see* **valgus**)

knuckle began as the Anglo-Saxon *cnucl* and is related to the Dutch *knokkel,* the diminutive of *knok,* "bone," hence a little bone.

koilo- is a combining form taken from the Greek *koilos,* "hollow or concave."

koilocyte is a hollow or empty cell, devoid of its normal cytoplasmic content (koilo- + Greek *kytos,* "cell or container").

koilonychia is a condition wherein the fingernails (and, in some cases, the toenails) assume a concave shape and are sometimes called "spoon nails." The term combines koilo- + Greek *onyx,* "nail."

kuru is a word of the Fore people of the eastern highlands of Papua, New Guinea, to denote tremor. It has been taken to name an exotic neuropathy that has excited biomedical interest far beyond its endemic location in

Melanesia. Kuru has been found to be due to a "slow virus," i.e., a virus that wreaks its havoc long after its initial infection. The disease in the primitive culture affected was transmitted by the eating of infected brain tissue. Fortunately, since cannibalism has declined in that area, so has the incidence of kuru. (*see* **scrapie**)

kwashiorkor in the language of Ghana means "displaced or strange child"; it can also mean "red boy." It has been taken to name a syndrome of severe nutritional protein deficiency characterized by changes in pigmentation of skin and hair, together with a potbelly due to **ascites**. When there is an associated calorie deficiency, the syndrome includes a marked wasting of muscle and subcutaneous fat, a condition known as "marasmic kwashiorkor."

kymograph was given in 1847 by Karl Friedrich Wilhelm Ludwig (1816-1895), an eminent German physiologist, as the name for an instrument on which moving or "wavy" lines could be recorded on a revolving drum. The name was contrived from the Greek *kyma*, "a wave," + *graphein*, "to write." In the early kymograph, a smoked paper was stretched around a rotating cylinder and etched with a fine needle.

kyphosis comes from the Greek *kyphos*, "bent or bowed," and usually refers to a bowing of the dorsal spine. It is a sign of osteopenia or bony depletion in the thoracic vertebrae, commonly seen in postmenopausal women and sometimes referred to as a "dowager's hump."

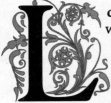**abium** is the Latin word for "lip." It is a neuter noun, so the plural (for a pair of lips) is labia. But here is where usage can be confusing. There is also a Latin feminine noun for "lip": singular *labia*, plural *labiae*. In anatomy the neuter noun is used, so that the two sets of opposing lips of the vulva (even though this is strictly a female organ) are properly called the **labia majora** (the larger, external lips) and the **labia minora** (the smaller, internal lips). A related Greek verb is *laphyssein*, "to swallow greedily, to devour." It would seem that these words, all pertaining to lips, originated in imitation of the sound produced by lapping fluid into the mouth.

labor is another word for parturition, the process of giving birth to a baby, and comes closer in meaning to the Latin noun *labor*, "a troublesome effort or suffering," than the common use of the word today as almost a synonym for ordinary work. The ancient meaning was implied in Jesus' entreaty, "Come unto me, all ye that labor and are heavy laden, and I will give you rest" (Matthew 11:28).

laboratory sounds as though it was conceived as a name for any place where work was done. But this is not the sense in which the word was used in ancient times or as it is used now. A place where people work at plucking chickens or at hammering out horseshoes is not a laboratory. The word comes from the Latin *elaborare*, "to work out, as a problem, and with great pains." An Old English spelling was *elaboratory* and designated a place where learned effort was applied to the solution of scientific problems. We have simply dropped the "e."

labyrinth is a near borrowing of the Greek *labyrinthos*, "a large structure with intricate passages intersecting each other." In Greek mythology the Athenians were at one time sorely oppressed by Minos, the king of Crete, who exacted from them an annual tribute of seven young men and seven young maidens. These unfortunate youngsters were condemned by Minos to be devoured by the voracious Minotaur, a monster with a human body and a bull's head. That the Minotaur was fed but once a year accounts for his appetite. The victims were placed in a labyrinth where the monster roamed, and from which there was no escape. A stop was put to this egregious practice by Theseus, the heroic son of the king of Athens. His device was a *clew* or **clue**, in its original meaning "a ball of string or yarn," which was kindly furnished by Ariadne, King Minos' daughter. By stringing the thread along his path, Theseus could readily find his way in and out of the labyrinth. This explains our use of clue for whatever leads to the solution of a problem. In anatomy "labyrinth" designates the lateral mass of the ethmoid bone and also the internal ear, both of which contain intricate passages.

laceration is a near borrowing of the Latin *laceratio*, "a tearing or a mangling." The word now serves for any cut incurred as an injury, but it retains its sense of forceful trauma. A cut made by a careful surgeon is an incision, not a laceration.

lacertus is a Latin word that to the Romans meant both "muscle" and "lizard," presumably because of the resemblance in shape. More specifically, the reference was to the biceps muscle in the upper arm. Now, in anatomy "lacertus" designates the fibrous expansion or attachment of certain muscles, particularly the biceps brachii and the lateral rectus muscle of the eye.

lacrimal originated in the Indo-European *dakru*, "a tear, as from a weeping eye." The same word was used by the Greeks. In archaic Latin this became *dacruma*, but in classical Latin the "d" was changed to "l" under Sabine influence, and to the Romans "a tear" was either *lacruma* or *lacrima*. The Anglo-Saxon derivative was *taehher*, whence the English "tear." In anatomy we put this together when we say "the lacrimal duct conveys the tears." An alternative spelling is **lachrymal**, which was an aberration arising from the medieval Latinists' custom of changing "c" to "ch" preceding an "r" (as in "pulchritude"); the "i" became "y" simply as a graphic variant. So "lacrimal" is the correct spelling, even though poetically we persist in using "lachrymose" to describe a person given to weeping.

lacteal refers to the fine, endothelial-lined lymphatic channels that convey fat-laden lymph from the absorptive intestinal mucosa. The appearance and consistency of such lymph suggests that of milk, hence the origin of the term in the Latin *lacteus,* "milky."

lactic acid was originally discovered in sour milk (Latin *lac*, "milk").

lactose is the sugar (a disaccharide that on hydrolysis yields glucose + galactose) that naturally occurs in milk. For an explanation of the suffix "-ose," *see* **glucose**.

lacuna is the Latin word for "a gap or hollow, a place where water tends to collect," such as a pit or pond. In anatomy the term is used to refer to any similar configuration as, for example, the tiny pits in compact bone. These minute apertures in bone, having been first described in 1691 by Clopton Havers (1657-1702), an English physician and anatomist, are also known as "Haversian canals." The lining of certain ducts, notably the urethra, is marked by small pits or lacunae.

lambdoid refers to whatever may be fancied in the shape of the capital Greek letter lambda, Λ, that looks like an inverted "V." Thus, the lambdoid suture of the skull and the lambdoid incision for gaining access to the epigastric viscera were so named.

lamina is the Latin word for "a thin plate," and **lamella** is the diminutive form meaning "a little, thin plate." A host of anatomic structures incorporates these terms in their names. For example, the platelike dorsal arches of the vertebrae are called "laminae," and the operation whereby they are removed is called a **laminectomy**.

lancet is a slightly shortened form of the French *lancette*, which was derived from the Latin *lancea*, "spear," and therefore is "a little spear." To lance a lesion, such as a boil, is to spear it.

lanolin is a fatty substance obtained from the wool of sheep. The name was concocted by combining the Latin *lana*, "wool," + *oleum*, "oil." As an emollient or unguent it is usually made up as a hydrous emulsion. It is commonly incorporated in cosmetic lotions aimed to soften or "moisturize" the skin.

lanugo is the Latin word for "down, meaning the small, fine hairs of plants." The lanugo of the fetus is the downy excrescence that appears about the fifth month of gestation.

laparotomy comes from the Greek *lapara*, "the soft parts of the body between the rib margins and the hips," that is, the flanks or loins. This, in turn, is related to *laparos*, "slack, loose, or relaxed." The suffix comes from the Greek *tomē*, "a cutting." "Laparotomy" was introduced as a term for an operation in 1878 by Thomas Bryant (1828-1914), an English surgeon. Purists insist that "laparotomy" should be used to designate only incisions in the flanks and not for those elsewhere in the abdomen, but the currency of usage has stifled their argument. Similarly, **laparoscopy** (+ Greek *skopein*, "to view") has been disdained in some circles as an improper term for looking into the abdominal cavity by means of an optical instrument, even though this instrument is inserted through the "soft parts" of the abdomen. This procedure was long known in the United States as "peritoneoscopy," but "laparoscopy," as the procedure is widely known and used in Europe and Japan, has rapidly gained supremacy.

larva is Latin for "mask or ghost." The Romans used the word to designate the specter of the dead, which they conceived as having the spirit but not the actual form of the living creature it represents. In this sense the term became applied to an early phase in the life of an insect or parasite before its true form became apparent (which is known by the Latin term *imago*). Regressing to its figurative sense, we may make reference to a "larval" form of a disease when we mean an early, undefined phase in its development. The same can be said for "larval" ideas.

laryngismus (*see* **trismus**)

larynx is a direct borrowing of the Greek term for "the upper part of the windpipe." This is related to the Greek verb *lary[n]ggixō*, "I bawl or bellow," from which the term **laryngismus** was derived, an allusion to the crowing sound issuing from a spastic larynx.

laser is an acronym (a word formed from initial letters or parts of a name or phrase, in sequence) derived from "*l*ight *a*mplification by *s*timulated *e*mission of *r*adiation." The laser is a device that converts, within a medium of crystal or gas, incident electromagnetic radiation of mixed frequencies to a discrete, coherent, highly amplified emission of visible light. As such, the laser is a means of transmitting intense, focused energy, and it is thus used therapeutically for coagulation and ablation of tissues.

latent is a slightly abbreviated form of the Latin adverb *latenter*, "secretly," and is related to the intransitive verb *latere*, "to lie hidden or concealed." Thus, latent syphilis is a "hidden" form of the disease.

latex is the Latin word for "a liquid or fluid substance," especially that from a hidden source, such as water from a spring or sap from a tree (*see* **latent**). In botany latex is the milky fluid extracted from certain plants, notably the rubber tree, which congeals on exposure to air or heat. In the laboratory, latex is any emulsion of fine particles of plastic substance that can be coagulated by certain constituents of serum. Thus, we have the "latex fixation test" for rheumatoid factor.

laudanum is an old designator of tincture of opium. Some scholars assert that the name is a derivative of the Greek *ladonon*, the resin obtained from an oriental shrub (not the poppy plant) that was known to the Persians as *ladan*. The claim is that this substance was confused with poppy juice, the source of opium. There is a more plausible, if not laudable, explanation. "Laudanum" was introduced into the pharmacopoeia by Aureolus Theophrastus Bombastus von Hohenheim (1493-1541), a Swiss physician who named himself Paracelsus to indicate that he was on a par with, if not superior to, the renowned Celsus. He claimed he had a secret remedy (which may or may not have contained opium) that he considered *laude dignum*,

"worthy of praise." It is curious to note that, much later, "heroin" was given its name because it was thought to be similarly laudable.

laughing gas was a name given to nitrous oxide in 1800 by Humphry (dubbed "Sir" in 1812) Davy (1778-1829), the remarkable English surgeon-apothecary-chemist, who investigated the curious psychotropic properties of the gas when it was inhaled. Davy went on to discover and isolate numerous elements, among them sodium, potassium, chlorine, and fluorine. Some say that Sir Humphry's greatest discovery was his assistant, Michael Faraday.

lavage comes from the Latin *lavare*, "to wash." Gastric lavage is another way of saying "a stomach washing." A lavatory, of course, is "a place for washing."

laxative is derived from the Latin *laxare*, "to extend, widen, open, or release." In the sense of loosening or relaxing the bowel, the term was not used by the Romans but came out of the Middle Ages, perhaps because those were such costive times.

Lazarus is the name attached to a syndrome or complex that includes the anxiety, depression, and sense of alienation suffered by some survivors of cardiorespiratory resuscitation (*Ann Intern Med*. 1972;76:135). These are patients who have been brought back from the perilous brink of death. The allusion, of course, is to the brother of Mary and Martha, whom Jesus raised from the dead (John 11:1-44). There is another, unrelated, biblical Lazarus, the diseased beggar shunned by the rich man who should have known better (Luke 16:19-31).

lecithin comes from the Greek *lekithos*, "the yolk of an egg." This name for the monoaminemonophosphatide was suggested by its early discovery in carp eggs. Its Greek origin would indicate the "c" in "lecithin" be pronounced as "k," yet almost invariably it is given a voiceless fricative "s" sound.

leech is the common name for a bloodsucking worm of the class Hirudinea, but it also is, or was, used to designate a physician. In fact the latter meaning came first, being derived from the Anglo-Saxon *lǽce*, "one who heals." Today, in Iceland a physician is a *laeknir*, and in Finland a *lāākari*. The Dano-

Norwegian is *laege*, the Polish *lekarz*. The bloodsucking annelid worm, in bygone days, was used medicinally, the idea being that the worm would consume corrupting substances from an inflamed lesion. Hence, the worm was given the name of "the healer" (*Ann Intern Med.* 1988;109:399). Still later, "leech" became an epithet for a person who clung to and extracted sustenance from another.

leiomyoma is contrived by a combination of the Greek *leios*, "smooth," + *mys*, "muscle," + *ōma*, "swelling"; hence, "a smooth muscle tumor." Such tumors commonly occur in the muscular wall of the uterus and were, and sometimes still are, mistakenly called **fibroids**.

leishmaniasis (*see* **kala-azar**)

lemniscus is an almost direct borrowing of the Greek *lēmniskos*, "a woolen ribbon or bandage," related to *lēmnos*, "wool." In anatomy a lemniscus is a band or bundle of neural fibers.

lens is the Latin word (the genitive is *lentis*) for the beanlike seed that we call "lentil." The only lens familiar to the ancients was that of the eye, and it was given the name of the bean because of its size and shape; its transparency had nothing to do with its naming. For those well acquainted with the lens of the eye but unfamiliar with lentil beans, examine the beans on your next visit to a grocery; you'll see the allusion is apt. The Greek word for the lentil bean is *phakos*, and by the same analogy that has been applied to the Latin *lens*, we have **phako-** as a combining form pertaining to the lens of the eye. **Aphakia** is an absence of the lens. Oddly, a **phakoma** is a minute, pale tumor seen microscopically in the retina in tuberous sclerosis; also it is the term applied to a patch of myelinated nerve fibers seen in the retina in neurofibromatosis. Another term is the misspelled "phaco-," as in **phacocele** (+ Greek *kēlē*, "hernia"), denoting a dislodged, misplaced lens.

lenta is the feminine form of the Latin adjective meaning "slow or sluggish." Subacute bacterial endocarditis was once known as "endocarditis lenta" because of its typically slow, lingering course.

lenticular can describe whatever is shaped like a lentil bean (*see* **lens**), particularly the nucleus found in the corpus striatum of the brain. It has nothing to do with the lens or the eye and was so named simply because of its shape.

lentigo is the Latin word for "freckle," related to the Latin *lens, lentis*, the legume bearing the small flattened bean we call "lentil." Indeed, what the dermatologist calls "lentigo" looks a lot like a freckle. It is a small, brown spot in the skin, resulting from the deposition of melanin pigment by an active focus of melanocytes near the basal layer of the epidermis. But to the dermatologist there is an important distinction. A freckle comes from exposure to the actinic rays of the sun, whereas **lentigines** (the plural) can be the result of various other causes. Conversely, a patch of white, depigmented skin is called **vitiligo**, a term derived from the Latin *vitium*, "a blemish or defect." To **vitiate** is to defile or make faulty. Incidentally, the suffix **-igo**, of Latin origin, once was used in a number of terms denoting conditions of disease in man, animals, plants, and even metals. Those medical terms that have survived are mostly related to dermatology, e.g., **lentigo, vitiligo, intertrigo**, and **impetigo**. Surviving terms related to other systems are **vertigo** and, as a slight variant, **lumbago**.

leontiasis is a rare form of hyperostosis, occurring as a fibrous dysplasia in younger persons or as a feature of Paget's disease of bone in the elderly, wherein the facial bones enlarge, giving the victim a countenance suggesting that of a lion. *Leo, leonis* is the Latin for "lion." Beethoven is depicted in his later years as having a somewhat leonine countenance, and it has been suggested the great composer might have been a victim of Paget's disease, which also could have contributed to his deafness.

leprosy comes from the Greek *lepros*, "scaly, rough, or mangy," hence, "the scaly disease." Gerhard Hansen (1841-1912), a Norwegian physician, correctly described the causative organism, *Mycobacteriae leprae*, and the condition is now properly known as **Hansen's disease**. In ancient Greece what we now know as leprosy probably did not exist. The "scaly disease" of the Greeks more likely was psoriasis. Aretaeus the Cappadocian described leprosy accurately in the second century A.D., but he called it "leontiasis" because of the facial deformity. There then followed a confusion of names, and in the translation of Arabic writings the Greek *lepra* became attached to what is now recognized as Hansen's disease. The term "leprosy," then, doubly deserves to be abandoned, not only because of its unjust connotation of despicableness, but also because it had been misplaced nosologically.

lepto- is a combining form taken from the Greek *leptos*, "fine, slender, or delicate." Thus, the **leptomeninges** (+ Greek *mēni[n]gx*, "membrane") are the thin, delicate membranes, comprising both the pia and the arachnoid, that envelope the brain and spinal cord. *Leptospira* (+ Greek *speira*, "coil") is a genus of finely coiled spirochetes.

lesbian (*see* **tribadism**)

lesion comes from the Latin *laesio*, "an attack or injury," which is related to the verb *laedere*, "to strike, hurt, or wound."

lethal (*see* **lethargy**; *also* **mortal**)

lethargy is a state of overpowering apathy or drowsiness, and it comes from the Greek *lēthargos*, "forgetful." In Greek mythology Lethe was the name of a river that flowed in the netherworld of Hades. The souls of the dead were obliged to drink of its water and so become oblivious of everything said or done during their span on earth. One might assume that the word **lethal**, meaning deadly, was of analogous origin. Not quite. "Lethal" is from the Latin *letum*, meaning "death or destruction." The "h" was put in the English word in the 17th century because of confusion with the Greek *lēthe*, "oblivion." Our word, then, should be "letal," but no one would recognize it.

leucine is an **amino acid** so called because of its color or lack thereof. This is one of the few names related to the Greek *leukos* (*see* **leuko-**) wherein "c" always appears.

leukemia is marked by a neoplastic proliferation of any one of the species of leukocyte. The term combines **leuko-** + Greek *aima*, "blood."

leuko- is sometimes spelled "leuco-" (although "k" is preferred to "c") and is a combining form, usually a prefix, taken from the Greek *leukos*, "white," also "light, bright, brilliant, and clear." The

apostle Luke, patron saint of physicians, owes his name to the same source.

leukocyte is a cellular element of blood (+ Greek *kytos*, "cell"), specifically of the multinucleate type, that when unstained appears white. **Leukocytosis** is an excess of white cells in the circulating blood.

leukoplakia is characterized by white patches or plaques on a mucous membrane (leuko- + Greek *plakoeis*, "flat, broad").

leukorrhea is a white vaginal discharge (leuko- + Greek *rhoia*, "a flow").

leukotrienes constitute a class of biologically active substances formed from arachidonic acid by the lipo-oxygenase pathway. They are so called because they act on leukocytes and contain three or more double bonds.

levarterenol is also known as norepinephrine and marketed as Levophed. It is the L- (for levo-) isomer (and the pharmacologically active form) of the chemical mediator liberated by mammalian postganglionic adrenergic nerves.

levator comes from the Latin *levare*, "to lift." There are a number of levator muscles in the body, and they all serve to lift whatever structure into which they are inserted. Muscles that lower attached structures are called **depressors**, a term derived from the Latin *depressus*, the past participle of *deprimere*, "to press down" (from *de-*, "down from," + *primum*, "above all").

levo-, **lev-** are prefixes taken from the Latin *laevus*, "on the left side." Purists insist "levo-" be spelled "laevo-," and they are correct insofar as the term has nothing to do with the Latin *lev-* (related to "lifting") or *lēv-* (related to "smoothness").

levulose is the name given by Claude Louis Berthollet (1748-1822), a French physician and chemist, to fructose (the sugar of fruits) because it caused polarized light to be rotated to the left. (*see* **glucose**)

L-forms are pleomorphic, poorly stained organisms found in cultured colonies of various bacteria. They are aberrant derivatives of the parent organisms—not contaminants—and most will eventually revert to their original forms. The initial "L" is taken from the Lister Institute in London, where the nature of these aberrant forms was first reported in 1935.

libido is the Latin word for "desire, longing,

fancy, lust, or rut." In psychoanalysis the term is applied to the motive power of the sex life; in Freudian psychology, to psychic energy in general.

lichen is a near borrowing of the Greek *leichēn*, "a tree moss." In botany a lichen is a compound plant composed by symbiotic union of a fungus and an alga, and it grows as an excrescence on rocks or trees. The term was used by the Greeks in reference to a blight or canker on olives, and hence came to be applied, in ancient medicine, to various skin eruptions, probably most often ringworm. Now, the medical term is used almost exclusively as part of **lichen planus** (the second word is Latin for "flat"), an inflammatory skin or mucosal disease characterized by an excrescence of flat, white plaques.

licorice is a confection and has little to do with medicine except that it is sometimes used as a flavoring agent to disguise the disagreeable taste of an active ingredient, as in cough syrups. Licorice is a leguminous plant, *Glycyrrhiza glabra*, and its name comes from the Greek *glyky[s]*, "sweet," + *rhiza*, "a root," therefore, "the sweet root plant." In Late Latin the initial "g" was dropped to form *liquiritia*, and in Middle English this became *lycorys*. Incidentally, most people think of licorice as being black. The black color is charcoal powder added only by confectional convention and has nothing to do with the flavor. A person who eats a lot of licorice might, to his dismay, pass a black stool, simulating melena. A candy-conscious doctor can be reassuring.

lienteric refers to a type of diarrhea wherein the feces contain particles of undigested food, indicating rapid passage through the gut. The word is a combination of the Greek *leios*, "smooth," + *enteron*, "the intestine"; thus, "a slippery gut." Obviously, "lienteric" should be spelled "leinteric," but it isn't. And it has nothing to do with *lien*, the Latin word for "spleen."

ligament is derived from the Latin *ligare*, "to bind or tie," and refers to the tough bands of connective tissue by which various structures are bound together or supported.

ligature can be anything used as a tie, especially in surgery, and to **ligate** is to tie. Oliver Wendell Holmes, the 19th century Boston savant, wrote in his *Medical Essays*, "I would never use a long word where a short one would answer the purpose. I know there are professors in this country who 'ligate' arteries. Other surgeons only tie them, and it stops the bleeding as well." The word "obligation," in the sense of a pledge, comes from the Latin *ob*, "on account of," + *ligare*, and thus means whatever one is bound to do for a particular reason. Another related word is "religion," which can be viewed as a bond or pledge. To return to things medical, an **obligate** parasite is one that is so bound that it cannot live apart from its host, whereas a **facultative** (Latin *facultas*, "opportunity, feasibilty") parasite can choose its environment and still exist by adapting to varying conditions.

limbus is the Latin word for "fringe, hem, or border." Thus, the limbus of the cornea is the border where it joins the sclera. **Limbo** was, in ancient theology, a supposed place, not quite hell and not quite heaven, that was the abode of infants who died without baptism and of the righteous who died before the coming of Christ.

liminal is derived from the Latin *limen*, "threshold." As in the relation of "lumen" to "luminal," the second vowel of the derived adjective changes from "e" to "i." A liminal stimulus is just barely perceived by the senses, and a **subliminal** stimulus is "below the threshold" and not perceived at all. To eliminate is to discard "beyond the threshold," and whatever is preliminary, as, for example, a tentative diagnosis, is something considered "before crossing the threshold."

linea is the Latin word for "line, string, or thread." To the Romans, according to Professor H. A. Skinner, the *linea alba* or "white line" was the mark made by lime or chalk across a track behind which chariots lined up for the start of a race. In anatomy the linea alba is the longitudinal white streak of fibrous tissue between the rectus abdominis muscles.

lingual is derived from the Latin *lingua*, "tongue," and is related to the verb *lingere*, "to lick or lap up." To pronounce the Latin word is almost to imitate licking with the tongue. For the Greeks, "to lick" was *leichein*, also an imitative sound. A related word is "language," the utterance of which requires an active use of the tongue. A colloquial term for the spoken word, especially that peculiar to a certain group, is **lingo**, recorded in English as early as 1600; it is close to the Latin.

lingula is used in anatomy as a term for anything shaped like a little tongue, e.g., the projection from the lower portion of the upper lobe of the left lung. The term is the diminutive of the Latin *lingua,* "tongue."

liniment comes from the Latin *linere,* "to smear on or to anoint." In ancient practice as today a liniment was a particularly thin, liquid ointment.

linitis plastica (*see* **syphilis**)

lipid is any fatty substance (*see* **lipo-**), insoluble in water and soluble in common organic solvents.

lipo- is a combining form taken from the Greek *lipos,* "animal fat or vegetable oil."

lipofuscin is a lipid-containing, granular pigment observed in various tissues and often attributed to cellular senility. It is sometimes called "wear-and-tear pigment." The name was contrived by hybridization of the Greek *lipo-* + the Latin *fuscus,* "dark brown," because of its color. The latter Latin term gives a clue to the origin of **obfuscate**, meaning to muddy up or make murky. (*see* **fuchsin**)

lipolysis is a dissolution of fat (lipo- + Greek *lysis,* "a loosening").

liter is the American spelling of the French *litre,* proposed in 1793 as a convenient unit of capacity, being that of a cubic vessel measuring 10 centimeters on a side (or, more accurately, the volume occupied by 1 kilogram of pure water at its temperature of maximum density and under standard atmospheric pressure). The term was suggested by *litron,* an obsolete French measure of capacity. This came from the Late Latin *litra* and the classical Latin *libra,* a unit of weight approximating 12 ounces. Twelve ounces compose 1 pound according to the troy or apothecaries scale, and this accounts for "lb" as an abbreviation for "pound," taken from the Latin *libra.*

litho- is a combining form taken from the Greek *lithos,* "stone."

lithotomy is the operation of "cutting for the stone" (litho- + Greek *tomē,* "a cutting") and originally referred to incision of the urinary bladder. Hippocrates, in his famous oath, required his disciples to forswear "cutting for the stone," leaving that practice to "such as are craftsmen therein," presumably meaning urologists. The condition of stones in the gallbladder is **cholelithiasis** (from the Greek *cholē,* "bile").

lithotripsy (*see* **sassafras**)

litmus comes from the Old Scandinavian *litmosi,* "dye moss," being a combination of *lit,* "color or dye," + *mossi,* "a moss or lichen." Litmus is a coloring matter obtained from certain lichens that exhibits the helpful property of turning blue in an alkaline solution ($pH>7$) and red in an acid solution ($pH<7$). For convenience in the laboratory the dye usually is impregnated in paper, a slip of which is immersed in the fluid to be tested for alkalinity or acidity. **Litmus test** is now sometimes used figuratively for any trial to determine which of two opposing conditions might be valid.

livedo reticularis is a mottled purple or dusky blue discoloration of the skin seen in hypoxic conditions (from the Latin *lividus* [*see* **livid**] + *reticulum,* "a network").

liver is the name of the largest solid organ in the body, generally acknowledged to be essential to life. Its name would seem to be related to the verb "to live." Perhaps it is. Its Anglo-Saxon predecessor was *lifer.* In German the organ is *die Leber,* and "to live" is *leben.* But scholars are not sure of the connection. It has been suggested that the Indo-European root word for the liver was *yekurt,* which became the Greek *hēpar* (from which we have hepatic, hepatitis, hepatomegaly, and similar combined forms) and the Latin *jecur.* The Latin term, oddly, has no descendent in Romance languages, being replaced by a Latin adjective *ficatum,* "stuffed with figs." It would seem the Romans combined liver and figs in a single dish. *Ficatum* became the Italian *fegato,* the Spanish *higado,* and the French *foie.* To the ancient Babylonians the excised liver of a sacrificed animal was an organ of divination wherefrom they read all sorts of portents. Ironically, the ancient people had not an inkling of the truly astonishing metabolic function of the liver. In fact, the liver fell into disrepute when it was found not to be the wellspring of blood and lymph, an earlier supposition. It remained for Claude Bernard (1838-1878), the renowned French physiologist, to establish the liver in its rightful place as a vital organ, "a veritable laboratory of life," as he put it. It is appropriate that *la maladie de foie* has become, in effect, the national disease of France.

livid is a derivative of the Latin *lividus*, "the color of lead," and describes the bluish-gray hue of hypoxic blood in the skin. Interestingly, the Latin *lividus* also means "jealous, envious, or spiteful." Presumably, this is an allusion to the complexion of persons consumed by these emotions. Because an ashen complexion often clouds the face of a person beset by shocked wrath, we may say, "He was livid with anger."

lobe comes from the Greek *lobos*, "a small, rounded projection," first applied to the floppy lower appendage of the external ear. This led to the Late Latin *lobus* and its diminutive *lobulus* (from which we have taken **lobule**). The lobes of the brain, lung, and liver were hardly mentioned as such in English until the 16th century.

lochia is the fluid that seeps from the vagina during the first week or so after childbirth. The term is derived from the Greek *locheia*, "childbirth," being related to the Greek verb *locheuō*, "I bring forth or I bear."

lockjaw (*see* **trismus**)

locum tenens is a Latin phrase that, translated literally, means one who "holds the place" (from *locus* + *tenere*, "to hold") and refers to a doctor or other professional person who temporarily carries on the practice of an absent colleague.

locus is Latin for "a place or site." The term is used in the names of various specific anatomic locations, particularly in the central nervous system.

loin (*see* **psoas**)

long in the tooth is an old phrase descriptive of aging. It refers to the observation that the gums tend to recede with age, thus exposing more of the teeth. The expression has been used of both horses and people. This also explains the admonition, "Don't look a gift horse in the mouth."

lordosis is an almost direct borrowing of the Greek *lordos*, "bent backward." Such a posture results in an exaggerated anterior convexity of the lumbar spine. The term has nothing to do with a haughty or lordly bearing. The English "lord," incidentally, originally was *hlafweard*, "guardian of the bread."

lotion (*see* **ointment**)

lozenge refers to the shape and not to the content or purpose of a medication so formulated. The French *losange* means "diamond-shaped." The origin probably was the Old Gothic *lausa*, "a flat stone," + *-inga*, the Germanis suffix indicating "pertaining to." In Portuguese *lousa* is "a tombstone." Now, in pharmacy, a lozenge is a tablet of any shape intended to be dissolved in the mouth for its topically soothing effect.

lues is the Latin word for "infection, contagion, plague, or pestilence," and may have come from the Greek *lua*, "a dissolution." To the Romans *lues* meant any sort of virulent, contagious disease. The more specific term *lues venerea* was taken to mean any disease acquired by the act symbolizing devotion to Venus, the goddess of love. It was not until 1835 that Philippe Ricord established syphilis as an entity distinct from gonorrhea. He accomplished this in a series of notorious experiments on Parisian prostitutes. Thereafter, lues was regarded as syphilis. "Lues," despite its final "s," is singular, not plural.

lumbago is an old-fashioned term for any rheumatic pain in the region of the loins. An explanation of the suffix "-ago, -igo" can be found in the entry for **lentigo**.

lumbar comes from the Latin *lumbus*, "the loin," and refers to anything pertaining to the lower paraspinal region. The lumbar vertebrae are situated between the loins.

lumbricoid is derived from the Latin *lumbricus*, "a worm," and refers to whatever has the appearance of a worm. *Lumbricus* in zoology is the name given to a genus of annelids, including the common earthworm. *Ascaris lumbricoides*, the scientific name for a parasitic enteric worm, would seem to be a redundancy; the Greek *askaris* means "an intestinal worm." The small, elongated **lumbrical** muscles in the hand and foot are so called because of their wormlike shape.

lumen is Latin for "light," including the light

that comes from a window or aperture. When sectioning a hollow viscus, one can see light through the opened space. Hence, "lumen" came to be a term designating that space. In the adjectival form **luminal** the "e" becomes an "i." Luminal was once a trade name chosen for phenobarbital presumably as a reflection of the Greek *phainein*, "to bring to light." It must have seemed a bright idea to someone at the time.

lunatic as a term for a person mentally disturbed comes from the Latin *luna*, "moon." Such use relates to the old belief that mental disorder was a consequence of being "moon-struck." Another derivation would seem to be the slang word "loony." However, there is another explanation. The expression "crazy as a loon" refers not to the large, diving, fish-eating bird but rather to the archaic "loon" that meant "a worthless, stupid fellow" and may have been derived from the Icelandic *luinn*, "beaten." One who had been beaten nearly senseless might well act strangely.

lung may have originated in the Sanskrit *laghu*, which meant "light" in the sense of "without weight." It is likely that the ancients were impressed by the lightness of lung tissue in contrast to the density of other viscera. In almost all languages the term for the lungs is related to the word for "lightness." For example, the Russian *legkoe*, "lung," is related to *lëgkii*, "light."

lupus is Latin for "wolf." The use of the wolf's name in the designation of various diseases reflects differing allusions. **Lupus vulgaris** (the latter word is Latin for "common") refers to tuberculosis of the skin wherein the infection appears to eat away at the skin, as by the gnawing of a wolf. **Lupus erythematosus**, a skin disease wherein the malar areas become inflamed and pigmented, was so named because it seemed to impose on its victim a lupine or wolflike countenance.

lutein is a yellow pigment or lipochrome. The term comes from the Latin *luteus*, "mud-colored," *lutum* being Latin for mud or clay. The corpus luteum is the yellow body or nodule that marks the site of a mature ovarian follicle from which an ovum has been discharged.

luxation is derived from the Latin *luxare*, "to put out of joint or to dislocate." It is akin to the Greek *loxos*, "crosswise." A **subluxation** is a less than complete dislocation. If the joint hurts, and you're not sure it is really dislocated, you can gravely pronounce the injury a "subluxation."

Lyme disease is a multisystem affliction consequent to a tickborne spirochetal infection. The name memorializes the first report of a cluster of cases recognized in the vicinity of the town of Old Lyme, Connecticut (*Arthritis Rheum.* 1977;20:7), an example of eponymic derivation.

lymph is a slightly shortened version of the Latin *lympha*, "clear water, especially that found in flowing springs." *Lympha* is a pseudoetymologic formation influenced by the Greek *nymphē* (wherein the "n" was exchanged for an "l"), the word for "a bride or marriageable girl." As a proper name, Nymphe was applied to goddesses of lesser rank who presided over springs, lakes, and forests. The association seems to have been with a sense of moisture. In ancient anatomy the lymphatic vessels were so named because, although they were thought to be veins, they were observed to carry a watery fluid rather than blood. The nodes intimately associated with these vessels were called "lymphatic glands" or, more correctly, "lymph nodes." The idea of *lympha* became incorporated in the humoral system of pathology, and a supposedly cool, moist temperament became known as the phlegmatic or lymphatic type. There was a time when a sluggish disposition was attributed to an overgrowth of lymphoid tissues. A person so perceived was said to be in **status lymphaticus**.

lymphocyte is the name given to certain mononuclear cells within lymph nodes and found elsewhere. The term originated with Paul Ehrlich (1854-1915), the famous German bacteriologist and immunologist.

lys- is a combining form taken from the Greek *lysis*, "a loosening or setting free." The term is used as a prefix, as in **lysosome** (*see* **soma**) and in **lysozyme**, a basic protein that functions as an antibacterial enzyme; as a suffix, as in hydrolysis, the breakdown or release of components of a substance by the addition of water (the H^+ going to one resultant part and the OH going to the other); or by itself, as in the **lysis** or "loosening" of fibrous adhesions.

Macerate comes from the Latin *maceratus*, the past participle of *macerare*, "to make soft or tender." The adjective *macer* means "lean and skinny" and also "thin or poor," as a depleted soil. Macerated skin is that made soft and friable by excessive moisture or oiling. A macerated fetus is one that has degenerated and disintegrated after dying in the uterus. **Emaciation**, with the prefix *e- (ex-)*, "out of, or as a result of," is the condition consequent to depletion.

macro- is a prefix taken from the Greek *makros*, "long in space or time." In medicine the term usually denotes an extended distance and, more particularly, a large size. Thus, a **macrocyte** is an extraordinarily large cell, and **macroscopic** means large enough to be seen by the naked eye. However, recently we encounter **macrobiotic** (+ Greek *bios*, "life") as applied to diet or exercise, the notion being that, properly applied, these activities can prolong life.

macula is the Latin word for "a small spot or blemish." The "-ula" ending denotes a diminutive emphasis. In dermatology a macula is a small, flat, unraised spot or blemish in the skin (in contrast to a papule, which is a raised spot). The **macula lutea** (from the Latin *luteus*, "mud-colored or yellow") is the spot at the posterior pole of the retina where the keenest vision is registered.

mad as a hatter is an expression used to describe a person more than slightly daft. It usually reminds one of Lewis Carroll's Mad Hatter, an amusing character encountered in *Alice's Adventures in Wonderland*, but the phrase was well known earlier. Its origin is disputed. Some say it began as "mad as an atter," the "atter" being an Anglo-Saxon word for adder, thus referring to the viper whose bite was thought to transmit madness. The alternative explanation, more plausible and medically more interesting, is that mercurous chloride was used in making felt for hats and that hatmakers or "hatters," inhaling the vapors, would eventually become victims of mercury poisoning. Among the symptoms of chronic mercury poisoning are tremors of the eyelids, lips, tongue, and fingers, due to cerebellar cortical atrophy.

magnesia is borrowed from the name of a town situated in the once wealthy kingdom of Lydia, the domain of the fabulous Croesus. The area is now part of northwestern Turkey. From a small mountain near this town was obtained an ore that included what we would now call magnesium carbonate. **Magnesium hydroxide** is the familiar "milk of magnesia," commonly used as a laxative agent. Apparently, there was another ore of different composition obtained from the vicinity of Magnesia that exhibited unusual properties; it was lodestone, then known as the Magnesian stone, and led to our word "magnet."

malady is an Anglicization of the French *maladie*, "an illness." This is derived from the Latin adverb *male*, "badly" (the Latin word is pronounced "mah-ley" and has nothing to do with "male," in the sense of the masculine gender). This provides an opportunity to give an example of false etymology. The fanciful story is told that the word "marmalade" goes back to the frequent illnesses suffered by Mary, the unhappy and unfortunate queen of the Scots. When Mary complained, the cry of her French-speaking courtiers would ring through the castle, "*Marie est malade!*" ("Mary is sick!"). The remedy was to be found in a nice dish of preserved fruit, and this took its name as an antidote for "Mary's malade." This story, as clever as it might be, has not a *soupçon* of truth in it. "Marmalade" comes from the Portuguese *marmalada*, "a quince jam," and goes back to the Latin *melimelum*, "a kind of apple," and to the Greek *melimēlon*, a combination of *mel-*, "honey or a sweet," + *mēlon*, "a fruit."

malaise is a French word descended from the Old French *mal-*, "bad or ill," + *aise*, "ease"; hence, "ill at ease." In medicine "malaise" can describe any vague feeling of bodily or mental discomfort.

malar comes from the Latin *mala*, "the cheek-bone." To the Romans this also meant the facial cheek itself, and it has been suggested that the term is related to the Latin *malum*, "an apple," presumably because of a fancied resemblance of a rosy, rounded cheek to a ripe apple.

malaria comes from the Italian wherein *mal-* means "bad" and *aria* is "air." The Italian expression used in the 18th century was *mal'aria*. The belief was that the disease then called "intermittent fever" was caused by *mal'aria* or noxious air emanating from marshlands. The connection with swamps was correct, but mosquitoes, not vapors, carry the cause of malaria. If one wishes to avoid *mal'aria*, one might consider moving to Buenos Aires, where the air is said to be good.

male is a borrowing of the French *mâle*, a step away from the Old French *masle*, which came from the Latin adjective *masculus*, "manly." **Female**, although it looks like it might be related to "male" because of its spelling, it is not; its origin is quite different. (*see* **female**).

malignant comes from the Latin adjective *malignus*, "spiteful, mean, stingy, or malicious," this being derived from a combination of *mal-*, "bad," + *[g]nascor*, "to be born." Thus, "malignant" literally means "born to be bad," and this comes very close to the sense of the word as it is used in pathology. A malignant neoplasm is one that is genetically predetermined to cause trouble. In English there are, among others, two pairs of nearly equivalent words: "benign/benignant" and "malign/malignant." Curiously, in medicine (and more particularly in pathology) we have chosen to use the shorter of the former pair and the longer of the latter pair to contrast the behavior of certain diseases, especially neoplasia. We speak or write of "benign" (rather than "benignant") tumors in contrast to "malignant" (rather than "malign") tumors. The choice is little more than a matter of custom. (*see* **benign**)

malingerer denotes one who feigns illness, often as a ruse to obtain an advantage or to avoid an obligation. The word comes from the French adjective *malingre*, "sickly or loathesome," and is a combination of *mal-*,

"bad," + the Old French *haingre*, "thin, emaciated." Presumably, "to malinger" came to its present meaning from the practice of soldiers who excoriated themselves, particularly by gouging ulcers on their legs, and thus appeared to have an incapacitating affliction. In modern soldiery the self-inflicted "shot in the foot" is a prime example of malingering.

malleus is the Latin word for "hammer or mallet." The diminutive form, *malleolus*, means "a little hammer." Inexplicably, in anatomy the malleus, one of the tiny middle-ear ossicles that is shaped like a hammer (*see* **incus**), is considerably smaller than the **malleolus**, a bony prominence on either side of the ankle, that seemed to someone to look like the protruding head of a hammer.

maltose (*see* **glucose**)

mammary is an adjective derived from *mamma*, which is both the Latin and Greek word for the breast, particularly that of a woman. The word is imitative of the "mama" sound uttered by a mewling infant seeking the nourishing breast. Every mother marvels when she hears that sound. "The baby has learned my name!" Little does she know that her name came from the sound and not the other way around. Mammals are vertebrate animals that suckle their young. **Mammillation**, a word derived from the diminutive of *mamma*, refers to a small excrescence that bears a fancied resemblance to a little breast.

management (*see* **treatment**)

mandible is a transliteration of the Latin *mandibula*, "the lower jaw." The word comes from the Latin verb *mandere*, "to chew"; the suffix *-bula* indicates "the means of." Ancient anatomists used **maxilla** for both the upper and lower jaws, and only much later did the "inferior maxilla" become the "mandible."

mania is the Greek word for "madness," being related to the verb *mainmai*, "to rage, to be furious, to rave in anger." A manic disorder is one characterized by an abnormally expanded emotional state, excessive elation, and heightened verbal and motor activity. The mythical Furies, who pursued and punished doers of unavenged crimes, were called Maniai. They were said to drive men mad.

manifest means "clearly evident," and a manifestation of disease is a readily apparent feature. "Manifest" comes from the Latin *manifestus*, a combination of *manus*, "hand," + *festus*, "struck." Anything that strikes the hand or is struck by the hand is clearly evident. A palpable tumor is certainly manifest.

mannitol is a nutrient alcohol, $C_6H_8(OH)_6$, also used as a diuretic, that takes its name from *manna*, the Aramaic term for a vegetable exudate. The biblical manna (Exodus 16:13-36) was the sustenance miraculously granted the Israelites to allay their ordeal in the flight from Egypt.

manometer is a word in which the "o" reveals the origin of the term. If the second vowel were "i" or "u," the first part would have to come from the Latin *manus*, "hand," but this is not the case. The "mano-" of "manometer" is taken from the Greek *manos*, "scanty or sparse." The second component of the word, "-meter," comes from the Greek *mētron*, "a measure." The first manometer called by that name was a device used early in the 18th century to record the decreasing pressure of rarefied or "scanty" air in a chamber from which the air had been extracted. Later, the term was applied to any instrument capable of measuring the pressure or tension of gases or liquids.

manu- is a combining form, usually a prefix, that denotes relation to the hand. It is derived from the Latin *manus*, "the hand."

manual as an adjective describes what can be done with the hands, and as a noun means a set of instructions (also called a **handbook**) telling what to do with the hands in performing a given task. These terms have nothing to do with the size of such a book, in the sense of being easily held in the hand. This explains why a so-called handbook (and particularly the German *Handbuch*) can, in some cases, be such a ponderous volume.

manubrium is another anatomically proper name for the breastbone, so called because the shape of the bone resembles the handle of a sword (manu- + Latin *hibrium*, from *habere*, "to hold").

marasmus is derived from the Greek *marainein*, "to quench, to extinguish" and also "to waste away, to languish." In former times, the term was used to describe the pitiable state of infants who became emaciated and wasted

from no known cause. Insofar as causes are now increasingly well defined and remedies are more available than before, "marasmus" is seldom heard nowadays. However, the adjectival form **marantic** is occasionally used.

marrow means the pith, the core, or the central substance of anything. The Latin equivalent, *medulla*, is used to refer to the pith of the kidney and brain, while "marrow" is used to refer to the pith of hollow bones. "Marrow" can be traced to the Anglo-Saxon *mearh* and the Sanskrit *majjan*, both of which referred alike to the marrow of bones or the pith of trees. "Spinal marrow" is an archaic term for the spinal cord, which was once believed, incorrectly, to be the marrow of the vertebrae.

marsupial comes from the Greek *marsippos*, "a bag or pouch." Formerly, the Latin *marsupium* was applied to various anatomic pouches, such as the peritoneal cavity and the scrotum. In surgery **marsupialization** refers to the operation whereby an external opening is provided for drainage of an internal cyst. An example would be the suturing of an opening in a pancreatic cyst to a stoma in the anterior abdominal wall, thus forming a sort of draining pouch. Such an operation is not currently favored; internal drainage by gastric or enteric anastomosis is preferred.

masochism is a perversion wherein self-induced pain or humiliation gives a sensation of pleasure. The term is taken from the name of Leopold von Sacher-Masoch (1836-1895), an Austrian writer who made a sufferer of this sadly distorted condition the protagonist of one of his novels. Masochism is to be distinguished from **sadism**, a perverted penchant for inflicting pain on another person, usually in a sexual context. This term is taken from the name of a French writer, Count Donatien Alphonse François de Sade, who lived from 1740 to 1814. He preferred to be addressed as the Marquis de Sade, the name by which he was known before succeeding to his father's title in 1767. During service with the army he acquired a reputation for vicious practices. His literary works were marked by unrelieved obscenity. Because of his scandalous behavior, he was confined for 27 years of his life to various institutions, including the Bastille, as a mentally deranged prisoner.

massage comes from the Greek *massein*, "to work with the hands, as in kneading dough," and probably is related to the Greek *maza*, "barley bread," and perhaps to the Hebrew *massāh*, "unleavened bread." Some patients given to colloquial speech refer to palpation, as that of the abdomen, as "mashing." This is not traceable to the Greek but rather to the Middle English *mēshen*, the crushing of cereal grains in water to provide a "mash" as a food for animals or a substrate for fermentation.

masseter is the name of the jaw muscle that brings the lower teeth of the mandible into contact with the upper teeth of the maxilla. It is so called from the Greek *masēter*, "the chewer." The redundant "s" in the English term may have been a copyist's error.

mast cell was so named by Paul Ehrlich (1854-1915), the renowned German immunologist and bacteriologist, who first used the term *Mastzelle* in 1879. The German *mästen*, "to fatten," is related to "mast," an Old English word for food, especially as fodder for animals. This, in turn, can be traced to the Sanskrit *mēda(s)*, "fat" (which, by another track, gives us "meat"). Ehrlich was impressed by the densely packed basophilic granules he observed in the cytoplasm of what he called *die Mastzelle*, at first mistaking the granules for particles ingested by phagocytosis. To him, the cell looked "well fed."

masticate comes from the Greek *mastazein*, "to chew or to gnash the teeth," and from this came the name *mastiche* for the resinous gum of an evergreen shrub. Yes, the ancients too had chewing gum. Though the proper Latin word for chewing is *mandere*, the Romans used *masticare* specifically for the enjoyment of chewing gum. The Greek *mastiche* also accounts for the word "mastic," a gummy substance used as a filler in masonry and as a styptic in dentistry.

mastitis is an inflammation of the breast. The first portion of the term comes from the Greek *mastos*, "the breast of a woman." An earlier Greek form was *mazos*, from which is derived "amazon," meaning literally "without a breast." According to Herodotus, the Greek historian, there was a mythical race of female warriors who lived in Scythia. To avoid impediment in drawing their bows, these formidable women were said to have deliberately cut off their right breasts. Hence, they came to be known as "Amazons." It seems that early Spanish explorers, attracted to this myth, were intrigued by the notion that such women warriors abounded in the New World. Despite the fact that the immense South American river had already been named by its original discoverer the *Rio Santa Maria de la Mar Dulce*, another Spanish adventurer, known as Orellano, fancied that he was engaged in battle by warrior women while descending that river, and so he rechristened it *"Amazonas."* Incidentally, a similar illusion that the west coast of North America was inhabited by a band of belligerent women under the rule of a Queen Califia is said to have led to the naming of what is now our most populous state.

mastoid refers to the smooth, rounded eminence of the temporal bone behind the ear. This was fancied to resemble a female breast. Hence, its name was taken from the Greek *mastos*, "breast," + *eidos*, "like." At one time this structure was known by the Latin term *processus mammiformis*.

materia medica is a now archaic term meaning, literally, "the stuff of medicine," and more particularly the nature and use of drugs, now called "pharmacology." The Latin *materia* is used in the sense of "the stuff of which anything is composed." If *materia* sounds like the Latin *mater*, "mother," the resemblance is more than coincidental. In bygone times there were but two departments in the medical curriculum, that of "physic" wherein one learned of the natural course of disease, and that of "materia medica" wherein one learned how to change it.

matrix is the Latin term for any female animal kept specifically for breeding and is related to the Latin *mater* and the Greek *mētēr*, both meaning "mother" and used in reference to the uterus as "the mother of the fetus." From this evolved a sense of matrix as a mold or enclosing mass in which anything is formed or shaped. The bony matrix is the groundwork in which bone is formed. The Latin *matrix* also was a public roll on which one's parentage was registered. Later, the diminutive *matricula* came to be a brief description of the members of a university. Those so listed could be said to have "matriculated."

maxilla is the Latin word for "jawbone." It sounds like a diminutive, and it may be, but of what no one is sure. It relates to the Greek *mastakos*, "that with which one chews." The ancients used *maxilla* for both the upper jaw and the lower jaw. Later, the lower jaw became known as the **mandible**, and "maxilla" was restricted to the upper jaw.

measles as the name for the familiar childhood disease is always used in the plural. The reason is that the child so afflicted is covered by many little red spots. The name originated with the Old High German *māsa*, "a spot." This was taken into Middle English as the diminutive plural *maselen*, "many little spots." There was another wholly unconnected Middle English word, *mesel*, "a wretch" and later, "a leper." This came from the Latin *miser*, "wretched." There should be no confusion between *maselen* and *mesel*.

meatus is the Latin word for "motion or movement," but it also means "a channel" and is related to the verb *meare*, "to go or to pass." "Meatus" is used in the sense of a channel when referring to the external auditory meatus, the passage leading into the ear.

meconium is almost a direct borrowing of the Greek *mēkōnion*, which was the dark, viscid juice obtained by pressing the poppy plant. The Greek name for poppy is *mēkōn*. Because the bowel discharge from newborn infants was thought to resemble poppy juice, it was given the same name.

median comes from the Latin *medius*, "the middle." The median nerve extends along the middle of the forearm to the hand. In statistics the median is the number in the exact middle of a list of numbers representing values arranged in ascending or descending order.

mediastinum sounds like a near borrowing of the Latin *mediastinus*, but to the Romans this meant "a servant or a drudge." In anatomy the mediastinum is a partition between bilateral pleural cavities. Despite the apparent disparity in usage of the term, there is, in a way, a connection. The word is derived from a combination of the Latin *medius*, "middle," + *stare*, "to stand." The anatomic medi-

astinum can be said to "stand in the middle" of the thorax, while the servant "stands in the middle" when he acts as an intermediary for his master.

medicine is taken almost directly from the Latin *medicina*, which to the Romans meant almost the same as "medicine" means to us. This word, in turn, is related to *mederi*, "to heal." Both in ancient times and now, the same word—*medicina* or medicine—was and is used to refer both to the science of healing and to the means of healing, that is, what we also call "drugs." Although no scholarly authority makes the connection, one is tempted to think of the "medi-" in "medicine" as being related to the Latin *medius*, "middle," in the sense of "coming between," as in "mediator" and "medium." Surely the practitioner of medicine tries to intervene in a helpful way between the patient and his or her affliction.

medulla is the Latin word for "the marrow," in the sense of the core or central substance of anything, and is related to the Latin *medius*, "middle." Thus, the adrenal medulla is the "core" of the adrenal gland. Andreas Vesalius (1514-1564), the renowned Flemish anatomist who taught at Padua, also used the Latin *medulla* as a name for the spinal cord, taking his cue from the Greeks, who called it *myelos rachitēs*, "the marrow of the spine," presumably because the spinal cord occupies a channel within the spinal column. In the 18th century the term "medulla oblongata" (the latter word meaning "rather long") was limited in reference to that part of the brainstem extending from the pons to the spinal cord proper.

mega- is a combining form, used either as a prefix or incorporated in a suffix, derived from the Greek *megas*, "great or big." In Latin this became *magnus*. Thus, **megacardia** refers to an enlarged heart, **hepatomegaly** refers to an enlarged liver, and a **megacyte** is an abnormally large blood or tissue cell. (For **megakaryocyte**, *see* **thrombocyte**.) Today, one occasionally hears "mega" used as a separate adjective, as in "mega doses" (exceedingly large doses of any medication) or "mega workup" (an exceedingly extensive diagnostic investigation).

meiosis is a special type of cell division pertaining to the maturation of gametes or haploid reproductive cells. When the male and female gametes join, the newly formed nucleus receives half its complement of chromosomes from each of the parent cells. The resulting somatic cells of the offspring are thus normally diploid. *Meiosis* is Greek for "diminutive."

melan- is a combining form derived from the Greek *melas*, "black."

melancholy is a gloomy, depressed emotional state which, according to humoral pathology, was thought to result from an excess of "black bile" (melan- + Greek *cholē*, "bile").

melanin is the dark pigment that tints the skin, the hair, the choroid coat of the eye, and the substantia nigra ("black substance") of the brain (*see* melan).

melanuria is the passage of dark urine (melan + Greek *ouron*, "urine") that can be produced by a variety of substances, including blood, melanin, and homogentisic acid.

melena describes feces rendered tarry, in consistency as well as color, by its content of blood that has become black as it traverses the gut after internal bleeding. The term is taken from the Greek verb *melainein*, "to darken or grow black." (*see* **hemotochezia**)

melitensis (*see* **brucellosis**)

mellitus (*see* **diabetes**)

membrane comes from the Latin *membrana*, "a skin or parchment." This, in turn, has been thought to relate to the Latin *membrum*, "a member," in the sense of a part of the whole, as a limb is a "member" of the body. It was the *membrana* that covered and delineated a *membrum*. Later, "membrane" was applied to any skinlike covering or supporting tissue.

men- is a prefix taken from the Greek *mēn*, "a month," and *mēnē*, "the moon." The cyclic changes observed in the moon provided one of the earliest measures of time, about 29.5 days. Hence, a month is really a "moonth." In Latin a month is *mensis* (plural *menses*), and *menstruus* means "monthly."

meninges is the plural of the Greek *mēninx*, "a membrane," and the earliest writers used this term for membranes found anywhere in the body. Later, the term was restricted and used in the plural for the three membranes that envelop the brain and spinal cord.

meniscus is a near borrowing of the Greek *mēniskos*, "crescent-shaped." The root word, obviously, is the Greek *mēnē*, "moon." The capillary effect on fluid in a tube, such as a pipette, produces a concave or convex shape at the top of the fluid column; this is known as a "meniscus." The articulating cartilages at the proximal end of the tibia at the knee joint are crescent-shaped and, as such, were given the name "menisci."

menstruation and the adjective **menstrual** reflect the early observation that a woman's cyclic vaginal bleeding nearly coincides with the period of lunar phases (*see* men-). Colloquially, some women still refer to their "monthlies." Because these usually occur predictably, they are often called "periods." **Menorrhagia** (+ Greek *rhēgnymi*, "to burst forth") is an excessive vaginal bleeding that occurs at regular monthly intervals. (**Metrorrhagia** is uterine bleeding, usually prolonged and occurring at irregular intervals; here the "metro-" is taken from the Greek *mētra*, "the uterus.") **Menopause** (+ Greek *pausis*, "cessation") signals the end of a woman's menstruation and, hence, her fertility.

menstruum is a Medieval Latin word once used by alchemists to designate a solvent, and even today one occasionally hears of a solvent medium being so called, e.g., Pitkin menstruum, a medium for the administration of heparin. What has this to do with **menstruation**? In centuries past the product of uterine flow or *menstrua* (in classical Latin the neuter plural was always used) was fancied as the medium by which the male and female elements (i.e., the sperm and the ovum) were united, or "dissolved," into a single being that gained form as the fetus.

mental really represents two terms and can refer to the mind or to the chin, depending on which Latin word is considered the origin. In common and most frequent usage, "mental" refers to the mind and as such is derived from the Latin *mens*, "the mind or intellect." Just as properly, but in another sense, "mental" is derived from the Latin *mentum*, "the chin." The mental artery goes not to the brain but, as a branch of the maxillary artery, to the skin and subcutaneous tissues of the chin.

menthol is a common ingredient of liniments, a volatile oil that gives off a minty odor and lends a tang to the ambiance of locker rooms. The Latin word for mint is *mentha*, closely related to the Greek *mintha*. In Greek mythology Minthē was the name of a nymph who caught the roving eye of Pluto. In a fit of jealousy Proserpine, Pluto's wife, transformed the nymph into an herb that was then known by her name. The Reverend Cobham Brewer, writing a century ago, pointed out that as Pluto was, in his right, god of the underworld, Minthē was saved by her transformation—presumably "from a fate worse than death"—and thus became an agent of healing.

mercury is a metallic element, unique in being liquid at room temperature. Mercury is the name of a deity in Roman mythology (known to the Greeks as Hermes) who served as a celestial messenger, but more than that was, in his own right, god of science and commerce, patron of travelers and rogues, vagabonds, and thieves—a curious combination of interests. Probably because Mercury was thought of as swift and elusive in his duties his name was attached to the shiny, slippery substance that was long known as "quicksilver." To the Greeks the element was known as *hydrargyros*, combining *ydōr*, "water," + *argyros*, "silver," and from this comes the chemical symbol "Hg."

mercyism (*see* **rumination**)

mesen-, meso- are combining forms, usually appearing as prefixes, taken from the Greek *mesos*, "middle." Thus, the **mesencephalon** (+ Greek *enkephalos*, "brain") is the midbrain. The **mesenchyme** (+ Greek *enchyma*, "instillation") is that embryologic tissue, situated in the **mesoderm** (+ Greek *derma*, "skin"), the middle germ layer between the ectoderm and the entoderm, that gives rise to connective tissue and to constituents of the vascular and musculoskeletal systems. The **mesentery** (+ Greek *enteron*, "intestine") would seem to be the "middle intestine." This, of course, is not so. Rather, the Greek *enteron* originally referred to the viscera generally. The mesentery, then, is properly named as the supporting membrane situated in the midst of the viscera.

mesmerism is so called from Franz Mesmer (1734-1815), a Viennese doctor of medicine. The newly discovered properties of magnet-

ism had become popular at the time, and Mesmer evolved the theory that a similar force could exercise a profound effect on the human body. This supposed force, known as "animal magnetism," purportedly could be transferred from one person to another. The practice of summoning and exerting this force, widely promoted by Mesmer, was a form of hypnotism, thus "to mesmerize" became part of the language. Both Mesmer and mesmerism fell into disrepute when French authorities, commissioned to investigate the man and his method, issued an unfavorable report. (*see* **hypnosis**)

meta- is a Greek preposition that can mean "among, between"; "after, above, beyond"; or "by way of change." It is in these last two senses that "meta-" is incorporated in a host of scientific names.

metabolism is a contrived term, combining meta- + Greek *ballein*, "to throw," that was introduced in 1839 by Theodor Schwann (1810-1882), an eminent German anatomist and physiologist, to designate the chemical changes whereby nutriment is converted (or "thrown into a different position") to energy and living tissues.

metacarpal describes the small bones situated in the hand "beyond" the wrist (meta- + Greek *karpos*, "wrist"). Their counterparts in the foot are the **metatarsal** bones. The analogy may be apt, but the etymology is a bit off the mark. "Metatarsal" came into use much later than "metacarpal." The tarsal bones owe their name to the Greek *tarsos*, which means "a flat surface"; *tarsos podos* means "the flat of the foot." The metatarsal bones are situated beyond the tarsal bones, but they are not exactly beyond the flat of the foot.

metachromasia signifies a condition wherein certain abnormal cells appear to differ in color or intensity from their normal counterparts when treated with a given stain (meta- + Greek *chrōma*, "color").

metamorphosis is a change in configuration, as from a caterpillar into a butterfly (meta- + Greek *morphē*, "form").

metaplasia is a process whereby a change takes place "beyond" the normal adult form (meta- + Greek *plassein*, "to shape or to mold"), as when, in response to injury, gastric mucosa assumes a form resembling intestinal mucosa.

metastasis is a word used by the ancient Greeks to mean "removal from one place to another" (meta- + Greek *stasis*, "a placing"). The term was introduced into Late Latin to designate a shift of disease from one part of the body to another. Now it is used almost exclusively in reference to the spread of malignant neoplasms to sites distant from their primary source.

metatarsal (*see* **metacarpal**)

meteorism is the condition wherein the gut is distended by excessive gas, most of which is swallowed air. The term comes from the Greek *meteōros*, "suspended in midair or raised aloft." To the patient afflicted with meteorism, his abdomen feels as though it were a balloon. He may also feel as though he were about to take off, like a meteor.

meter (*see* **metric**)

methemoglobin is a term (wherein the "t" and the "h" are pronounced separately) that was introduced by Ernst Hoppe-Seyler (1825-1895), a German biochemist, for the change (thus the prefix "met-") that occurs in hemoglobin when its iron content has been oxidized from the ferrous to the ferric state, from which oxygen cannot be readily released.

methyl designates the radical CH_3 as a component of various organic compounds, a simple prototype substance being **methanol** (CH_3OH), originally called "wood alcohol," being first distilled from a woody substrate. The term "methyl" is attributed to Johann Jakob Berzelius (1779-1848), a Swedish chemist, who combined the Greek *methy*,

"wine," + *ulē*, "wood." Chemists were well grounded in classical languages in those days.

metr- is a combining form taken from the Greek *mētra*, "uterus." Thus, the **endometrium** is the lining of the uterus, the **myometrium** is the muscular wall of the uterus, and **metrorrhagia** (+ Greek *rhēgnymi*, "to flow from") is bleeding from the uterus at times other than regular menstruation.

metric is borrowed from the Greek *metron*, "a measure, rule, or standard." What we know as the metric system is a product of the French Revolution. Before this momentous political upheaval, no European country had any uniform system of measures or weights. In 1790 the revolutionary assembly charged the *Academie des Sciences* with the task of devising a sensible and universally usable system, which they completed in 1799. Except for minor corrections in later years, the basic concept remains. The genius of the system is that it is designed on a base of 10, i.e., it is a "decimal system," and its derived units can be calculated merely by shifting a decimal point. The entire system is based on only two "natural" units: the **meter**, as a measure of length (originally intended to be 1/10,000,000 the distance of the earth's surface from the equator to either pole), and the **gram**, as a measure of weight or mass (being that of pure water at maximum density, sufficient to fill a cube whose edges are 0.01 meter). All other units are therefrom derived. Some are named in the table below.

PREFIX	ABBREVIATION	DERIVATION	POWER OF 10	EQUIVALENT
tera-	T	Greek *teras*, "monster"	10^{12}	trillion
giga-	G	Greek *gigas*, "giant"	10^9	billion
mega-	M	Greek *megas*, "large"	10^6	million
kilo-	k	Greek *chilioi*, "thousand"	10^3	thousand
hecto-	h	Greek *hekaton*, "hundred"	10^2	hundred
deca-	da	Greek *deka*, "ten"	10^1	ten
deci-	d	Latin *decimus*, "a tenth"	10^{-1}	one tenth
centi-	c	Latin *centum*, "a hundredth"	10^{-2}	one hundredth
milli-	m	Latin *millesimus*, "a thousandth"	10^{-3}	one thousandth
micro-	μ	Greek *mikros*, "small"	10^{-6}	one millionth
nano-	n	Greek *nanos*, "dwarf"	10^{-9}	one billionth
pico-	p	Italian *pico*, "small"	10^{-12}	one trillionth
femto-	f	Danish *femten*, "fifteen"	10^{-15}	one quadrillionth

metrorrhagia (*see* **menstruation**)

miasma is a direct borrowing of the Greek word for a supposedly noxious vapor arising from contaminated soil and thereby the cause of disease endemic to certain areas. Miasma was once thought to be the cause of **malaria**. When the true cause of malaria and similar afflictions became known, the concept of miasma fell into disrepute. The term is thought to be outmoded, but perhaps it can be revived and again found useful in the light of recently evident environmental concerns.

micro- is a combining form, usually used as a prefix, that is a near borrowing of the Greek *mikros*, "small, petty, trivial." The number of medical terms incorporating "micro-" is not small.

microbe is a concoction of micro- + the Greek *bios*, "life," proposed in the late 19th century to designate any minute, living organism.

microscope is a term said to have been invented in 1628 by Johannes Faber (1574-1629) by combining micro- + Greek *skopein*, "to view." Faber's offering surely was an improvement on *vitrum pulicare*, "flea glass," as the earliest lenses were known by those fascinated by a magnified view of scurrying fleas. A **microtome** (micro- + Greek *tomē*, "a cutting") is an instrument for cutting ultrathin sections of tissue for examination under a microscope.

microvilli (*see* **villus**)

micturate (*see* **urine**)

midwifery refers to the performance of a midwife, a person who assists a woman at childbirth. The name is an Anglo-Saxon combination of *mid-*, "together with," + *wif*, "a woman." A midwife, therefore, can be of either sex. The one who is being assisted is the wife, not the one who is assisting. In current and common parlance, a midwife is a nurse or other practitioner specially trained and experienced in attending women at childbirth. But many years ago in some medical schools the head of the obstetrics department held the title "professor of midwifery."

migraine is a common and severe head pain that has been long recognized as typically occurring on only one side of the head at a time. The term began as the Latin *hemicrania* which was derived from the Greek *hēmi-*, "half," + *kranion*, "the skull." In Medieval Latin this was shortened to *migraena* and

came into French as *migraine*.

miliary is often used in descriptive pathology to describe lesions that are of the size of millet seeds, e.g., those of "miliary" tuberculosis. But how many doctors have ever seen a millet seed? Millet is a cereal grass cultivated through the centuries for food and fodder. Its seed is about 2 millimeters in diameter. The Latin word for millet is *milium*, hence the derived adjective. **Miliaria** is a skin eruption characterized by numerous papules, approximately the size of millet seeds. It is caused by abnormal retention of fluid in sweat glands and often is marked by extravasation of sweat into adjacent layers of the skin, with attendant inflammatory reaction. (*see* **sudamen**)

minim was formerly used in pharmacy and therapeutics as the term for "a small drop." It came from the Latin *minimus*, "the smallest or the least." Small doses of liquid medicines were prescribed in minims. It became obvious that all drops are not of the same size, and in the mid-19th century the London College of Physicians defined a "minim" as $1/60$ of a dram or $1/480$ of a fluid ounce. Today, some liquid medicines are dispensed with their own standard dropper to ensure a proper dose.

miosis (*see* **mydriasis**)

mithidratism is the technique of inducing immunity to the effects of a poison by administering at first minute amounts and then gradually increasing the doses of the poisonous substance. This is somewhat akin to desensitizing an allergic person by injecting increasing amounts of the antigen that causes the reaction. The term is taken from the name of Mithridates, king of Pontus, an ancient country bordering on the Black Sea. As a precaution against being poisoned Mithridates cautiously and diligently conditioned himself to the effects of some noxious substance (which one is not known). As it turned out, Mithridates was defeated in war and captured by the Roman general Pompey in 67 B.C. To evade the ignominy of his plight, Mithridates tried to commit suicide by taking poison but failed. As a last resort he bid his slave run him through with a sword. So much, then, for being excessively cautious.

mitochondrium is a combination of the Greek

mitos, "a thread," + *chondros*, "a cereal grain" or any coarsely granular substance. The term was introduced in 1902 by Karl Benda (1857-1933), a German physician, as a name for the granular structures with threadlike membranes found in the cytoplasm of cells.

mitosis was suggested in 1882 as a term for cell division by Walther Flemming (1843-1905), a German cytologist. The term was taken from the Greek *mitos*, "a thread," the allusion being to the threadlike formation of nuclear chromatin as it becomes conspicuous in a cell prepared to divide.

mitral as a descriptive term for the bicuspid valve between the left atrium and ventricle of the heart is so used because the two cusps of the valve resemble a bishop's miter or headdress. The Latin *mitra* referred to a cloth band that could be worn either as a girdle or as a snood or headband. These terms perhaps are related to the Greek *mitos*, "a thread," as in woven cloth.

mnemonic comes from the Greek *mnēme*, "memory." Mnemonics is the art of improving memory, and mnemonic devices are those that aid in recollection. Medical students through the ages, required to commit to memory a vast store of information, have been among the cleverest users of mnemonic devices. (An example is given in the entry for **carpal**.) The problem is that sometimes one remembers the mnemonic device but forgets what it represents. An **amamnesis** (+ Greek *ana-*, "again") is a recollection and a word that can serve as a fancy term for a medical history, as opposed to a **catamnesis** (+ Greek *kata-*, "back down"), which is a retrospective follow-up history.

moiety comes by way of the French *moitié* from the Latin *medietas*, "the middle or the mean." Originally, "moiety" meant "half," but now it can refer to any designated portion, e.g., the carbohydrate moiety of a glycoprotein.

molar is the name for a tooth that grinds. It comes from the Latin *mola*, "millstone." Thus, the molar teeth are distinguished from the incisor teeth, which are designed for a different purpose. Ask anyone whose molar teeth have been extracted how well he can chew with only front teeth.

mole can mean a number of things: a dark spot on the skin, a uterine mass, a chemical mass,

a breakwater or pier, or a small burrowing animal. The mole of the skin comes from the Gothic *mail*, "a wrinkle or blemish." The mole that is a fleshy mass forming in the uterus as a result of degeneration or abortive development of an embedded ovum comes from the Latin *moles*, "a mass or pile." From this same Latin source comes "mole" as a word for the massive pile of stone forming a breakwater or pier and also for the term designating the mass in grams of a chemical compound numerically equivalent to its molecular weight. In this last instance we have the odd sequence of a standard term converted to its diminutive, then back again to its standard form. From the Latin *moles* came "molecule," which was then abbreviated as "mole."

molecule is taken almost directly from the New Latin *molecula*, the diminutive of *moles*, "mass," i.e., a mass of exceedingly small size.

molluscum as in molluscum contagiosum comes from the Latin *mollis*, "soft or spongy." Originally, the Latin *molluscum* referred to a soft fungus growing on trees, and also to a sort of nut with a soft shell. The phylum Mollusca includes snails, squids, and octopuses. To **mollify** is to soften or smooth, and **mollycoddle** means to pamper or make soft. Somehow the image of mollycoddling an octopus does not readily come to mind. In pathology **molluscum contagiosum** is a spongy excrescence of the skin caused by a transmissible virus.

monad in biology is a single-celled organism, particularly a primitive protozoan. A **pseudomonad** is any of the ubiquitous, rod-shaped, gram-negative, flagellated bacteria of the phylum Pseudomonad, commonly found in dank soil or decaying matter. The name was given, supposedly, to distinguish these organisms from monads or protozoans previously described. Included in this phylum is the genus *Pseudomonas*, certain species of which are pathogenic and often recognized as a cause of opportunistic infection in humans.

mongolism (*see* **idiot**)

moniliasis is an exudative inflammation of the skin or mucous membranes consequent to infection by the fungus *Candida albicans* (and, in some quarters, better known as "candidiasis"). The genus in which the fungus is classified was known formerly as *Monilia*, this name being taken from the Latin *monile*, "a necklace." Under a microscope the organism appears arrayed as a string of beads. The speckled white exudate, especially as it occurs in the mouth or throat, has long been commonly referred to as **thrush**. Possibly, this is an allusion to the speckled throat and breast of a familiar songbird, the thrush. The disease known as **sprue** gets that name from the Dutch *spruw* or *sprouw*, as the monilia-induced thrush is called in Holland. The connection is that patients afflicted with sprue can become severely debilitated and thus liable to infection by the monilial fungus.

mono- is a prefix derived from the Greek *monos*, "single," and denotes reference to one thing or part, especially a basic unit. A **mononuclear cell** contains a single nuclear clump. Occasionally, one hears "mono" as a nickname for the disease known as infectious **mononucleosis**.

monoclonal (*see* **hybridoma**)

monomania is a psychosis limited to a single delusion (mono- + the Greek word for "madness").

monster is sometimes construed as being related to "huge," but its use in reference to size reflects only a subsidiary meaning. In mythology a monster is a fabled creature that hideously combines animal and human forms. In pathology a monster is an infant born with a grotesque anomaly, such as an absence or excess of limbs or other misshapen form. Whatever its use, "monster" comes from the Latin *monstrum*, "a divine omen, portent, or warning," this being related to the verb *monere*, "to warn." Fortunately, the belief has long dissipated that delivery of a deformed infant is a sign of divine wrath.

mons veneris is the rounded prominence covering the pubic arch just above the female external genitalia. *Mons* is Latin for "hill or mountain"; *veneris* refers to Venus, the Roman goddess of love and whatever may appertain thereto. (*see* **venereal**)

morbid is an adjective derived from the Latin *morbus*, "sickness or disease." What we now call "pathology" formerly was known as "morbid anatomy."

mordant describes a substance used to intensify the staining of tissue sections for microscopy. Examples include alum, aniline, certain oils, and phenol. The term is taken from the Latin *mordere*, "to bite."

morgue is the French name originally used for a place where captured prisoners were first examined, then later for a place where the bodies of persons recently dead could be viewed and identified; it is not related to the Latin *mors*, death. The term comes from the Old French verb *morguer*, "to regard solemnly." Knowing the derivation of "morgue" can remind us of the proper demeanor when attending a necropsy.

moribund is a near borrowing of the Latin *moribundus*, "at the point of death." The Latin word is equivalent to the verb *mori*, "to die," + *bundus*, an adjectival suffix meaning "tending to or bound for."

moron is a term codified about 1905 by two Frenchmen, Alfred Binet and Theodore Simon (a physiologist and a physician, respectively), who were charged by the authorities responsible for the care of the feebleminded with the task of devising tests to determine the levels of mental retardation. According to the Binet-Simon scale, the mental ages of retarded adults are: 1 to 2 years, "idiot"; 3 to 7 years, "imbecile"; and 8 to 12 years, "moron." Perhaps Binet and Simon were inspired in their choice of the last term by their compatriot, the 17th-century French playwright Molière, who gave the name Moron to the fool in one of his plays. In any event, the name can be traced to the Greek *moros*, "dull, sluggish, slow in wit."

morphine is the name given to the principal alkaloid of opium in 1805 by a German apothecary, Adolf Serturner (1783-1841), doubtless inspired by an acquaintance with Morpheus, the mythologic god of dreams. In the parlance of show business, Morpheus "created, designed, and produced" nocturnal fantasies. The Greek word *morphē* is cited under **morphology**.

morphology combines the Greek *morphē*, "form, shape, or appearance," + *logos*, "a discourse." In biology "morphology" properly refers to a study or treatise on the form or structure of an organism or its parts, as contrasted with physiology, a study of its function. Whatever is

amorphous is without shape or form.

mortal means subject to death, in contrast to **immortal**. Somatic cells are inexorably mortal, whereas reproductive cells are potentially immortal. "Mortal" comes from the Latin *mors*, "death." This brings to mind several similar words. **Fatal** (from Latin *fatum*, "prophecy or doom") means capable of causing death or disaster. One can speak of "a fatal mistake" without necessarily implying a consequence of death. **Deadly** means capable of killing, as in "a deadly disease." **Lethal** describes an agent of death and is derived from the Latin *lefum*, "death or destruction" (not from the Latin *lethe*, "forgetfulness," the source of **lethargy**).

mortar (*see* pestle; *also* **trituration**)

morula is the diminutive of the Latin *morum*, "a berry," usually a mulberry or a blackberry. As an allusion to its berrylike shape, the cluster of blastomeres formed by cleavage of a fertilized ovum is called a "morula."

mosquito (*see* **Anopheles**)

mountebank is an epithet for a quack doctor and comes from the Italian *montambanco*, related to a combination of *montare*, "to mount," + *banco*, "bench," literally "one who mounts a bench" to proclaim his nostrums. If what a mountebank had to say carried the weight of truth, he wouldn't have to make such a fuss about it.

mucosa is a convenient shortening of the Latin *membrana mucosa*, which refers to any membrane or surface made slimy by a covering of mucus. (*see* **mucus**)

mucus is the Latin word for "a semifluid, slimy discharge from the nose." The Greek *muktēr* is "the nose or snout." Incidentally, the colloquial, vulgar term "snot" comes from "snout," literally. In current usage "mucus" designates a clear, viscid fluid exuded from any epithelial surface. Some people, slipshod in their spelling, tend to confuse "mucus" (the noun) and "mucous" (the adjective).

multi- is a combining form, usually a prefix, that comes from the Latin adjective *multus*, "many or abundant." The medical terms so formed are, indeed, multiple. One example is **multipara** (+ Latin *parere*, "to give birth to"), the term for a woman who has given birth to more than one child.

mumps probably is related to the Icelandic *mum-pa*, "to eat greedily, to fill the mouth too full." A major feature of mumps is visible swelling of the parotid glands, and this makes the afflicted person appear to have a large mouthful. A related word is **mumble**, meaning to speak indistinctly, as if one's mouth were full of marbles. However, "mumps" also has been attributed to the Old English verb *to mump*, which meant to appear sulky or sullen. This, too, could describe the countenance of a patient with mumps.

Münchhausen syndrome was so named by Dr. Richard Asher (*Lancet.* 1951;1:35), an exceptionally perceptive and articulate English physician, to describe the startling and often bizarre presentation by arch-malingerers who feign catastrophic illness by citing all sorts of outlandish and improbable symptoms. Baron Karl Friedrich Hieronymous von Münchhausen (1720-1797), a German soldier, adventurer, and extravagant raconteur, became the protagonist of a further embellished narrative of impossible adventures, written in English in 1785, by Rudolf Eric Raspe, a German author. In 1850 the word "Münchhausenism," meaning exaggerated tales, was applied to the writings of Herodotus, the ancient Greek historian.

murmur is a Latin as well as an English word and has the same meaning in both languages. To the Romans *murmur* also could mean "growling or rumbling." A related word is the Sanskrit *marmaras*, "noisy, as the rustling wind." The onomatopoeic quality of the word is enhanced by its reduplication of sounds. When French clinicians in the early 19th century described what they heard from the heart, all sounds were called by the French word *bruit*. It was Joseph Skoda (1805-1881), an Austrian physician, who clearly distinguished normal heart tones from adventitious murmurs.

Murphy's law is often cited in medical circles, in one or another of its several versions: (*a*) nothing is as easy as it appears; (*b*) any job will take longer than you think; or (*c*) if anything can go wrong, it will. The last version is heard most often. Strange to say, no one knows who Murphy is or if there ever was an actual Murphy. According to Robert T. Nagler, as quoted by William and Mary Morris in their *Dictionary of Word and Phrase*

Origins (New York, NY: Harper & Row; 1977), "Murphy's laws were not propounded by Murphy but by another man of the same name (the first law); and although I have spent many years at the task, I have been able to discover nothing about the life and career of this great philosopher (the second law)." Nagler concludes that Murphy may have been the fellow who undertook one evening to stroll along a deserted country lane, taking the precaution to walk on the left side of the road so as to face oncoming traffic, then was struck down by a motorist from England who had just arrived that day in this country (the third law).

muscarinic refers to the parasympathomimetic action of certain cholinergic agonists. The origin of the term is in the Latin *musca*, "a fly." The prototype is **muscarine**, a natural alkaloid isolated in 1869 from a species of poisonous mushroom called *Amanita muscaria*. *Amanita* is an ancient Greek name for a kind of fungus; *muscaria* refers to its hairy appearance. The Latin *muscarium* means, literally, "pertaining to flies," but to the Romans a *muscarium* was specifically a sort of flyswatter made up of hairs from a horse's tail. If a horse can get rid of flies with a flick of his tail, the Romans could follow suit. So, the hairy mushroom that looked a little like a flyswatter was found to contain a poisonous alkaloid that was given the name of the flyswatter.

muscle comes from the Latin *musculus*, the diminutive of *mus*, "a mouse," hence, literally, "a little mouse." The use of *musculus* for muscle, and that is what it meant to the Romans, is usually explained by the allusion to rippling of muscles under the skin as the scurrying of little mice; or perhaps it was fancied that the shape of dissected muscles resembled that of small rodents. This may seem farfetched, but the fact is that pre-Galenic anatomists had little knowledge of the function of muscles. Indeed, Plato and Aristotle, among other ancient authorities, conceived of muscular tissue as simply another form of flesh serving as a cover for the body. This brings us to two Greek words: *mys* means both "mouse" and "a muscle of the body," while *myō*, a different word, means "I close," especially the lips and the

eyes, thus implying a muscular function. The combining form **myo-** may be owed to either of these Greek words.

mutation is derived from the Latin *mutare*, "to move, shift, change, or alter." In biology a **mutant** is an offspring whose **phenotype** ("pheno-" comes from the Greek *phainein*, "to show"), or outward expression of its heredity, differs from that normally expected of its **genotype** ("geno-" comes from the Greek *gennaō*, "I produce"), or genetic disposition of its parents. The genetic theory of mutation was advanced in 1886 by Hugo de Vries (1848-1935), a Dutch botanist. Previous to de Vries' explanation, such aberrant individuals were recognized but poorly understood and were called "sports." **Sport** is a contraction of the Middle English *disporter*, "to amuse oneself, as from being removed from labor." This, in turn, is derived from the Latin *dis-*, "away," + *portare*, "to carry." This accounts for "sport" as a diverting game and for "sport" as a mutant; in both there is a sense of being "carried away."

mycelium comes from the Greek *mykēs*, "fungus," + *hēlos*, "an ornamental nail or stud." Presumably, the array of fungal filaments or **mycelia** was thought to resemble a collection of decorative nails. The combining prefixes **myc-**, **myco-**, and **mycet-** appear in a number of biologic terms and denote a relationship to fungus.

mydriasis is a Latin term meaning an unnatural dilatation of the pupil of the eye. Such a dilatation can be induced by an anticholinergic drug, such as atropine, or by an intense, endogenous, adrenergic (sympathomimetic) stimulus. The latter phenomenon could explain the origin of the term in the Greek *mydros*, "a red-hot mass." The Greek phrase *mydrous airein cheroin* can be translated as "to grasp masses of red-hot iron," as an ordeal. Surely under such trying circumstances the pupils of the eyes would be dilated. In contrast, **miosis** is an excessive contraction of the pupil of the eye, the term being a near borrowing of the Greek *meiōsis*, "a lessening." This is in no way related or connected to "myopia" or nearsightedness.

myelin (*see* **myelo**)

myelo- is a combining form taken from the Greek *myelos*, "the marrow or inmost core."

In medicine this can refer either to the marrow of bone or to the "marrow" of the central nervous system, viz., the brain, the peripheral nerves, and especially the spinal cord. It is easy to conceive of bone marrow as the core of hollow bones. But the application of the term to the central nervous system is more difficult to appreciate unless one looks at these structures through the eyes of ancient observers. Then, the spinal cord might appear to be the **marrow** of the spinal canal, and the brain the marrow of the skull. By tradition, therefore, **myelitis** can be either an inflammation of the spinal cord or an inflammation within bone (though the latter is usually qualified as **osteomyelitis**). **Myelophthisis** (myelo- + Greek *phthisis*, "a wasting") can be either degeneration of the spinal cord or withering of cellular production in bone marrow. On the other hand, **myeloma** (+ Greek *-ōma*, "tumor") is restricted as a designation for neoplasia arising in constituents of bone marrow, not of nervous tissue. But sometimes tradition persists despite logic. What we call **myelin** is actually the substance of a fatty sheath covering nerve fibers and clearly not the core of nerve tracts.

mylohyoid is a muscle whose name tells us that it extends from the lower jaw to the hyoid bone. The first part, "mylo-," comes from the Greek *mylē*, "a mill" (the lower jaw is part of a mill wherein the teeth are grinders). "Hyoid" is a Greek way of saying "U-shaped," and that describes the hyoid bone.

myo- is a prefix denoting a relation to muscle and can define a structure (as in "myocardium" or "myometrium") or tell the origin of a substance (as in "myoglobin"). **Myotonia** is a spastic condition of skeletal muscle (myo- + Greek *tonus*, "tension").

myopia is the technical term for nearsightedness and, as such, is a somewhat special case. This clearly is a combination of the Greek *myō*, "I close," + *ōps* (the "ps" being the Greek letter *psi*), which means "the eye." This adds up to "shut eye." Observe the nearsighted person as he tries, without glasses, to look at a distant object. He squints. It is the squint or closing of the lids that suggested the term "myopia."

myringo- is a combining form taken from the Late Latin *myringa* that appeared as a term for the eardrum or tympanic membrane, probably as a corruption of the Greek *mēninx*, "membrane." Although there are many membranes in the body, the combining form "myringo-" in medical parlance refers only to the **tympanic membrane** of the ear.

myringotomy is the operation of incising the eardrum (myringo- + Greek *tomē*, "a cutting"). It is said this operation was introduced by a Parisian quack doctor as a remedy for deafness, presumably to let sound gain easier access to the ear. Only later did myringotomy gain respectable status as a means of providing drainage for suppurative collections in the middle ear.

myxedema is contrived by combining the Greek *myxa*, "mucus," originally used in reference to the discharge from the nose, + *oidēma*, "a swelling up." It was Sir William Gull (1816-1890), an English physician, who first described in 1873 the peculiar swelling of subcutaneous tissue associated with thyroid insufficiency, as observed in a "cretinoid state" in adults. In 1877 William Ord (1834-1902), an English surgeon, proposed the term "myxoedema" (the British spelling) for this "mucoid dropsy."

Nape has served since the Middle Ages as a term for the back of the **neck**. Perhaps it can be traced to the Old German *noppe*, "to pluck," insofar as the back of the neck is a convenient place to grab and hold a man or animal. Sometimes we refer to the "scruff of the neck." "Scruff" comes from the Gothic *skruft*, "hair of the head." Alternatively, "nape" could be related to the Old Frisian *hals-knap*, "the bump on the neck," and the Anglo-Saxon *cnaep*, "the top of the hill" (from which also comes "knob"). Whether "nape" originally referred to the external occipital protuberance at the posterior base of the skull or to the protuberant spine of the seventh cervical vertebrae is uncertain. The anatomic adjective **nuchal** is derived from the Arabic *nukha'*, "the back of the neck."

narcissism is taken from the name of the mythologic Narcissus, son of Cephisus, the river god, and the nymph Liriope. Narcissus was a handsome but heedless youth, much taken with himself, who attracted then shunned the woodland nymphs. One forsaken nymph prayed that Narcissus would himself learn how it felt to be spurned. And so he did. One day, kneeling by a sylvan pond, Narcissus saw his own reflection mirrored in the placid water. Not recognizing the image as his own but imagining it to be a gorgeous inhabitant of the pond, he reached out to embrace the reflection. With the water thus disturbed the image disappeared, only to return when the water was still. The more he looked, the more Narcissus became enamored of his own visage; the more often the figure eluded his grasp, the more frustrated he became. And thus Narcissus languished and

died, shunned by his own image. His place at the edge of the pond was taken by a lovely white flower that is still known by his name. Psychiatrists refer to narcissism as a warped sexual attraction to oneself.

narcosis comes from the Greek *narkē*, "numbness or torpor." A narcotic drug is one that numbs or induces torpor. **Narcolepsy**, combining "narco-" + the Greek *lēpsis*, "a seizure," is the term used for a condition marked by sudden, uncontrollable compulsion to sleep.

nares is the Latin plural term for the paired external openings to the nasal cavity. If you wish to use the Latin word for just one nostril, it is the singular *naris*. **Nasal** is an adjectival formation taken from the Latin *nasus*, "the nose." To the Romans *nasus* always meant the external nose or snout, but now "nasal" refers to whatever pertains to the nose, inner as well as outer.

nausea is an almost direct borrowing of the Greek *nausia*, "seasickness." Quite logically this comes from the Greek *naus*, "ship," which also yields "nautical" and, by way of the Latin *navis*, "navy." Only later did "nausea" acquire the broader meaning of that disagreeably queasy feeling that often precedes vomiting, such as can occur on land and in the air as well as at sea.

navel is an ancient word, traceable in various forms through all Teutonic languages, with the same meaning today. The Anglo-Saxon *nafe* was the center or hub of a wheel where the axle was inserted; its diminutive *nafela* was the name given to the belly button, probably because it looked like a "little hub" and was situated in the center of the abdomen. (However, "nave" as the central part of a church is derived from the Latin *navis*, "a ship.") To the Greeks the navel was *omphalos* (from which we take our combining form **omphalo-**, "pertaining to the navel") and to the Romans it was **umbilicus**, the anatomic term we use as a noun today.

navicular is taken from the diminutive of the Latin *navis*, "a ship," hence "a little ship." Early anatomists used "navicular" for any structure they fancied to have a shiplike shape. The navicular bone in the wrist was so named. But some classically minded anatomists preferred the Greek, so they called it the **scaphoid** bone (from *skaphē*, "a light boat or skiff," + *eidos*, "like").

neck comes by way of the Middle English *nekke* from the Anglo-Saxon *hnecca*, originally "the nape of the neck" (*see* **nape**). Whereas we now think of the neck as the entire structure interposed between the head and the torso, the original term referred to the back or nape of the neck. The Teutonic *hnakkon* conveyed the sense of a projection, as in the Gaelic *cnoc*, "hill."

necropsy is the proper term for postmortem examination and should be used rather than "autopsy" (*see* **autopsy**). The Greeks did not have a word like "necropsy," but they would have understood the term, taken as it is from the Greek *nekros,* "corpse" + *opsis,* "a viewing"; hence, literally, "an inspection of a dead body." The Germans render it *Leichenbeschauung,* "a corpse-beholding or corpse-showing."

necrosis is a transliterated borrowing of the Greek *nekrosis,* "becoming dead," from *nekros,* "a dead body or corpse." In pathology necrosis is the lethal degeneration of cells or tissues rather than death of the entire organism; also, necrosis implies an induced degeneration rather than a natural dissolution of spent cells, which is known as **apoptosis**.

negative (*see* **positive**)

nematode is a name by which certain round worms are known, concocted from a combination of the Greek *nēma,* "a thread," + *eidos,* "like," hence "threadlike." The Nematoidea is a multitudinous order of intestinal worms characterized, in most species, by an intricate, threadlike alimentary tract. The reference, then, is not to the shape of the worm but to the worm's own innards.

neo- is a combining term, usually a prefix, taken from the Greek *neos,* "new, young, fresh, or recent." The prefix serves a variety of medical terms. In neuroanatomy it designates those structures that are considered to represent more recent, advanced evolution, e.g., the neopallium and the neothalamus. "Neo-" is sometimes added to the tradenames of drugs to convey the idea that something new (and presumably better) is being purveyed.

neoplasm means literally "new growth" (neo- + Greek *plasma,* "that which is formed") but in the sense that the abnormal proliferation is among cells that have reverted to a primordial or "young" configuration; the implication is not that the tumor or growth itself is recent.

nephro- denotes that which pertains to the kidney and is taken from *nephros,* the Greek word for that organ. Although the Greek term is used as a combining form, the Latin *renes* is the source of the adjective **renal**. To the Greeks **nephritis** would have been any kidney condition (*see* **-itis**), whereas we have restricted the term to denote an inflammatory disease. Similarly, **nephrosis** to the Greeks would have meant simply "pertaining to the *nephros,*" whereas to us it means any noninflammatory, nonneoplastic disease of the kidney. The surgical excision of a kidney is **nephrectomy** (nephr- + Greek *ektomē,* "a cutting out").

nephrolithiasis is the presence of concrements in the kidney (nephro- + Greek *lithos,* "stone").

nephrosclerosis describes a degenerative process, usually of vascular origin, that is marked by pervasive scarring or "hardening" of the kidney (nephro- + Greek *sklēros,* "hard").

nerve is descended from the Greek *neuron* and the Latin *nervus,* both of which have physical and metaphysical meanings. The Greek and Latin terms, in a physical sense, mean "a sinew, tendon, thong, string (as a bowstring), or wire." But in a metaphysical sense the terms also mean a sort of "strength, force, or energy." Our word "nerve" is used in a dual sense, too. There is a big difference when we say, "He has nerves" (an unlikely, superfluous remark, inasmuch as we all possess these structures) and when we say, "He has nerve!" or "He is nervous." (There was a time when "nervous" was used to indicate a capacity for sensibility or sensitivity, as in the 18th century when the Rev. Dr. Douglas, bishop of Salisbury, defended Samuel Johnson as "an elegant and nervous writer.") In ancient anatomy, the Greek *neuron* was used as a name for any white, cordlike structure; thus, tendons and nerves were confused (and this confusion persists in what we still call an **aponeurosis**). Aristotle and Galen were among the first to restrict *neuron* to the nerves. The Greek word gives us our noun **neuron**, any conducting cell of the nervous system, as well as **neuro-**, a combining form that designates anything pertaining to nerves. Just as the ancient Greeks and Romans usually did not distinguish bandlike structures, so tendon, ligament, and nerve were encompassed by the Anglo-Saxon *sionu*, the origin of our modern English **sinew**. Present-day cognates include the German *Sehne* and Danish *sene*, both meaning "tendon," whereas the Dutch *zenuw* means "nerve."

neuron (*see* **nerve**)

neuter (*see* **female**)

neutrophil combines the Latin *neuter*, "neither," + the Greek *philos*, "fondness or affinity." This hybrid term, meaning literally "fond of neither," was given by Paul Ehrlich (1854-1915), the renowned German microbiologist, to those blood corpuscles that appeared attracted neither to the acidic stains (as were the oxyphils or eosinophils) nor to the basic stains (as were the basophils). Neutrophils have an affinity for neither. If Ehrlich had been as strict a linguist as he was a cytologist, he would have stuck with Latin and called his cell a "neutramor" or "neutraffin," but he wasn't, and didn't, and neither do we.

nevus is a near borrowing of the Latin *naevus*, "a body mole, especially a birthmark." It has been suggested that the word is related to the Latin *nativus*, "inborn or congenital." Certain moles or blemishes, particularly the striking vascular lesions, are clearly evident at birth, and it is logical they would be so named.

nicotine is so called after the name of a French ambassador to Portugal, Jean Nicot, Sieur de Villemain (1530-1600), who was presented with a sample of tobacco seeds brought from the New World by Portuguese sailors. The genus of the plant was named *Nicotiana* in his honor. In 1560 he literally planted the seeds of the tobacco industry in France and thus achieved immortality of a sort. In the latter years of the 19th century physiologists observed that the alkaloid nicotine in small initial doses stimulated, then in larger subsequent doses blockaded autonomic ganglia and the endplates of

skeletal muscle. This is exhibited also by acetylcholine and has been termed the "nicotinic effect."

nightmare is readily understood in its first part, "night," but what about the "mare"? This has nothing to do with a female horse, but rather comes from the Anglo-Saxon *maere*, an imaginary demon or evil spirit said to descend on sleeping persons. More specifically, a *maere* was conceived as a male demon intent on having his way with a sleeping woman. The Romans, too, had a word for a nightmare, and it was *incubus*, from the Latin verb *incubare*, "to lie upon." Incubus also came to be the name of a male demon given to nocturnal visitations with sleeping women. A female demon of similar proclivity was known as Succuba, her name being taken from the Latin *succubare*, "to lie under."

nigra is the feminine adjectival derivative of the Latin *niger*, "black, dark, or swarthy." Thus, the substantia niger is a layer of dark, pigmented substance separating the tegmentum from the cerebral peduncles in the brain. **Nigricans** means "of a dark hue, almost black." (*see* **acanthosis**)

nihilism is derived from the Latin *nihilum*, "nothing, not a bit of," this being a combination of *ni*, "not," + *hilum*, "a trifle." The term refers to an attitude of despair, assumed by almost all doctors at one time or another when no remedy seems available. This is "therapeutic nihilism." On occasion such an approach can be of benefit to the patient when he is spared the possible adverse effect of **nostrums**. Writing at a time when the dangerous use of nostrums was prevalent, Oliver Wendell Holmes (1809-1894), the noted Boston physician and savant, put it well: "I firmly believe that if the whole materia medica, as now used, could be sunk to the bottom of the sea, it would be better for mankind—and all the worse for the fishes." Happily, we now practice our art in a more enlightened era when, for most conditions, safe and effective therapy is at hand. But even now, on occasion, a little therapeutic nihilism—and a little less therapeutic hubris—can serve us well.

nipple is the derived diminutive of the Anglo-Saxon *neb* or *nib*, "a beak or nose," hence literally "a little beak." It is not farfetched to imagine the pigmented projective of the breast as "a little beak." The word "nibble," meaning to peck away at, comes from the same source.

nitrogen can be traced through the French *nitre* to the Latin *nitrum*, the Greek *nitron*, and the Hebrew *nether*, all of these being related to the Latin *natron* and the Arabic *natrun*. In ancient times *nitrum* and *natron* were sometimes used interchangeably for any sort of chemical salt that was used as a cleanser. The actual chemical constituents of these salts were unknown in those days. Probably *natron* was often a crude sodium carbonate, whereas *nitron* may have been saltpeter (potassium nitrate). It was not until the 18th century that the distinction between sodium and potassium became clear. The name "natron" was then assigned to sodium carbonate and "nitron" to the nitrate. Meanwhile, the gas we know as nitrogen was identified as a constituent of air in 1772 by Daniel Rutherford (1749-1819), a Scottish physician, who called it "mephitic [noxious] air." To Joseph Priestley (1733-1804), the noted English clergyman, author, and chemist, the residue after removing oxygen from air was "dephlogisticated air" ("phlogiston" being a supposed substance released during combustion but now known to be nonexistent). To early French chemists this residue was known as *azote* (from the Greek *a-*, "not," + *zoein*, "to live") because it was found not to support life. They had observed that when a lighted candle and a mouse were both placed in a sealed glass jar, and the oxygen was consumed in the flame of the candle, the candlelight was extinguished, and the mouse expired. From *azote* comes the medical term **azotemia**, meaning an accumulation of nitrogen in the blood. Finally, Henry Cavendish (1731-1810) found that the same gas as azote could be produced from nitre (potassium nitrate); hence, it was given the name "nitrogen," concocted from nitro- + the Greek *genos*, "a descendent."

nociceptor combines elements of the Latin adjective *nocens*, "injurious" and the Latin verb *capere*, "to capture" in order to denote a neural sensory cell that signals tissue injury, particularly that which initiates a pain impulse. (*see* **proprioception**)

node is a near borrowing of the Latin *nodus*, "a knot or a knob," this being probably related to the Sanskrit *gandh*, "to grasp" (from which "handle" descends). Surely a subcutaneous bump, be it bone, scar, or lymph node, could feel like a knotted rope or the knot in the wood of a tree. If the bump was small, it was called by the diminutive **nodule**, "a little knot."

nomenclature is taken from the Latin *nomenclator*, "a name caller," this being a combination of *nomen*, "name," + *clamare*, "to proclaim." In Roman times a *nomenclator* (the poet Martial used a variant spelling, *nomenculator*) was a servant or slave who accompanied his master and identified those whom they met, especially during a political campaign. It is hoped this small volume can serve the reader as well, by helping to identify words encountered in the pursuit of medicine.

nondisease is a term introduced in 1965 by C. K. Meador of the University of Alabama in a delightful essay, "The Art and Science of Nondisease" (*N Engl J Med.* 1965;272:92-95). The author cited numerous circumstances wherein symptoms appeared to be present, but the disease they were thought to represent was not. Dr. Meador concluded by admonishing, "The treatment of nondisease is never the treatment indicated for the corresponding disease entity." In this statement lies the ultimate value of the science of nondisease.

nor- as a chemical prefix is an abbreviation of "normal" and customarily denotes the parent compound in a pair of related substances. An example is **norepinephrine**, a naturally occurring catecholamine having a powerful adrenergic effect. Its homolog is **epinephrine**, whose structure bears an additional methylene group (CH_2). Both compounds have similar but not identical properties.

normal comes from the Latin *norma*, actually "a carpenter's square" or, figuratively, "a rule or standard." In medicine "normal" is defined as that which conforms to the common or established type. Whatever deviates from this standard is called **abnormal** (from the Latin *abnormis*, "irregular or unorthodox," this being a combination of the Latin *ab-*, "away from," + *norma*, "the standard"). In statistical usage "normal" often is considered to be the average or mean, give or take two standard deviations. On a Gaussian or bell-shaped curve, this accounts for approximately 95% of presumably normal subjects. For example, this is the way the "normal" range is established for values of various blood-chemistry determinations in printouts issuing from multichannel analyzers.

nose is a modern version of the Anglo-Saxon *nosu* and is related to the Latin *nasus*, both meaning "the nose." This term and its antecedents refer to the external, midline projection from the face. Each of the two openings is called a **nostril** and this term, as unlikely as it may seem, is related to our common word "thrill." The Middle English *thrillen* originally meant "to pierce." To be thrilled was to be more than touched but "pierced with emotion." "Nostril" used to be spelled "nosethirl" and literally meant "a hole pierced in the nose."

noso- is a prefix taken from the Greek *nosus*, "disease" and has come to be attached to a variety of medical terms thereby indicating a reference to disease.

nosocomial can describe any affliction, usually an infection, acquired by a patient while otherwise under medical supervision (noso- + the Greek *komeion*, "to take care of").

nosology is not the province of one who deals with noses; it is the proper term for the science of disease, especially its classification. The term was contrived by tacking the familiar "-logy" (Greek *logos*, "a study or discourse") onto "noso-."

nosomania is the delusion by a patient that he or she suffers from a given disease (noso- + Greek *mania*, "madness").

nosophobia is the dread of a particular disease, real or imagined (noso- + Greek *phobos*, "fear").

nostalgia is a sort of sickness that is commonly experienced but for which there is no medical remedy. The word combines the Greek *nostos*, "homecoming," + *algos*, "pain"; thus, a sentimental longing to go back to one's origin. In plain English this is "homesickness." By extension "nostalgia" has come to mean a bittersweet yearning for circumstances as they were in the past.

nostrum now means a worthless remedy and comes directly from the Latin as the neuter form of the adjective *noster*, meaning "our own." The explanation is that a proprietary concoction whose secret formulation was obscured as "our own" probably has little actual efficacy. Many of the so-called patent medicines flamboyantly purveyed in years past were eventually recognized as nostrums. However, there was a time when "nostrum" was a proudly proclaimed label. In the 17th century a flock of presumed experts descended on London, each claiming to be the sole producer of a concoction that could cure victims of the plague. Each declared he had a nostrum, presumably to establish proprietorship, as well as to flaunt his facility with Latin.

notochord is the name given to the rod-shaped, primitive axis of the embryo, and it is derived from a combination of the Greek *notos*, "the back," + *chordē*, "a string of gut, especially the string on a lyre." Thus the notochord is "the string of the back." Strangely, this is almost the only biomedical term related to the Greek word for the back.

noxious is a near borrowing of the Latin *noxius*, "harmful or injurious." The Indo-European root word probably was *nek*, "death," but the sense became softened a bit as the word descended to later tongues.

NSAID (*see* salicylate)

nuchal (*see* nape)

nucleus began as the Latin word for "a little nut or kernel," this being the diminutive of *nux*, *nucis*, "nut or nut tree." To the Romans *nucleus* usually referred to the kernel or pit of a fruit, then by extension to the hard core or central body of a mass. That there was a central body in the blood corpuscles of fish had been noted by Anton van Leeuwenhoek (1632-1723), the pioneer Dutch microscopist. But it was not until the early 19th century that "nucleus" appeared in English writings as a name for the "kernel" of a cell. When finer structural details became apparent, the nucleus was found to contain a still smaller body, and the term **nucleolus** was coined (there being no such Latin word). Thus, in "nucleolus" we have a diminutive of a diminutive.

nullipara is contrived as a combination of the Latin *nullus*, "not at all," + *parere*, "to give birth." The term is used in obstetrics and gynecology to designate a woman who has never borne a viable child.

numb and **nimble** seem strange word-fellows, but that is what they are. They both are descended from the Anglo-Saxon *niman*, "to take or seize" (the "b" was added later). So, to catch something you have to be nimble, but if you are caught you may be rendered numb. Numbness in a medical sense probably was thought of as a sort of seizure.

numbers derived from classical sources are often incorporated in medical terms. The following table gives combining forms used as numerating prefixes and includes a few that pertain to relative quantity.

ENGLISH	LATIN	GREEK
one (1)	uni-	mono-
two (2)	bi-	di
three (3)	ter-	tri-
four (4)	quadri-	tetra-
five (5)	quinque-	penta-
six (6)	sex-	hexa-
seven (7)	septi-	hepta-
eight (8)	octo-	octo-
nine (9)	novem-	ennea-
ten (10)	decem-	deka-
eleven (11)	undecim-	endeka-
twelve (12)	duodecum-	dodeka-
hundred (100)	cent-	hecto-
thousand (1000)	milli-*	kilo-*
one and one half (1½)	sesqui-	
whole	omni-	holo-
equal	equi-	homo-
many	multi-	poly-
more	super-	hyper-
less	sub-	hypo-

The Latin prefix milli- usually indicates thousandths; the Greek kilo- usually indicates thousands.

nummular describes a type of skin eruption, as in nummular eczema, in which the affected patches are coin-shaped. The term is taken from the Latin *nummus*, "a small coin."

nurse is derived from the Latin *nutrix*, "a nurse." In the plural *nutrices* this meant "the female breasts." The Latin verb *nutrire* means "to suckle or nourish an infant" but also, by extension, "to bring up or to take care of." Originally, a nurse was a woman hired to suckle a baby—what we would call today a "wet nurse." Later, the name was given to an attendant who cared for any sick or helpless person. The Latin term became the French *nourrice* and the Middle English *nurice*.

nutrition apparently trickled down from the Indo-European root *(s)nau*, "drips," which conveyed a sense of flowing or wetness. From this descended, by various paths, the Greek *nektar*, a wine used at sacrifices, regarded as "the drink of the gods" (whence "nectar") and the Latin *nutrire*, "to suckle" (from which we get nourish, nurse, nursery, and nurture). From the Middle English *snaken*, "to bite," we have "snack." To the Romans the idea of nourishment as a means of promoting growth was expressed as *nutrimentum*. To them this meant both food for the body and, by extension, support in general. Today we still use "nourish" in both a literal and a figurative sense. We nourish our bodies by the assimilation of food, but we can also nourish a thought or idea. But we restrict "nutrition" to the sense of providing food, in one form or another, by mouth or parenterally.

nyctalopia is a contrived combination of the Greek *nyct-*, "night," + *aloas*, "obscure or blind," + *opsis*, "vision." The term refers to impaired vision in dim light or at night. It is symptomatic of deficiency of vitamin A.

nymphomania first appeared in the English medical literature about 1800 as a term for a morbid, uncontrollable, sexual desire in women. It is not related to an actual Greek word but was concocted by combining the Greek *nymphē*, "a bride or maiden," + *mania*, "madness." Among the more attractive creatures of Greek mythology, the nymphs were lovely maidens who combined certain divine and human features. The Greeks were fond of believing that there were nymphs abounding in the woods (the Dryads) and in the hills (the Oreads), cavorting about springs and streams (the Naiads), and abiding in the sea (the Nereids). Nymphs were playful and sexually seductive. In a more down-to-earth sense, a Greek *nymphē* was any marriageable woman. Early anatomists applied the Latinized *nympha* as a term for the **clitoris** and, in the plural, *nymphae* to the labia minora. The male counterpart is **satyriasis**.

nystagmus comes from the Greek *nystakēs*, "nodding or drowsy." The meaning has changed from that of a drooping of the head or eyes as a sign of sleepiness to that of repetitive, involuntary movement of the eyeball in a horizontal, vertical, or rotatory direction. It was Johannes Purkinje (1787-1869), a Bohemian physiologist, who first associated nystagmus with vertigo. Later, nystagmus was recognized as a sign of vestibular disease by Robert Bárány (1876-1936), a Viennese otologist who was awarded a Nobel Prize in 1914 for his studies on the physiology and pathology of the vestibular apparatus.

**O and "H" antigens** distinguish agglutinins that react with either somatic (O) or flagellar (H) antigens exhibited by certain bacteria. The distinction is applied in the Widal test, named for Fernand Widal (1862-1929), a French physician, for antibodies to components of typhoid bacilli. Originally, *Proteus vulgaris* was studied as a prototype of flagellated microorganisms that, when cultured on an agar medium, spread as a thin film ("H" stands for the German *Hauch*, "film"); nonflagellated organisms, however, were observed to grow in compact, discrete clumps ("O" stands for the German *ohne Hauch*, "without, or not as, a film").

obese is a near borrowing of the Latin adjective *obesus*, meaning "fat, plump, swollen, or coarse." This, in turn, is the past participle of *obedere*, "to eat upon." The ancients knew that whoever was fat probably had eaten to excess. (*see* **adipose**)

obligate (*see* **aerobe**)

obstetrics is a transliterated borrowing of the Latin *obstetrix*, "a midwife." Note the feminine ending "-trix," as in the agent nouns "cicatrix" and "matrix." The term comes from the Latin *obstare* (*ob-*, "in front of," + *stare*, "to stand"). Thus, an *obstetrix* was a woman who stood in front of the mother-to-be and assisted in delivery of the baby. A venerable professor of obstetrics from Cleveland, Ohio, marked his retirement by moving to a balmy hideaway in the West Indies. To announce his intent to withdraw from active practice, he had printed a new letterhead proclaiming himself "Obstetrician to the Virgin Islands."

obstipation (*see* **constipation**)

obtunded refers to a dulled mentality. It comes from the Latin verb *obtundere*, "to beat upon or to stun." Anyone who has been beaten upon, as by the ravages of disease, is likely to be mentally dull or insensible.

obturator comes from the Latin *obturare*, "to block up or to plug." The obturator of a needle or catheter is the insertable shaft that plugs the lumen. The **obturator foramen** in the pelvis is the large opening in the innominate bone that is almost occluded by a tough, fibrous membrane. **Obturation ileus** is a plugging of the bowel, as by an errant gallstone.

occasional (*see* **periodic**)

occiput is a direct borrowing of the Latin term for the back of the head. The word is a combination of *ob-* (which here becomes "oc-") + *caput*, "head." The Latin *ob-* has all sorts of prepositional meanings, among which are "in front of" but also "against" in the sense of opposite to or other than. Thus, the occiput is that aspect of the head opposite the front.

occult is from the Latin *occultus*, the past participle of *occulere*, "to cover up or to hide." Occult blood, as in feces, is present but hidden from view and can be discerned only by chemical tests.

ochronosis is a sign of a rare metabolic disorder now known as alkaptonuria. The disease is characterized by deposition, mainly in cartilage, of a yellow-brown pigment (a homogentisic acid polymer). Thus, "ochronosis" signifies "the yellow disease," the name being contrived from the Greek *ochros*, "yellow," + *nosus*, "disease." But be careful. The pigmented cartilage, showing through the skin, as in the pinna of the ear, often appears blue or slate-gray. So if you see blue, think of the yellow disease.

ocular refers to the eye, the Latin word for which is *oculus*. It is interesting to note that we use the English noun "eye," but for an adjectival form we resort to the Latin derivative "ocular." The explanation is that in Old English there were few adjectives. When a modifier was needed, the noun was used, as in "eyeball" or "eyelid." This sufficed in common usage, but scientists insisted on something more highfalutin. One could say "eye nerve," but somehow "ocular nerve" sounds better. Many "eye doctors" prefer to be called "oculists." Other Old English nouns for which classical adjectives have been adopted are *mouth* (oral), *nose* (nasal), *mind* (mental), *moon* (lunar), and *star* (stellar).

odontoid describes anything fancied to be in the shape of a tooth and is derived from the Greek *odous (odont-)*, "tooth," + *eidos*, "like." The odontoid process is a toothlike projection from the body of the axis, the second cervical vertebra, on which rotates the atlas, the first cervical vertebra.

odyno- is a combining form taken from the Greek *odynē*, "pain." **Odynophagia** (+ Greek *phagein*, "to eat") is painful swallowing. An **anodyne** (Greek *a[n]-*, "without") is an old word for a drug that relieves pain.

oenophile is derived from the Greek *oinos*, "wine," + *philos*, "affinity or love," and refers to a person not only fond of wine but generally regarded as a connoisseur of the grape. An oenophile does not become of professional concern to physicians until he becomes an **oenomaniac** (+ the Greek word for "madness"), that is, one who is overly wild about wine.

officina is a Latin word that first meant a workshop or storeroom but later was restricted to a place for the preparation and storage of drugs. The derived adjective **officinalis** came to mean "pharmaceutical." Hence its incorporation in the names of certain herbals, e.g., *Althea officinalis*, the marsh mallow (its mucilaginous root was once used in confectionery); *Nasturtium officinalis*, watercress; and *Hirudo officinalis*, a medicinal leech. The English "officinal" is no longer used, probably because writers and typesetters so often omitted the "n," thus altering its meaning.

-oid is a suffix taken from the Greek *eidos*, "that which is seen, the form or shape of something, the sort or kind." It has been hooked on to numerous classical terms to form adjectives or nouns, thereby conferring either of two senses: (*a*) having the appearance of, as in *scaphoid* (like the hull of a boat); or (*b*) almost, but not quite, like, as in *carcinoid* (a tumor resembling, but not really, a carcinoma).

ointment can be traced to the Latin *ungere*, "to anoint or to apply oil." A more direct derivative is **unguent**, meaning "a healing salve."

The Old French *oignement* was "an anointing" but also could designate the substance thereby applied. This was taken into Middle English as *oinement*. Later, a "t" was interposed between the syllables, either to facilitate pronunciation or to make the word sound more like "anoint." In pharmacology an ointment, having an **oleaginous** base, is usually distinguished from a lotion or cream, which has a watery base. **Lotion**, incidentally, is taken from the Latin *lotio*, "a washing," related to *lavere*, "to wash."

olecranon is an almost direct borrowing of the Greek *ōlekranon*, "the point of the elbow." This combines *ōlenē*, "the arm from the elbow to the wrist," (whence the Latin *ulna*) + *kranos*, "helmet." Apparently, someone thought the proximal end of the larger bone in the forearm looked a little like a helmet. (*see* **ulna**)

oleum is the Latin word for "oil," being related to the Greek *elaion*. Originally, the Greek and Latin terms referred specifically to olive oil. Later, the terms were used generically for any natural oil.

olfactory comes from the Latin *olfactare*, "to sniff at," this being related to the transitive verb *olfacere*, "to smell." In the Latin *olere*, "to smell of," as in the English "to smell," the verb can function as both transitive and intransitive. The combination of *olere* + *facere* (Latin, "to make") intensifies the transitive sense of the verb. The second cranial or olfactory nerve serves the sensitive receptors of smell in the nasal cavity. **Smell**, incidentally, is an old, old word that can be traced back, almost unchanged, to its Teutonic roots. Because most oils are volatile and therefore odoriferous, one can postulate a relation between words for oils and smells.

oligo- is a combining form, usually a prefix, taken from the Greek *oligos*, "few or scanty."

oligodendroglia are ectodermal, nonneural cells that form part of the adventitial structure of the nervous system. Linear projections of the cells suggest sparse branches of a tree (oligo- + Greek *dendron*, "tree," + *glia*, "glue"). If the cells become neoplastic, a fourth Greek component is added to form **oligodendroglioma**.

oligodontia is an insufficiency in the number of teeth due to a developmental failure of dental eruption (oligo- + Greek *odous*, "tooth").

oligohydramnios refers to a paucity of amniotic fluid surrounding the fetus, usually taken to be less than 300 milliliters (oligo- + Greek *hydōr*, "water," + *amnion*, "fetal sac").

oligomenorrhea is abnormally infrequent or scanty menstruation (oligo- + Greek *mēn*, "month," + *rhoia*, "a flowing").

oliguria (oligo- + Greek *ouron*, "urine") is diminished formation or excretion of urine.

-oma is taken from the inseparable Greek suffix *-ōma*, which, as explained by Professor H. A. Skinner, was used in the back formation of nouns from verbs. An example of the Greek sequence would be *adēn*, "a gland"; *adenoō*, "I form a gland"; *adenōma*, "a gland formation." In its early medical application "-oma" could refer to any swelling or tumor. Later, it became restricted to neoplasms. Dr. John Dirckx points out that the stem to which "-oma" is attached can indicate a site (as in hepatoma), a physical feature (as in psammoma), a histologic component (as in epithelioma), a chemical constituent (as in cholesteatoma), a product (as in insulinoma), a cause (as in ameboma), or an eponym (as in schwannoma). I once heard a medical student facetiously refer to a proliferating workup of a patient as a "testoma."

omentum is the Latin word that Celsus used for the fatty caul or cap that covers most of the abdominal viscera. The origin of the term is obscure. Some authors relate it to the Latin *operimentum*, "a lid or cover," assuming "omentum" to be a contraction therof.

omphalos is the Greek word for "the navel." In a figurative sense, *omphalos* meant "the center of anything." Thus, the word referred to the boss or decorative knob at the center of a warrior's shield or to the knob in the middle of a yoke. In medicine the word is not used alone but only as a combining form, as in **omphalocele** (+ Greek *kēlē*, "tumor or hernia"), a protrusion of the intestine, enclosed in a thin-walled sac, through a defect in the umbilicus.

onanism refers to the practice of "coitus interruptus" (wherein the penis is withdrawn from the vagina before ejaculation) and also to masturbation. The term immortalizes the name of a man whose fate is told in the Old Testament, Genesis 38:7-10, as follows:

And Er, Judah's firstborn, was wicked in the sight of the Lord; and the Lord slew him. And Judah said unto Onan, Go in unto thy brother's wife and marry her, and raise up seed to thy brother. And Onan knew that the seed should not be his; and it came to pass, when he went in unto his brother's wife that he spilled it [his semen] on the ground, lest that he should give seed to his brother. And the thing which he did displeased the Lord; wherefore He slew him also.

onco- is a combining form, usually a prefix, derived from the Greek *o[n]gkos*, "a bulk or mass" and, later, "a tumor." By custom the Greek "g" (gamma), when preceding "k" (kappa), becomes "n" as a word moves from the classical to a modern vocabulary. Also, the Greek "k" becomes the English "c." Hence, the scientific combining form is "onco-." **Oncology** (+ Greek *logos*, "a study or treatise") is the science of neoplasia.

oncogenes are the chromosomal components that, when activated, produce malignant transformation in cultured cells and cancers in living organisms (onco- + Greek *gennaō*, "I produce").

oncotic as used in the sense of "pertaining to or caused by swelling" is derived from the Greek *o[n]gkos*, "a mass." Thus, oncotic pressure is that exerted, as an osmotic property, by colloids in a confined system. An example is the oncotic pressure exerted by small protein molecules, mainly albumin, in circulating blood.

ontogeny refers to the sequential development of an individual organism. The word is a combination of the Greek *on* (genitive *ontos*), "that which actually exists, a being," + *genos*, "descent," in the sense of origin. This is in contrast to **phylogeny**, the development of a whole kind or type of organism. The Greek *phylon* means "a race, stock, or tribe."

oö- is a combining form taken from the Greek *ōon*, "egg," and denotes a relationship to an ovum. The diaeresis (¨) placed over the second "ö" indicates it is to be pronounced distinctly from the first "ō" and that "oö" is not a diphthong. Note that the Greek ō and o- are two different letters: omega (ω) and omicron (o).

oöcyst is the encapsulated, fertilized form of the

malaria parasite in the stomach of a mosquito, just waiting for its chance to infect a person (oö- + Greek *kystis*, "bladder").

oöphoro- is a combining form contrived by putting together the Greek *ōon*, "egg," + *phora*, "a bearing or producing," and thus it is an apt reference to the ovary. **Oöphoritis** is an inflammation of the ovary, and **oöphorectomy** (+ Greek *ektomē*, "a cutting out") is the surgical removal of the ovary.

ooze (*see* **exude**)

operculum is a direct borrowing of the Latin word for "a lid or cover." In anatomy various structures are called "opercula" because they cover something. For example, the dental operculum is the hood of gingival tissue overlying the crown of an erupting tooth.

ophthalmo- is a combining form taken from the Greek *ophthalmos*, "the eye." A common error in spelling is to omit the first "h." To avoid this lapse, it helps to remember that the "-phth-" represents a sequence of the Greek letters φ and θ (phi and theta). **Ophthalmia** can refer to any disease of the eye, but usually it is restricted to an inflammatory condition ("ophthalmitis" is seldom used by ophthalmologists). The suffix *-ia* was used by ancient medical writers to denote any morbid condition of a given structure. Another example is "pneumonia."

opisthotonus is a posture of recumbent, rigid hyperextension wherein the head and legs are bent backward and the trunk is bowed forward. This is the position of tetanic muscular spasm observed in severe meningitis and in tetanus. Obviously, all muscles are spastic, but the stronger extensors predominate over the flexors. The term combines the Greek *opisthen*, "backward," + *tonos*, "stretching."

opium originated in the Greek *opos*, "the juice, sap, resin, or gum of trees or plants." Opium, extracted from the juice of the poppy plant (*Papaver somniferum*), was known to the ancients as a drug. Homer described it as "the healing draught that drowns all pain and sorrow." It has also been long known that opium and its congeners can cause a lot of pain and sorrow.

opsonin is an antibody that renders bacteria and other cells particularly susceptible to phagocytosis. The term was proposed in 1903 by Sir Almroth Wright (1861-1947), professor of pathology at Saint Mary's Hospital in London, who cleverly took it from the Greek *opōnion*, "vituals." The Greek *opsōnein* means "to buy provisions." Thus, Sir Almroth fancied that opsonin rendered bacteria available to satisfy hungry phagocytes. George Bernard Shaw offered a more savory account in his play *The Doctor's Dilemma*, published in 1906. He has a principal character, Sir Colenso Ridgeon (whose persona is unmistakably that of Sir Almroth Wright), explain: "Opsonin is what you butter the disease germs with to make your white corpuscles eat them. . . . The phagocytes won't eat the microbes unless the microbes are nicely buttered for them." Alas, the real Sir Almroth Wright had his detractors who, behind his back, snidely referred to him as "Sir Almost Right."

optic is derived from the Greek *optikos*, "pertaining to sight," which originated in *optos*, "visible."

optometrist is a specially trained person who measures eyesight (Greek *optos*, "what is seen" + *mētron*, "a rule or measure") and prescribes corrective lenses, which then are produced and purveyed by an **optician**.

oral (*see* **os**)

orbicularis is a diminutive of the Latin *orbis*, "ring." This name applies to the flat muscles (not sphincters) that surround certain apertures, such as the mouth or eye.

orbit comes from the Latin *orbita*, "the track or rut made by a wheel." The Latin *orbis* could be applied to almost anything circular, including a wheel. In the Middle Ages *orbita* came to be used as a name for the eye socket.

orchi- is a combining form derived from the Greek *orchis*, "testicle" and is incorporated in medical terms such as "orchitis" and "orchiectomy" (commonly spelled "orchidectomy"). Incidentally, the highly prized and much admired flower we call "orchid," bears a name that can be literally translated as "like a testicle." Pliny the Elder, the 1st century Roman author and naturalist, pointed out that the bulbous double roots of the plant resemble testicles.

organ is a derivative of the Greek *organon* and

the Latin *organum*, both meaning "an instrument or implement." The Greek word is related to the verb *ergein*, "to do work." In biology the etymologic sense of organ then is of function rather than structure. The concept is not of what an organ is but of what it does.

orgasm comes from the Greek *orgainein*, "to swell," which, in the case of fruit, means to swell until it ripens, or, in the case of animals, to swell with lust or to be in heat. In English the word was first used to describe any turgid fit of anger or passion. Later, it was applied specifically to the climax of coitus.

ornithosis is a viral disease of birds that is transmissible to man. The origin of the term is in the Greek *ornis*, "bird." If a parrot transmits the disease, it is **psittacosis**, from the Greek *psittakos*, "a parrot."

orphan is derived from the Greek *orphanos*, "the state of being left without parents," and, by extension, "bereft or destitute." The term **orphan diseases** has been applied to those conditions bereft of needed attention by researchers, not for lack of interest but because such diseases are so rare that funding agencies, particularly those of government and commerce, are reluctant to provide the support required for research. Drugs that are postulated or proved to be effective in the treatment of these rare diseases are called **orphan drugs** because pharmaceutical manufacturers are, in some cases, loath to produce medications from which will be derived only a negligible commercial return.

ortho- is a combining form, usually a prefix, originating in the Greek *orthos*, "straight or erect."

orthodontics is the practice of straightening misaligned teeth (ortho- + Greek *odous*, "tooth"). (*see* **tooth**)

orthopaedics is, literally, the practice of "straightening a child" (ortho- + Greek *paes* or *pais*, "child"). Now, by spelling this term with "ae" rather than just "e," a bag of worms has burst. Some people might look upon "orthopaedics" as archaic pedantry, but it is not. To spell it "orthopedics" would relate the term to the Latin *pes, pedis*, "foot." This is incorrect on two counts: (*a*) the practice was never intended to be restricted to "foot straightening"; and (*b*) to link the

Greek *ortho-* and the Latin *pedis* would create a mongrel word. Those who still might want to argue are referred to an exhaustive discussion in the journal *Medical Communications* (1981;9:93-99). Even more to be condemned is the use of "orthopod" as a slang term for one who practices orthopaedics. This makes no sense at all.

orthopnea as it is usually spelled by American authors (the British spell it "orthopnoea") is a classical sign of left ventricular cardiac failure. *Orthopnoia* (Greek *ortho-* + *pnoia*, "breath") was used by Hippocrates to describe the plight of patients who breathed easily only when in an upright posture.

orthostatic describes an upright posture (ortho- + Greek *statos*, "standing"). Orthostatic hypotension is a sharp drop in blood pressure when assuming an erect position.

os is one of two Latin words, both spelled the same and both neuter nouns. One means "mouth," and the other means "bone." There is a difference in classical pronunciation: the "o" in *os*, "mouth," is pronounced as in "hope," while the "o" in *os*, "bone," is pronounced as in "often." The genitive of the Latin *os*, "mouth," is *oris* and describes whatever pertains to the mouth; from this we have the adjective **oral**. In anatomy the classical noun is occasionally used, as in "the cervical os," meaning the mouth of the uterine cervix. The genitive of the Latin *os*, "bone," is *ossis*, and from this we derive the adjective **osseus** to designate whatever pertains to bone. This Latin *os* is related to the Greek *osteon*, "bone," and it is the Greek that provides the combining form **osteo-**.

os calcis (*see* **calcaneus**)

-ose (*see* **glucose**)

-osis is a suffix of Greek origin that denotes "a condition of," as in "nephrosis" (thus providing a distinction from inflammation, as in "nephritis"), and also "an increase in," as in "leukocytosis." It is comparable to the Latin *-osus*, "abounding in or having the quality of," from which is derived the English suffix "-ous," as in "cancerous" or "poisonous."

osmosis is derived from the Greek *ōsmos*, "a push or impulse," this being related to *ōtheō*, "I thrust, push, or shove." Osmosis is the passage (or "shoving," if you will) of a solvent through a semipermeable membrane from a solution of a lesser to a greater concentration. The result is a trend to equilibration. The term was introduced in 1854 by Thomas Graham (1805-1869), an English chemist.

osteo- is a combining form taken from the Greek *osteon,* "bone," and appears in terms such as osteitis, osteoblast, osteoclast, and osteomyelitis.

osteoblast is a cell, derived from a particular line of fibroblasts, that has acquired the capacity to form bone (osteo- + Greek *blastos,* "germ or sprout"). The name was given by Carl Gegenbaur (1826-1903), a German anatomist.

osteoclast is a term contrived by linking "osteo-" and a derivative of the Greek *klastos,* "broken." Originally, an osteoclast was an instrument designed to artificially fracture bony structures. According to Professor H. A. Skinner, Rudolf von Kölliker (1817-1905), long an esteemed professor of histology at Würzburg, called the cells observed to resorb bone "osotoclasts" to avoid confusion with the name of the surgical instrument. Later, when "osteoclast" in its early meaning became outmoded, the term reverted as a name for the multinucleated cells that nibble away at bone.

osteomalacia is a degenerative softening or weakness of bone (osteo- + Greek *malakia,* "softness"), especially in the sense of bone weakened by demineralization and particularly that owing to depletion of calcium such as observed consequent to vitamin D deficiency.

osteomyelitis is an inflammation, usually due to infection, that can involve all components of bone and not the marrow alone, as the term might suggest (osteo- + Greek *myelos,* "marrow").

osteopathy could be taken to mean any bone disease (osteo- + Greek pathos, "suffering"), as it once was and yet might be. But now the term usually refers to the system of therapy founded in 1874 by Andrew Still (1828-1917), an American medical practitioner, and based on the supposition that most diseases are caused by bony deformation and can be cured by manipulation of the skeletal structure. There remain extant in the United States several schools that grant a DO degree (doctor of osteopathy), but their curriculum now closely approximates that of medical schools generally.

osteopenia is sometimes used as a generic term encompassing a weakening of bone structure of any cause (oseto- + Greek *penēs,* "poor or poverty-stricken"). Now, since the advent of a technique by which the density of bone can be accurately measured, "osteopenia" more specifically designates diminished bone density within 1 standard deviation of normal.

osteoporosis is an excessive sponginess of bone resulting from impaired formation of bone matrix (osteo- + Greek *poros,* "passage"), due either to suppressed **osteoblastic** activity or to excessive **osteoclastic** activity. More specifically, the term designates a condition wherein bone density measures 2 or more standard deviations less than normal.

ostium is the Latin word for "an opening, a door, or a mouth." The plural is **ostia.** The coronary ostia are the openings at the root of the aorta that lead into the left and right coronary arteries that supply the heart muscle. The suffix **-ostomy** designates an entrance, usually artificial, constructed into the wall of a viscus, e.g., a gastrostomy or a colostomy. A distinction is made between "-ostomy" and "-otomy," the latter meaning "a cut into." Incidentally, Ostia was the name of a town at the mouth of the Tiber River, which served as an ancient Roman port.

oto- is a combining form taken from the Greek *ōtos,* genitive of *ous,* "the ear." An example of its use is **otosclerosis** (+ Greek *sklēros,* "hard or tough"), an abnormal formation of new bone around the oval window of the ear, immobilizing the stapes and resulting in a progressive loss of auditory acuity.

ouabain is the Gallicized version of the Somali name *wabayo* for the plant *Strophanthus gratus,* an extract of which yields a glycoside exhibiting cardiotonic properties similar to those of digitalis. **Strophanthin,** the glycoside, was introduced to pharmacology in 1890 by Sir Thomas Fraser who discovered its medicinal properties while investigating African arrow poisons. The name of the plant, a woody vine indigenous to tropical Africa, combines the Greek *strophos,* "a twisted band," + *anthos,* "a flower."

ounce (*see* **dram**)

ovary is a near borrowing of the Late Latin *ovarium,* "a receptacle of eggs." Ancient writers did not use this term but rather referred to "the female testis or gonad." The term "ovary" became generally adopted after the writings of Reijnier de Graaf (1641-1673), the Dutch anatomist. The Greek *ōon*, "egg" (which became the Latin *ovum*), led to *ōophoros* (+ Greek *pherein*, "to carry"), literally "an egg bearer." Classically, this term referred, in general, to animals that bear eggs. From *ōophoros* was derived the combining form **oöphor-**, since used specifically to refer to the ovary and incorporated in such terms as oöphoritis and oöphorectomy.

oxalic is a chemical designation that has nothing to do with oxygen but comes from *oxalis*, the Greek name (*oxys*, "sour") for the sorrel plant from whose succulent leaves a sour or acid juice was obtained.

oxygen is a word introduced as a result of the seminal discoveries by Antoine Laurent Lavoisier (1743-1794), the celebrated French chemist. Curiously, the word signifies a mistaken concept in that it was contrived from a combination of the Greek *oxys*, "sharp, as an acid," + *gennaō*, "I produce." Originally, it was thought that the newly discovered "vital air" conferred the property of an acid when it was combined with another radical and, thus, was an "acid producer." It was not until 60 years later, in 1837, that Justus von Liebig (1803-1873), the renowned German chemist, showed that the essential component of acids was actually hydrogen (which, if anything, more aptly deserves to be called an "acid producer").

oxyntic comes from the Greek *oxys*, "sour," and was applied, in the 1880s, by an English physiologist, John Langley (1852-1925), to the acid-producing (or parietal) cells of the gastric mucosa.

oxytocic was contrived by combining the Greek *oxys*, "sharp or quick," + *tokos*, "a bringing forth, a birth, a time of delivery." Hence, an oxytocic is any agent that hastens childbirth.

oxyuriasis is a fancy name for pinworm infection. The pinworm *Enterobius vermicularis* is a member of the family Oxyuridae, so called from the Greek *oxys*, "sharp or pointed," + *oura*, "tail."

Pabulum is a substance that gives nourishment, especially a simple, soft food suitable for infants. It is a Latin word for food, probably derived from the first part of *pascere*, "to feed," + *-bulum*, a suffix indicating "the means of." Once there was a baby food purveyed under the name Pablum. A similar but unrelated word for an infant's food is **pap**, said to be imitative of a baby's muttering. By extension, both "pap" and "pabulum" have come to mean any insipid intellectual exercise or instruction.

pachy- is a combining form, usually a prefix, taken from the Greek *pachys*, "thick or clotted." **Pachycephaly** is an abnormal thickness of the bones of the skull (pachy- + Greek *kephalē*, "the head"). **Pachyderma** is an abnormal thickening of the skin (pachy- + Greek *derma*, "skin"). **Pachymeninx** is a seldom used alternative term for the dura mater (pachy- + Greek *meninx*, "membrane"), yet sometimes encountered as in **pachymeningitis**. **Pachynychia** is an abnormal thickening of the fingernails or toenails (pachy- + Greek *onyx*, "nail, claw, or hoof"). Incidentally, the gemstone onyx, a type of chalcedony, was given its name because of its veined translucency, similar to that of an animal's hoof or claw.

pacinian corpuscles are the highly discriminating end-organs of sensory nerves in the skin of the hands and feet. Their name memorializes Filippo Pacini (1812-1888), an Italian anatomist who published a detailed description in 1840. Pacini was not the first to observe these structures, but later authorities, notably Friedrich Henle and Albert von Kölliker, were sufficiently impressed by Pacini's work to establish the eponym.

pagophagia is a perverted craving for the eating of ice. The term incorporates the Greek *pagos*, "anything stiffened or hardened, such as frozen water," + *phagein*, "to eat." Pagophagia is a form of pica and is symptomatic of iron deficiency.

pain comes through the French *peine* from the Latin *poena*, "a penalty or punishment." The derivation of "pain" sadly reflects the old belief that suffering was divinely decreed as penance for sinful acts. This idea still lurks in the minds of some patients who bewail their fate by asking, "What have I done to deserve this?"

palate is the name of the arched partition that separates the oral and nasal cavities. The term is derived from the Latin *palatum*, which means the same thing but was extended figuratively to "taste" in the sense of discriminating between what is palatable and what is unpalatable. Scholars debate the origin of the Latin term for the roof of the mouth, but probably it is related to the Latin *pala*, "a shovel or spade," in part because of its shape and in part because it helps convey food into the gullet. **Palatine** describes what relates to the palate, as in "palatine tonsils."

paleo- is a combining form taken from the Greek *palaios*, "old or ancient." In neuroanatomy it is used as a prefix to denote structure of a phylogenetically older rank. The cerebral **paleocortex**, having to do largely with the sense of smell, is an example.

palindromic is used in medicine to describe a recurring disease or symptom, particularly one marked by complete remissions. The word is a near borrowing of the Greek *palindromos*, "a running back again." Palindromic rheumatism is a recurring polyarthritis that results in no permanent joint deformity or functional impairment. More intriguing are the palindromes that are words, phrases, or sentences that read the same backward as forward. Among the best known (and, one might guess, probably the first) is "Madam, I'm Adam," said to be Adam's manner of introducing himself to Eve. Willard Espy, ever playful with words, contributes a remarkably extended palindrome that suggests a dispute between dermatologists: "Straw? No, too stupid a fad. I put soot on warts." The award for the perfect palindrome goes to the San Diego

Zoological Society for the copyrighted title of its journal, *ZOONOOZ*. It reads the same upside down, too.

palliate is derived from the Latin *pallium*, "a coverlet or cloak." More specifically, this was a garb worn by scholars in ancient times. It consisted of a rectangular woolen cloak draped over the left shoulder, thus partly covering the body. When we seek a palliative treatment for a disease, we do not provide a complete remedy or cure but rather treat it partially and as far as possible with the means at hand, so that its manifestations are not fully evident.

pallid is a near borrowing of the Latin *pallidus*, "pale or sallow," said to be related to the Greek *polios*, "gray-white, particularly of the hair as a sign of aging." The globus pallidus is a pale, gray portion of the corpus striatum in the brain. Persons exhibit **pallor** when the normally rich red blood coursing through the capillaries no longer shows through the skin. To be appalled by some shocking circumstance means to grow pale. The shock stimulates a reaction in the sympathetic nervous system that entails constriction of the cutaneous arterioles.

palpate comes from the Latin *palpare*, "to stroke or to pat." The sense of the Latin word is to touch and feel lightly, and this is precisely the manner in which palpation, as part of the physical examination of a patient, should be undertaken. I well remember the wise advice given by one of my medical school instructors years ago: "When palpating the abdomen, get friendly with it before you get familiar."

palpebral refers to the eyelid, which the Romans called *palpebra,* from the Latin intransitive verb *palpitare,* "to quiver." The eyelid is a structure given to fluttering.

palpitation is a disagreeable consciousness by the patient of his own heart throbbing, typically with abnormal intensity or irregularity. The term is taken from the Latin *palpitare,* "to throb or quiver."

palsy is an old, almost archaic term for paralysis. Indeed, it is an Anglicized contraction of the French *paralysie.* For some reason, its use persists in the designation "Bell's palsy," a peripheral facial paralysis caused by a lesion of the seventh cranial nerve. The eponym is owed to Sir Charles Bell (1774-1842), a Scottish anatomist and neurologist who described the condition in 1830.

pampiniform is taken from the Latin *pampinus*, "a tendril," a slender coiling extension from the stem of a climbing plant by which it attaches to an adjacent structure. The pampiniform plexus in the male is the rich network of veins from the testicle and epididymis that invests the spermatic cord; in the female it is the plexus of ovarian veins in the broad ligament. (*see* **varicose**)

pan- is a prefix borrowed from the Greek *pan*, this being the neuter form of *pas*, "all, the whole of."

panacea comes from Panaceia, the name of one of the daughters of Asklepios, the Greek god of healing. Another daughter was Hygieia. Both daughters dutifully followed their father's calling, but their paths took different turns. Panaceia became the patroness of clinical medicine or what we might call "critical care medicine." She advocated the use of specific remedies as indicated by the occurrence of particular needs. Hygieia was concerned rather with preserving health or what might be called "preventive medicine." As it turned out, the goddesses competed more often than they cooperated. "Panacea" is taken to mean "a universal remedy," which has been long and widely sought but of which no example exists in modern medicine. To the ancient Greeks, *panakeia* (a combination of *pan-*, "all," + *akos*, "remedy") was an all-healing herb.

panangiitis is an inflammation affecting all coats of a blood vessel (pan- + Greek *a[n]ggeion*, "a vessel").

panarteritis is an inflammation of all coats of an artery (pan- + Greek *artēria*, "a conduit") and **panphlebitis** (pan- + Greek *phleps, phlebos*, "a vein") means inflammation of all coats of a vein. In these designations it is important to point out that "pan-" refers to the whole of the individual vessel involved and not to all the vessels throughout the body. **Polyarteritis** and **polyphlebitis** are terms indicating inflammation affecting numerous vessels at the same time.

pancreas is a near borrowing of the Greek *pa[n]gkreas*. Remember that the Greeks pronounced their letter "g" (gamma) as "n" in "ng" when it preceded palatal consonants. The term is a combination of *pan-*, "all," + *kreas*, "flesh," and was used by Herophilus to describe the "all meaty" structure of the gland. The pancreas is, indeed, a thoroughly fleshy gland, though of a rather firm consistency.

pandemic describes the circumstance wherein nearly all of a given population are affected by a certain disease at the same time (pan- + Greek *dēmos*, "people").

panhysterectomy is a surgical extirpation of the whole uterus, including its cervix (pan- + Greek *hystera*, "the uterus," + *ektomē*, "a cutting out").

panic is an expression of acute, often extreme, anxiety in which terror is of such intensity as to impair normal function. In an individual this is recognized as "a panic attack"; in a large group, this is **pandemonium**. "Panic" (but not "pandemonium," which can be roughly translated as "abode of all devils") is taken from Greek mythology and the name Pan for the god of woods, fields, and flocks. Pan was a demonic figure with a human head and torso and a goat's legs, ears, and horns, whose occasional caprice was to strike terror in people who ventured in rural areas, especially at night. Pan's name implies he was a god of all Nature.

pannus is a direct borrowing of the Latin word for "a piece of cloth." In pathology "pannus" has come to mean either (*a*) a superficial vascularization of the cornea accompanied by a granulomatous infiltrate or (*b*) an inflammatory exudate overlying the synovial membrane of a joint. In both instances the allusion is to a piece of cloth covering the affected structure. **Panniculus** is the diminutive of the Latin *pannus*. Originally, in anatomy, "panniculus" was applied to a variety of membranes. Currently, its use is usually restricted to the layer of fatty subcutaneous tissue. When we refer to an obese person as having "a heavy panniculus" we mean that he or she is well padded. To use "heavy" in the same breath as a diminutive of a term seems odd, but oddities abound in medical parlance.

pap (*see* **pabulum**)

papain is a naturally occurring vegetable enzyme capable of digesting protein. It is a product of papaya, an altered form of the Cariban Indian term for fruits of the genus *Carica*. Inasmuch as the ending "-in" indicates a product, the last three letters of "papain" should be pronounced as two syllables (the "-ai-" is not a diphthong).

papaverine is an alkaloid having the property of relaxing smooth muscle generally. Although in 1848 it was isolated from opium, it possesses none of the analgesic or soporific properties of the other opium alkaloids. Its name indicates that it is a derivative of the poppy plant *Papaver somniferum*. *Papaver* is the Latin name for the poppy plant.

papilla is the Latin word for "nipple or teat," being related to the verb *pappare*, "to consume pap (baby food) in the manner of an infant." In early treatises on anatomy "papilla" was restricted to designate the nipple of the female breast, but later the term was applied to various structures fancied to have a nipplelike appearance; for example, the small projections on the surface of the tongue that bear taste buds, the projections of the renal medulla into the pelvis of the kidney, and the mucosal projection from the luminal surface of the duodenum that serves as an exit for the biliary and pancreatic ducts.

papule is a near borrowing of the Latin *papula*, "a pimple." Dermatologists use "papule" to designate any small, circumscribed, solid elevation on the skin surface, as distinct from a **vesicle**, which contains a fluid substance, and a **macule**, which is flat and even with the skin surface. **Pimple** seems to have descended, as a diminutive and by a devious route, from the Greek *pomphos*, "a bubble or a blister."

par as in the expression "I've not been feeling up to par" is taken directly from the Latin word meaning "equal." It conveys the sense of comparison to a normal or usual standard.

para- is a combining form, usually a prefix, taken from the Greek preposition *para*, "along the side of, in comparison with, or during." The list of Greek words and their derivatives to which "para-" has become affixed is almost endless. Mention has been made of how Paracelsus took his name. (*see* **laudanum**)

paracentesis is the tapping of a body cavity, usually the abdomen and customarily at one side or the other, to relieve an abnormal accumulation of fluid (para- + Greek *kentēsis*, "puncture").

paracrine designates a newly recognized class of peptides that act as hormones but, rather than traveling in the general circulation as do endocrine substances, serve to stimulate immediately adjacent effector cells, as in the gastrointestinal mucosa (para- + Greek *krinein*, "to separate, to set apart"). Still another recently defined class is that of **autocrine** peptides that act upon their own cells of origin.

paralysis originated as the Greek *paralytikos*, meaning, literally, "the condition wherein one's side was lax" (para- + Greek *lysis*, "a loosening or disruption"), this being the plight of a person afflicted by **apoplexy**. Later, "paralysis" was extended to mean a loss of motor function in any part.

paranoia is a direct borrowing of the Greek word for "madness or mental derangement," the Greek *noein* meaning "to think." Probably the idea related to the figurative sense of one beset or "beside himself." Now to be paranoid is to suffer delusions of persecution.

paraphasia is the utterance of confused speech, particularly the use of senseless words inappropriate to the intended thought (para-, in the sense of "beside," + Greek *phasis*, "an expression"). The condition indicates a cerebral disturbance.

paraplegia was adopted from the Greek *paraplēgia* (para- + *plēgē*, "a stroke") and originally meant "a stroke on one side," but the medical meaning has now shifted to designate a paralysis of both legs and the lower part of the body consequent to a lesion of the spinal cord.

parasite denotes an organism that feeds along with its host. The original Greek *parasitos* (para- + *sitos*, "food") meant "eating at the side of another, as at the same table," but later the sense was changed to that of a poor friend or relation who boarded at the expense of another. "Parasite" was introduced into English as a biologic term in the early 18th century.

parasympathetic (*see* **sympathetic**)

paratyphoid (*see* **typhoid**)

pare- is a prefix equivalent to "para-" that is used when the final "a" of "para-" might be thought to conflict with a following letter.

paregoric when prepared according to the specifications of the *United States Pharmacopoeia* is a tincture of opium (equivalent to 0.04% anhydrous morphine) in which there is also benzoic acid, camphor, and anise oil. Though now paregoric is seldom prescribed and then usually to suppress diarrhea, formerly its principal use was as a sedative and analgesic agent. The name comes from the Greek *paregoreō*, meaning "I address in a consoling or soothing manner." In *paregoreō* we see the prefix "pare-" together with a derivative of *agora*, "a place of assembly for commercial or political purposes." Such a place could be a scene of raucous confusion, and anyone who could temper the tumult by a soothing speech would be highly regarded. Hence, paregoric, as a drug, was seen to address a paroxysm of pain in a soothing manner. And it can quell an uproarious bowel, too.

parenchyma refers to the essential functional elements contained within an organ, as distinct from its capsule or supporting structures. The term is a direct borrowing of the Greek word meaning "that which is poured in." This is explained by the ancient and erroneous belief that the inner substance of solid viscera, such as the liver, spleen, or kidneys, was infused and coagulated blood. Incidentally, the "y" in "parenchyma" is always pronounced as a short "i," not as "eye."

paresis is a direct borrowing of the Greek word for "a slackening" or, by extension, "a loss of strength." In modern medicine the term is used in two ways: (*a*) as another name for dementia paralytica, the chronic and inexorable condition marked by degeneration of the central nervous system consequent to syphilis; and (*b*) for a partial loss of motor function in a part, short of total paralysis. The latter is the more frequent use.

paresthesia is a morbid or perverted sensation, such as burning, tingling, formication, or itching, that may occur in a part "beside or along with" normal sensation (pare- + Greek *aisthēsis*, "perception").

parietal is a derivative of the Latin *parietalis*, "belonging to the wall," this being related to *paries,* "a wall that encircles." Ancient writers used *parietalis* to designate the wall of a body cavity. Thus, the parietal peritoneum lines the wall of the abdominal cavity, whereas the visceral peritoneum envelops the walls of internal abdominal organs.

parity (*see* **parturition**)

paronychia is an inflammation at the margins of the nailbed of the fingers or toes (par-, equivalent to "para-,"+ Greek *onyx,* "nail"). (*see* **whitlow**)

parotid describes the location of the large salivary gland situated beside (actually in front of) the ear (par-, equivalent to "para-,"+ Greek *otos,* "the ear").

paroxysm is the term for a sudden recurrence or exacerbation of a symptom (par-, equivalent to "para-," in the sense of "during," + the Greek *oxys,* "sharp or acute"). One can have a smoldering fever or a lingering cough, but a paroxysm is an abrupt, accentuated attack of that symptom.

parthenogenesis is reproduction by the development of a female ovum without benefit of fertilization by a male sperm. This remarkable event happens in certain lower animals but has not been known to occur in man (or, more properly, in woman). The term combines the Greek *parthenos,* "a virgin," + *genesis,* "coming into being." The Parthenon is an Athenian temple erected in the 5th century B.C. and dedicated to the virgin goddess Athena.

parturition is another word for the process of giving birth to a baby. It comes from the Latin *parturire,* "to be ready to bear young." The Latin *partus* is the past participle of *parere,* "to produce." **Parity** as an expression of a woman's fertility is a purely English invention and bears only a tortuous relation to the Latin *parere.*

Pascal's wager has been cited to support the position of a doctor who knowingly (or unknowingly) invokes a "hanging-of-the-crepe" strategy when dealing with the plight of a critically ill patient. By this strategy the doctor intimates—or, in effect, wagers—that the patient is sure to die. If the patient does die, the doctor is credited with an accurate prediction. If the patient is treated and miraculously survives, the doctor appears to have wrought a seemingly impossible victory over insurmountable odds. By "hanging the crepe," the doctor may feel he has set up an "all gain, no loss" condition. But has he? Blaise Pascal (1623-1662), the French philosopher of nature and religion, thought he had achieved a similar condition when he stated: "Let us weigh the gain and loss in wagering that God is. Let us estimate the two chances. If you gain, you gain all; if you lose, you lose nothing. Wager, then, without hesitation that He is." But, for a number of reasons explored in a perceptive essay by Dr. Mark Siegler (*N Engl J Med.* 1975;293:853), neither Pascal's wager nor the "hanging-of-the-crepe" strategy is unassailable.

patella is the Latin word for "a small pan, dish, or plate," this being related to the verb *patere,* "to stand open or to be accessible to." The small bone in the front of the knee came to be called the patella, though its shape is such that it would hardly make much of a saucer. "Kneecap" seems a better name.

patho-, -pathy are combining forms, a prefix and suffix, respectively, taken from the Greek *pathos,* "suffering or disease."

pathogenesis refers to the manner in which a diseased state or lesion evolves (patho- + Greek *genesis,* "bringing into being"). The pathogenesis of a given disease may include, but is not limited to, a consideration of initial cause.

pathognomonic is a near borrowing of the Greek *pathognomonikos,* "skilled in judging diseases." The Greek *gnōmōn* designated both "one who knows" and "the indicator pin on a sundial." A pathognomonic symptom or sign is one so characteristic that it clearly indicates, not merely suggests, a given disease.

pathology is properly a discourse or study of disease (patho- + Greek *logos,* "a treatise"). "Pathology" is commonly (and deplorably) used by some medical speakers and writers as a pseudoesoteric synonym for a given disease or a lesion itself. To state, "There's no 'pathology' there," when trying to say that no lesion exists, is ridiculous (unless, of course, one is referring to a school of medicine whose curriculum does not include a study of disease).

patient is derived from the Latin verb *patior,* which means "to suffer," both in the sense of feeling pain and of forbearance. Therefore, the two English uses of "patient"—one as a noun, "a person who suffers," and the other as an adjective, "to bear with fortitude"—are of common origin. The identity of the adjective and noun can lead to awkward, if not impossible, constructions: persons who suffer may lack forbearance, but to call them "impatient patients" sounds odd, if not non-sensical.

p.c. is an abbreviation of the Latin *post cibum* (*post*, "after," + *cibus*, "food") and is used on prescriptions to instruct the patient to take his medication after meals. The initials **a.c.** represent the Latin *ante cibum*, "before a meal."

pectinate is derived from the Latin *pectin* or the Greek *pekten*, both meaning "a comb." The Indo-European root *pek* meant "to pluck wool or hair." The pectinate line is the sinuous border marking the junction at the anus between the squamous epithelium of skin and the columnar epithelium of the rectum. It vaguely resembles the teeth of a comb. "Pectinate" is not to be confused with **pectin** (from the Greek *pektos*, congealed or curdled"), a carbohydrate substance used to produce a gel.

pectoral refers to the anterior chest and comes from the Latin *pectus*, "the breast." One can reflect on the Greek *pēktis*, an ancient sort of harp, and on *pēkte*, a cage to confine birds, and conjure up an allusion to the appearance of the bony thorax.

pectoriloquy is a term invented by René Théophile Hyacinthe Laënnec (1781-1826), the French clinician who also invented the stethoscope, to describe the sound of the patient's voice as transmitted by cavities in the lung, as detected by **auscultation** (Latin *pectus*, "chest" + *loqui*, "to speak").

pediatrics used to be spelled (and is still so spelled by the British) "paediatrics," which, though it looks stilted that way, serves to remind us that the prefix of "pediatrics" comes from the Greek *pais, paidos*, "a child," and not from the Latin *pes, pedis*, "a foot," or from the Latin *pedis*, "a louse." The suffix "-iatrics" is of Greek derivation and means "treatment of disease." **Pederasty**, meaning a perverted sexual relationship with children, especially with young boys, comes from

pais + the Greek *erastes*, "a lover."

pedicle is taken from the Latin *pediculus*, the diminutive of *pes, pedis*, hence "a little foot." The term was adopted in the 16th century as a name for the supporting stalk or stem of a fruit or flower and, soon after, as a name for the point of attachment for various organs of the body, e.g., the pedicle of the kidney. In Late Latin, **peduncle** was contrived as a distinguishing variant of *pediculus*, mainly because the latter term was also used as a name for the louse (because of its many little legs). In neuroanatomy a peduncle is a stalk-like bundle of fibers connecting different parts of the central nervous system. In pathology, any lesion having a stemlike point of attachment is said to be pedunculated.

pedigree is an English way of pronouncing and spelling the French *pied de grue*, literally, "the foot of a crane." Apparently, the graphic tracing of a family lineage reminded someone of the imprint of a crane's foot.

peduncle (*see* **pedicle**)

peliosis is taken from the Greek *pelios*, "leaden-colored, as the gray-blue of skin discolored by a bruise." It is likely the Greeks recognized a blemish of skin at the site of a bruise to be due to extravasated blood. **Peliosis hepatis** is a condition marked by extra-sinusoidal "blood lakes" in the liver, often attending debilitating disease or sometimes associated with the use of androgenic steroids. In the past, "peliosis" was used interchangeably with **purpura**.

pellagra is a disease characterized by "the 4 D's": dermatitis, diarrhea, dementia, and death. The Italians were impressed by the cutaneous and nervous manifestations of the disease, and the name "pellagra" was proposed by Francesco Frapolli in 1771, admixing the Latin *pellis*, "hide," + the Greek *agra*, "a seizing." Frapolli also was probably aware of the term *pellarella*, perhaps used for a similar condition that had appeared in the register of a Milan hospital as early as the 16th century. The solution to the ancient mystery of the cause of pellagra is a fascinating story (*Hospital Practice*. March 1978: 136-164). Its protagonist is a U.S. Public Health Service doctor, Joseph Goldberger (1874-1929), who found, by his determined research in the early 1900s, that the disease resulted from a lack of dietary niacin and could be cured by assuring an adequate intake of foods containing that vitamin.

pellucidum combines the equivalent of the Latin *per-*, "through," + *lucere*, "to shine." The septum pellucidum is the translucent membrane that separates the anterior horns of the lateral ventricles of the brain.

pelvis is the Latin word for "a basin or bucket," and is related to the Greek *pyelos*, "a tub or trough." Thus, "pelvis" aptly describes the basinlike structure at the bottom of the torso that is bounded by the pubis anteriorly, the hip bones laterally, and the sacrum posteriorly. The pelvis of the kidney is really the funnel-shaped expansion of the uppermost ureter and is more accurately an **infundibulum**. But, apparently to save syllables, everyone calls it a pelvis.

pemphigus is a generic term for a group of severe, sometimes fatal, skin diseases characterized by crops of blisters that, after they subside, leave pigmented spots in the skin. The term is taken from the Greek *pemphix*, "a blister." **Pemphigoid** (+ Greek *eidos*, "like") is the name given to a vesicular eruption in the skin that looks like pemphigus but is clearly distinguished as being benign.

-penia is a neo-Latin combining term taken from the Greek *penēs*, "poverty stricken." The word "penury," meaning a state of utter destitution, comes from the same source. ("Penalty" is unrelated, being derived from the Latin *poenalis*.) In pathology "-penia" indicates a lack or deficiency of something. **Leukopenia** is a deficiency of white blood cells; **neutropenia** specifies a deficiency of neutrophils, and **lymphopenia** specifies a deficiency of lymphocytes—not of lymph— and really should be **lymphocytopenia**. **Osteopenia** is a deficiency in bony substance that can include both **osteoporosis** (an impaired maintenance of the bony matrix) and **osteomalacia** (a demineralization of bone).

penicillin immediately suggests the name of an antibiotic agent, but there was a *penicillium* long before the celebrated discovery in 1928 by English bacteriologist Alexander Fleming (1881-1955) that staphylococci failed to grow in a culture medium contaminated by the fungus *Penicillium notatum*. The name is taken from the Latin *penicillum*, "a painter's brush," to which the fronds of the fungus bear a resemblance.

penis originally in Latin meant "a tail." The Romans showed a proclivity, apparently common through the ages, for having numerous names for the male reproductive organ. In addition to penis, Professor H. A. Skinner listed **clava** ("club"), **gladius** ("sword"), **radix** ("root"), **ramus** ("branch"), and **vomer** ("plow"). *Penis* became so closely associated with the male organ that the Romans enlisted *cauda* to designate an actual tail. The Latin *penis* is related to the verb *pendere*, "to hang down."

penumbra sometimes is used to refer to the shadowy margin of a condition, i.e., outlying circumstances as opposed to a central focus. For example, abdominal pain is a symptom that may occur in the penumbra of migraine. The word comes from a combination of the Latin *paene*, "almost" + *umbra*, "shadow." The Latin *paene* is not to be confused with the Greek *penēs*, "depleted," from which the suffix "-penia" is derived.

pep is a sprightly little word for "spirited animation and vigor," a quality many patients complain they lack. It is actually a contraction of "pepper." The allusion to the pungent spice is obvious. "Pepper" is a name of ancient lineage that can be traced back, through the Latin *piper* and the Greek *peperi*, to the Sanskrit *pippali*, all meaning "berry." Common pepper is made from the berries of the plant *Piper nigrum* and was probably known to the earliest people who inhabited the globe.

pepsin comes from the Greek *pepsis*, "a cooking," this being related to the Greek *peptein*, "to soften, ripen, cook, or digest." Pepsin is a proteolytic enzyme and, being an enzyme, one might think the term should end in "-ase." It should, and the correct name is **protease**. But pepsin was named before the suffix denoting enzymes became customary. The "-in" at the end means simply that pepsin has something to do with digestion.

per- is a combining form, usually a prefix, taken from the Latin preposition *per*, "through, throughout, or by means of," also used as an intensive.

per se is a much overworked Latin phrase (per + *se,* "itself") of which medical students and doctors alike become enamored. Why not simply say "in itself" or "of itself"?

percussion is a method of physical examination whereby a resonant part, such as the chest, is tapped to elicit a sound that varies according to the underlying consistency. The term is taken from the Latin *percutere,* "to strike,"(per + a derivative of *quatere,* "to cause to vibrate"). The diagnostic implications of percussion were first recognized about 1754 by Leopold Auenbrugger (1722-1809), chief physician at the Hospital of the Holy Trinity in Vienna, and published by him in 1761. But not until the publications in French by Jean Nicolas Corvisar in 1808 and by René Laënnec in 1816 did the method become widely applied.

perforate means to make a hole into or through something (per- + Latin *forare,* "to bore").

peri- is a prefix meaning "around or about" and is a direct borrowing of the Greek preposition of the same meaning, equivalent to the Latin *circum.* "Peri-" has been attached to a variety of words to make up a host of medical terms. It is essential to distinguish between "peri-" and "para-," the latter being the Greek for "beside." Thus, there is a significant difference between **periumbilical,** "around the umbilicus," and **paraumbilical,** "beside the umbilicus," when, for example, referring to the site of abdominal pain.

pericardium is the membrane forming the sac that envelopes the heart (peri- + Greek *kardia,* "heart").

perineum is a near borrowing of the Greek *perinaion* and refers to the area between the anus and the scrotum or the vulva. The first part of the Greek word is clearly *peri-,* but the origin of the last part is less certain; it could well be the Greek *inan,* "to excrete." The derived adjective is **perineal,** not to be confused with "peroneal."

periodic is actually two words, spelled the same but pronounced differently, and of separate origins. The less often used "periodic" is pronounced "per-i-*oh*-dik" and is the name of an oxidizing inorganic acid containing iodine ($H_5IO_42H_2O$). Here the "per-" is from Latin and used as an intensive, indicating a constituent element (iodine) in its highest oxida-

tive state. The more familiar "periodic" is pronounced "pir-ee-*od*-ik" and is derived from the Greek *periodikos,* "pertaining to a circuit," combining *peri-,* "around," + *hodos,* "way." The term is used in medicine to describe symptoms or afflictions that occur from time to time. However, "periodic" is properly restricted to conditions that recur at relatively fixed or predictable intervals. Related but distinct terms are **episodic** (Greek *epeisodios,* "entering on top of or in addition to"), **intermittent** (Latin *intermittere,* literally "to send between" but meaning more "to interrupt or to suspend"), **occasional** (Latin *occasionem,* "opportunity"), **sporadic** (Greek *sporadikos,* "scattered or isolated"), and **recurrent** (Latin *recurrere,* "to run back, to return"). "Episodic" refers to a self-limited circumstance that may occur singly or may be repeated at no necessarily fixed interval. Attacks of peptic ulcer distress are typically episodic. "Intermittent" emphasizes the interval rather than the incident. "Occasional" is used as an inexact term implying "from time to time." "Sporadic" suggests in time "once in a while" and in space "here or there." "Recurrent" stresses repetition; however, in anatomy, "recurrent" is used more particularly (and in a manner more faithful to its origin) to mean "running in a reverse direction," as does the recurrent laryngeal nerve. For further illustration a **tertian** or **quartan** (both from Latin numeration) fever, as in certain forms of malaria, recurs predictably every 3rd or 4th day, respectively, bearing in mind that the initial occurrence is counted as the 1st day, so a "tertian" fever actually recurs every other day. Fever that is intermittent is marked by varying afebrile intervals. A hectic fever, imprecise though the descriptor might be, is marked by high, afternoon "spikes" of temperature elevation, usually accompanied by flushing, chills, and drenching sweats.

periodontal (*see* **tooth**)

periosteum is the tough fibrous covering of a bone (peri- + Greek *osteon,* "bone").

peristalsis is literally a circumferential contracting, as occurs in the muscular coat of the intestine (peri- + Greek *stalsis,* from *stellein,* "to set up, to bring together, to contract").

peritoneum is the membrane stretched around

the abdominal viscera and the inner surface of the cavity containing them (peri- + Greek *tonos*, "a stretching").

perityphlitis (*see* **cecum**)

perleche is a French word (pronounced per-lesh') combining "per-," in the sense of excessive, + *lecher*, "to lick." In French the connotation is one of "overpolishing." The term describes a thickening and cracking of the lips, particularly at the corners of the mouth, consequent to drooling and excessive licking of the lips. "Perleche" has been applied specifically to the result of frequent licking of the lips as a symptom of oral moniliasis in children but more often the condition is seen in elderly, debilitated patients. The lesion is similar to that of **cheilosis** (from the Greek *cheilos*, "lip"), a chapped fissuring at the corners of the mouth, a condition commonly consequent to drooling and only rarely attributable to deficiency of riboflavin.

pernicious is an almost direct borrowing of the Latin *perniciosus*, "ruinous," derived in turn from the noun *pernicies*, "death-dealing disaster or calamity" and also "a pestilence or curse." The Latin word combines *per-* + *nex*, *necis*, "death." In lay language "pernicious" has been softened to "hurtful." But in medicine, before a remedy was found in liver extract and later in vitamin B_{12}, "pernicious anemia" was a fatal disease.

peroneal refers to the fibula or to the anterior, lateral aspect of the lower part of the leg, and to the muscles, blood vessels, and nerves serving that region. The adjective comes from the Greek *perone*, meaning "anything pointed for piercing," especially the tongue of a buckle or broach. This is an allusion to the shape of the fibula, whose name is the Latin word for "clasp or pin." The Latin term became firmly fixed to the leg bone itself, but the adjectival form remained Greek.

perspire is derived from a combination of "per-" + the Latin *spirare*, "to breathe," and would appear to have a connection to air rather than sweat. To the Romans, *perspirare* meant "to breathe through" or, as wind, "to blow constantly." When Romans sweated they called the moisture *sudor*. It was in the 17th century when **perspiration** took on the meaning of an effluvium from an external surface, such as the skin.

pertussis is a term wherein the "per-" indicates intensity and is coupled with the Latin *tussis*, "a cough," hence, "a violent cough." The term was introduced into English by Thomas Sydenham (1624-1689), the celebrated London physician, and thereafter became identified with the disease of children commonly known as whooping cough, the "whoop" describing the strident cough typical of the disease.

pes is the Latin word for "foot." It is incorporated in **pes anserinus** (Latin *anser*, "goose"), the parotid branches of the facial (seventh cranial) nerve said to resemble a goose's webbed foot. **Pes planus** (Latin *planus*, "flat") is literally "flat foot," whereas **pes vacus** (Latin *cavus*, "hollow or vaulted") is a foot with an abnormally high arch.

pessary comes through the Latin *pessarium* from the Greek *pessos*, the name given to an oval stone used by the Greeks in playing a game similar to our checkers. The same term was used for a round plug of lint that the Greeks used as a sort of vaginal tampon. Hippocrates is said to have advised insertion of half a pomegranate in the treatment of prolapsed uterus. The prototype of the ring-shaped pessary used in more modern times was devised by Rodericus a Castro (1546-1627), a Portuguese physician who practiced in Hamburg, Germany.

pestilence is taken from the Latin *pestis*, "plague," and denotes an epidemic of dire disease, typically infectious. A shortened and softened derivative is "pest" as a name for anyone or anything that is a nuisance (a word weakened as it passed through the Old French *nuisant*, softened somewhat from the Latin *noxius*, "injurious").

pestle is a small, club-shaped instrument, now almost obsolete, once used in pharmacies to convert friable solids into powders. The term is derived from the Latin *pistillum*, "a pounder," this being related to the Latin verb *pinsere*, "to pound." The pounding was done in a **mortar** (from the Latin *mortarium*, a vessel in which anything might be pulverized or kneaded) (*see* **trituration**), which also became the name of the contents, such as a mixture of calcined clay and crushed limestone used as an adhesive between stones or bricks in building. More often mortar is mixed on a flat palette. The traditional headdress that American students don only at graduation ceremonies resembles such a palette and is called a "mortarboard."

petechia is a near borrowing of the Italian *petechio*, "a fleabite." When numerous the minute, flat, red spots are "petechiae" and indicate focal bleeding in the skin as seen in various blood and vascular disorders. They resemble the punctate bites of fleas. A related term, but antecedent and implying greater virulence, is **impetigo**.

petit mal is a French term meaning, literally, "a little illness." The term is used in medicine to designate a minor form of epilepsy, typically occurring in young children and characterized by sudden, brief lapses in consciousness. In contrast **grand mal** designates the major tonic and clonic seizures of epilepsy.

petri dish (*see* **vital**)

petrous is an adjective derived from the Latin *petra*, "rock." The petrous portion of the temporal bone, wedged in at the base of the skull between the sphenoid and occipital bones, is composed of an unusually dense form of bone. The **petrosal nerves** and the **petrous ganglia** are so named because they are situated in or near the petrous portion of the temporal bone.

-pexy is a suffix taken from the Greek *pēxis*, "a fixing." In *pēxis* the "x" stands for the Greek letter xi, not chi, and should be pronounced like "z" but is not. The fix is more in the sense of fastening rather than repair, though one may think by fastening one has effected a repair. **Nephropexy**, for example, is an operation whereby a kidney, presumably loosened from its moorings, is restored by fixing it to its normal position. A somewhat related but distinct suffix is **-rhaphy**, from the Greek *rhaphē*, "a seam," meaning a procedure whereby separated parts are joined by a sutured seam.

pH is the symbol signifying the logarithm of the reciprocal of the hydrogen ion concentration of a given solution in gram atoms per liter. The pH of various body fluids, such as the blood, is a critical factor in determining health or disease. The "p" can be thought of as standing for either "potential," i.e., the hydrogen potential, or for "para," in the sense of "another expression for"; the "H," of course, stands for "hydrogen." Francophiles would insist the symbol is pure French, standing for *puissance hydrogène*, "the power of hydrogen."

phacocele (*see* **lens**)

phage is a sort of nickname for **bacteriophage**, a group of viruses that infect bacteria and cause their dissolution. The latter part of the term "bacteriophage" was concocted from the Greek *phagein*, "to devour," a graphic depiction though somewhat off the mark. A **phagedenic** ulcer is one that spreads rapidly, seeming to devour all surrounding tissue.

phagocytosis is the process whereby certain scavenger cells of the body ingest and destroy dead or foreign material such as bacteria. The concept and its name were introduced in 1884 by Elie Metchnikoff (1845-1916), the celebrated Russian pathologist. The term was contrived by combining the Greek *phagein*, "to eat," + *kytos*, "cell," hence an "eating cell."

phako-, phakoma (*see* **lens**)

phalanges is the plural of the Greek *phala[n]gx*, the name given by Aristotle to the bones of the fingers (and later extended to the bones of the toes) because they are arranged in ranks suggesting the military formation favored by Greek warriors in battle.

phallus is derived from the Greek *phallos*, primly defined in Greek lexicons as the *membrum virile* ("the manly member"). Apparently, lexicographers figure that if you are old enough to translate Greek, you are old enough to know this means the penis. An effigy of the *phallos* was borne in solemn procession in the Bacchic orgies as a symbol of the generative power of nature. In embryology the phallus is the primordium of the penis or the clitoris.

pharmacy comes from the Greek *pharmakon*, "a drug." The Greek term was used to designate remedies, particularly those applied externally as salves or ointments, and also charms or poisons. **Pharmacology** (+ Greek *logos*, "treatise") is the study of drugs, their sources, and their properties. **Pharmacopoeia** (+ Greek *poiein*, "to make") is an authoritative or official listing of drugs and their components. The first *U.S. Pharmacopoeia* was published in 1820. It was printed in both English and Latin and listed 217 drugs that were considered worthy of mention.

pharynx is a direct borrowing of the Greek word for "the throat," and designates a common passage, shared by the upper respiratory and alimentary tracts, extending from the back of the nasal passages and mouth to the larynx and esophagus. A related Greek word *phary[n]gos* could also mean "a ravine or gully."

pheno- is a combining form only slightly modified from the Greek *phainō*, "I bring to light, I show." This is best exemplified by **phenotype**, the visibly evident expression of the hereditary constitution of an organism (*see* **mutation**). A **phenomenon** today is almost exactly what *phainomenon* was to the Greeks, "a thing observed or brought to light." The use of "pheno-" in the designation of numerous organic chemical compounds is owed to the naming of the prototype **phenol** (+ Latin *oleum*, "oil"), literally "the shining oil" because of its derivation from coal oil, which was used in lamps. **Phenolphthalein**, a dye used as an indicator of pH and also as a purgative, indicates a relation to phthalic anhydride, the latter term being a shortening of the Greek *naphtha*, "a liquid bitumen."

pheochromocytoma is a catecholamine-producing tumor arising from cells related to the sympathetic nervous system, especially those in the adrenal medulla. The name can be dissected according to its contrived derivation: Greek *phaios*, "dark or dusky," + *chrōma*, "color," + *kytos*, "cell," + *-ōma*, "tumor." The explanation is that unfixed sections of such a tumor, when exposed to chromium salts, take on a dusky brown color because they are composed of chromaffin cells.

-phil is a combining form, usually a suffix, taken from the Greek *philos*, "loved." In some instances it denotes possession in the absence of affection. In scientific usage "-phil" conveys the sense of "affinity." Among the cellular components of blood, the basophil has an affinity for basic dyes, the eosinophil for eosin, and the neutrophil for neither. Another example in biology is **drosophila** as the name for the fruit fly, commonly used in the study of heredity. The drosophila was so named because, aside from its fondness for fruit, it is inclined to frolic in the dew (Greek *droso*, "dew").

philtrum is the name given to the vertical cleft between the base of the nose and the upper lip. Both the Greeks and the Romans had their love charms and love potions known in the singular as *philtron* and *philtrum*, in their respective languages. This feature of surface anatomy is so called, presumably, because in an attractive partner it invites kissing.

phimosis is a condition wherein the foreskin of the penis (or clitoris) is so tight it cannot be drawn back over the glans. The term originated in the Greek *phimos*, "a muzzle," such as used to keep an animal's mouth shut, and from the noseband on a horse's bridle.

phlebo- is a combining form taken from the Greek *phleps* (genitive *phlebos*), "vein," which could mean a vein of ore or a spring of water. The Greek root verb was *phlein*, "to gush or overflow." Hippocratic writers used *phleps* for blood vessels generally, including both arteries and veins. Probably it was the gushing of blood from a severed vessel that first suggested a name related to *phlein*. When the arteries were distinguished as such (under the mistaken impression they contained air), *phleps* was restricted to veins.

phlebotomy is an incision or puncture into a vein to permit the outpouring of blood (phlebo- + Greek *tomē*, "a cutting"). *Phlebotomus* is a genus of pesky flies that bite hard and suck blood, thereby transmitting "sandfly fever," kala-azar, and probably other diseases.

phlegm comes from the Greek *phlegma*, "a flame or heat." Ancient writers used the term in reference to inflammation generally. The Greek *phlegma* was incorporated into the archaic "humoral pathology," but oddly the term was assigned to the cold, moist "humor." From this came the custom of referring to the mucous secretion of the respiratory tract as "phlegm." Echoing the idea of cold and moist is the use of **phlegmatic** to describe a person of a sluggish or indifferent temperament, also known as "a cold fish" or "a wet blanket."

phlegmon designates an infiltrating inflammation that often leads to abscess and ulceration. (*see* **phlegm**)

phlogiston is an archaic term once used to designate the supposed component that produced fire in whatever was combustible. The term was first used in the 17th century, being taken from the Greek *phlogistos*, "set on fire."

Later, this dubious idea was adopted to explain the origin of inflammation in body tissues, especially that externally visible. Within living memory there was a concoction of glycerine, kaolin, and aromatics called Antiphlogistine which was purveyed as an anodyne and antiseptic preparation purported to suppress inflammation in skin lesions.

phlyctenule is a diminutive derivation from the Greek *phlyctaina*, "a blister or pimple." Once used in reference to papular or vesicular eruptions of various sorts, the term is now restricted to minute vesicles, often ulcerated, of the cornea or conjunctiva.

phobia is a near borrowing of the Greek *phobos*, "fear." Psychologists cite all sorts of morbid phobias or aversions, ranging from **acrophobia** (Greek *akron*, "peak"), a fear of high places, to **zoophobia** (Greek *zōon*, "a living creature"), a fear of animals. A few other phobias are listed:

> **agoraphobia** (Greek *agora*, "market place"), fear of venturing into any crowded place.
> **ailurophobia** (Greek *ailouros*, "a cat"), fear of felines.
> **anemaphobia** (Greek *anemos*, "wind"), fear of hurricanes.
> **bromidrosiphobia** (Greek *brōmos*, "stench," + *idrōs*, "sweat"), dread of body odors, real or imagined.
> **claustrophobia** (Latin *claustrum*, "a barrier or fence"), fear of being confined.
> **ergasiophobia** (Greek *ergon*, "work"), aversion to work (and perhaps a word to keep in mind when filling out disability forms).
> **noctiphobia** (Latin nox, noctis, "night"), fear of darkness.
> **nosophobia** (Greek *nosus*, "disease"), fear of illness
> **pantophobia** (Greek *pantos*, "all"), fear of everything.
> **photophobia** (Greek *phōs*, "light"), painful sensitivity to light.
> **stenophobia** (Greek *stenos*, "narrow [place]"), fear of caves.
> **taphophobia** (Greek *taphos*, "a grave"), fear of cemeteries or a fear of being buried alive.
> **triskaidekaphobia** (Greek *tries-kai-deka*, "thirteen"), superstitious aversion to 13 of anything.
> **tropophobia** (Greek *tropos*, "a turning"), fear of making decisions or changes.
> **xenophobia** (Greek *xenos*, "a stranger"), aversion to anyone or anything alien or foreign.

phrenic is an adjective derived from the Greek word that in the singular, *phrēn*, means "the mind or the seat of reason and of passion" and from which comes such turbulent words as frenetic, frantic, and frenzy. The plural, *phrēnes*, means "the muscular diaphragm," perhaps because that structure lies so close to the heart and spleen. Actually, the Greeks had a much more recognizable term, *diaphragma* ("a partition"), for the muscle that separates the chest from the abdomen. In any case, "phrenic" now is used for whatever pertains to the diaphragm, such as the phrenic nerves.

phrenology was a pseudoscience of the 19th century based on the belief that a person's character could be determined by closely observing the shape of his head, particularly noting any bumps. The term was taken, obviously, from the Greek *phrēn* + *logos*. The 19th century concept of "phrenology" is so absurd that the sensible Greeks would have been appalled by this abasement of their language.

Phrygian cap is the name given to an anatomic variant of the gallbladder wherein its fundus appears, by contrast radiography or in a dissected specimen, to fold over on itself. The name comes from the floppy, conical headdress worn by liberated slaves as a sign of their freedom in Phrygia, an ancient country in Asia Minor. This sort of cap, often hoisted on a pole, was displayed by the proletariat in the French Revolution. The Phrygian cap of a gallbladder usually has no clinical significance.

phthisis is an archaic name for tuberculosis and was used when, because of its devastating effect, tuberculosis was commonly known as "the consumption" (a fulminant course was called "galloping consumption"). The Greek *phthisis* means "a dwindling or wasting away."

phylogeny (*see* ontogeny)

physiatry is the science and art of physical therapy, i.e., the treatment of impairment, usually musculoskeletal, by mechanical means, such as exercise, massage, heat, and light. A **physiatrist** is one who practices physical medicine. The terms combine the Greek *physis*, "nature," + *iatreia*, "the art of healing." Though the derivation suggests a connection with "naturopathy," there is none, as any physiatrist will vehemently affirm.

physician is a designation for a practitioner of the healing arts and is used only in English-speaking countries. Everywhere else in the world such a practitioner is known, in one form or another, as a "healer." To the Greeks whatever pertained to nature or its laws was known as *physikos*, and *physikoi* were philosophers who pondered the origin and existence of material things rather than abstract or moral issues. The Greek *physikos* when taken into English provided two words: "physic" and "physics." The latter is that branch of science that deals with matter and energy, and its practitioners are known as "physicists." The former word is a now almost forgotten term for the practice of medicine, once used because doctors were supposed to know the nature of things. In Ireland the school of medicine at Dublin's Trinity College is still known as "The School of Physic." And at Harvard University there is still a Hersey Professor of the Theory and Practice of Physic. Strictly speaking, a doctor of medicine functions as a physician when he opines how, why, and what ails his patient. There was a time when he could do little else. Nowadays, there is much a physician can do to alter the course of "nature." In addition, there was another use of "physic," and that was as a colloquial term for a cathartic, probably because cathartics were among the few effective drugs that practitioners of "physic" at one time used. In a cathartic vein, it has been said that the ancient Egyptian equivalent of a physician was called *swnw* (pronounced "soo-noo") or "shepherd of the anus." In the pathophysiology of that time long ago, the anus was considered the repository for the various bodily humors, including a product of putrefaction called *okhedu*. The physician was charged with removing this deleterious residue by administering enemas to both the living and the dead.

physiology is an almost direct borrowing of the Greek *physiologia*, "an inquiry into the nature of things," this combining *physis*, "nature" + *logos*, "a treatise, discourse, or study." Through the centuries *physiologia* covered all that was known of natural science. As various specialized studies estab-

lished purviews of their own, "physiology" became restricted to that department of natural science that deals with the functions of living organisms and their parts.

physostigmine is an alkaloid whose principal property is inhibition of cholinesterase activity; thereby, it exerts a cholinergic effect. It is derived from the calabar bean, a product of the plant *Physostigma venenosum*. The botanical name is a combination of the Greek *physa*, "a bellows," + *stigma*, used here to refer to that part of the pistil that receives the pollen. This describes the shape of the flower. The Latin *venenosum* indicates it is potentially poisonous.

pia mater is a delicate membrane, the innermost of the three meninges that cover the brain and spinal cord. *Pia* is the feminine of the Latin *pius*; in this sense "tender," the feminine form being required to agree with *mater*, which is used here in the Arabic sense of "covering or protecting" (even though the Latin *mater* ordinarily means "mother"). The term serves to distinguish the inner, delicate membrane from the outer, tough, dura mater, between which is the weblike arachnoid network.

pica is the Latin word for "magpie," a bird noted for its indiscriminate gleaning of all sorts of odd objects for inclusion in its nest. Medically, pica is an inordinate craving for bizarre foods or the eating of substances not ordinarily considered as foods. The commonest cravings are for ice, clay, or cornstarch. Such craving is now recognized as a sign of iron deficiency.

Pickwickian syndrome was so named by Dr. C. S. Burwell and his coauthors (*Am J Med.* 1956;21:811) as a whimsical allusion to the sleepy fat boy of Charles Dickens' *Pickwick Papers*. The syndrome of obesity, plethoric facies, and reduced vital capacity, as seen in pulmonary alveolar hypoventilation associated with corpulence, was first described 20 years earlier by Dr. W. J. Kerr and Dr. J. B. Lagen (*Ann Intern Med.* 1936;10:569). Incidentally, the reference is not to the title character of *Pickwick Papers* but to Mr. Wardle's servant Joe, often called "The Fat Boy," who falls asleep whenever he stops moving, even when he is on his feet.

pill is a shortened, Anglicized version of the

French *pilule*, which is taken from the Latin *pilula*, the diminutive of *pila*, "a ball." Indeed, pills originally were spherical, a given dose of the active medicament being mixed with an excipient plastic substance, often lactose, then rolled by hand into a little ball that was finally coated with a varnishlike substance. Incidentally, the "pill-roller's tremor," often mentioned as characteristic of parkinsonism, was not mentioned as such by James Parkinson (1755-1824) in his "Essay on the Shaking Palsy," published in 1817, but was used as a vivid descriptor by later writers. The Latin *pila* is related to the Greek *pilos*, "wool, or hair made into a sort of felt." The balls used in play by the Romans were made of felt.

pilo- is a combining form taken from the Latin *pilus*, "hair, especially that which can be compressed as felt." (*see* **hair**)

pilocarpine is an alkaloid exhibiting cholinergic properties, originally obtained from leaves of the plant *Pilocarpus* (pilo- + Greek *karpos*, "fruit") *microphyllus*; presumably, the plant was thought to bear feltlike fruit.

pilomotor describes the erector muscles that, when contracted, elevate the hair and cause a puckering of the skin known as "goose flesh" (Latin, *cutis anserina*) or "duck bumps."

pilonidal describes an anomalous dermoid cyst occurring in the sacrococcygeal region, usually bearing a cluster of fine hairs (pilo- + Latin *nidus*, "nest").

pimple can be traced in English to the 15th century when it was first used to describe a scabrous skin eruption. Some say the word originated, through the Old English *piplian*, from the Latin *papilla*, "a nipple." (*see* **papule**)

pineal is a shortening of the Latin *pinealis*, "pertaining to the pine [tree]," or more specifically, "the pinecone." The small, cone-shaped structure, an outgrowth of the epithalamus in the brain, is called the "pineal body" because of its fancied resemblance to a little pinecone. Although the pineal body was known and described by ancient anatomists, its function remains uncertain to this day. It has been found to harbor a remarkable variety of neurotransmitter substances, and some say the pineal body is implicated in the regulation of circadian rhythms, as a sort of internal clock.

pinna is the Latin word for "feather or wing" and, by allusion, can easily be applied as a name for the winglike external ear that projects from either side of the head.

pinocytosis is the process whereby certain cells can imbibe fluids from their environment. They do this by forming invaginations in their cell walls, thus engulfing droplets of adjacent fluid. The term was contrived by combining the Greek *pinein*, "to drink," + *kytos*, "a cell."

piriform comes from a combination of the Latin *pirum*, "a pear," + *forma*, "shape." The term has been used to describe various pear-shaped structures and lesions. An example is the piriform fossa or sinus in the lateral wall of the laryngeal pharynx. Inexplicably, the term is sometimes misspelled "pyriform," thus utterly destroying its meaning. "Pyri-" would suggest a relation to the Greek *pyr*, "fire."

pisiform is derived from a combination of the Latin *pisum*, "a pea," + *forma*, "shape." The pisiform, as one of the carpal bones is called, might be said to resemble a large pea in shape and size.

piss (*see* **urine**)

pituitary comes from the Latin *pituita*, "phlegm," this being related to the Greek *ptuō*, "I spit." The Greek word is obviously and vividly imitative and a forerunner of the expletives "Ptooey!" and "Phooey!" The ancients entertained the notion that the brain secreted a mucoid substance that was discharged through the nose. Aristotle, no less, suggested that this was a cooling process, designed to allay an unduly hot temper. Indeed, Vesalius used the Latin *infundibulum*, "funnel," to describe the attachment of the pituitary gland to the brain. The idea that the pituitary gland elaborated a sort of spit was discarded in the 17th century, but the name stuck. A much less interesting but more accurate name for the gland is **hypophysis** (Greek *hypo*, "below," + *physis*, "a growth"), which simply tells us that the structure grows beneath the brain.

pityriasis is a word that Hippocrates and Discorides used to describe a scruffy excrescence on the skin. The scurf or dandruff resembled the husks of cereal grain, known in Greek as *pityron*. We still use "pityriasis," much as did the ancient writers, for a group of scaly diseases of the skin, though we usually designate specific types by modifying terms, such as pityriasis rosea.

placebo is the first person singular of the future tense of the Latin *placere* and is literally translated "I will please." In medicine a placebo is any relatively inert substance given, in a form that resembles a medicament, merely for the purpose of pleasing or gratifying the patient (or, sometimes, the doctor who gives it). In that strict sense placebos are rarely, if ever, knowingly prescribed, except in the conduct of controlled therapeutic trials wherein a drug of purported effect is to be compared with an inactive dummy. In this regard all seasoned clinicians and investigators are well aware of the phenomenon of "a placebo effect" whereby as many as one third of subjects given an inactive substance in the guise of medication will report a favorable or beneficial result.

placenta is the Latin word for "a cake" and is related to the Greek *plakous*, "a flat cake." A derivative is "plaque." This is descriptive of the shape of the placenta in the gravid uterus, where it serves as a communication, by way of the umbilical cord, between the fetus and its mother. To the ancient Greeks what we call the placenta was known as *ta deutera*, and to the Romans as *secundae*, both terms meaning "the second thing" expelled after childbirth, in the manner of the common English "afterbirth." A **placenta praevia** (Latin *praevia* being the feminine of *praevius*, "leading the way") is a placenta that develops in the lower part of the uterus at or near its outlet and, at the time of delivery, tends to precede the fetus. **Abruptio placentae** (Latin *abruptio*, "breaking off") is premature detachment of the placenta from the uterine lining.

plague is a derivative of the Greek *plēgē*, "a blow or stroke." The Latin *plungere* means "to beat or strike" and "to bewail or lament." In reference to devastating pestilence, the image is both that of a divine stroke of retribution and the lamentation that this evokes. Originally, the term was applied to any destructive epidemic disease, particularly that marked by fever. The **black plague** of the 14th century was so called because the

extensive subcutaneous hemorrhage of its victims gave their bodies a dark-blue hue. In some areas the pestilence was known as the **bubonic plague** (Greek *boubōn*, "swollen groin") because of the characteristic inguinal adenopathy or **buboes**. This disease, which still occurs sporadically in various parts of the world, is now known to be the result of infection by facultatively anaerobic bacteria transmitted to man from rodents by fleas. The causative organism was isolated by Alexandre Yersin (1863-1943), born a Swiss but later naturalized as a French citizen, who had been summoned to Hong Kong in 1894 to investigate an outbreak of plague. Yersin named the organism *Pasteurella pestis* in honor of Louis Pasteur, his French patron. In 1970 the name was changed to *Yersinia pestis* as a tribute to its discoverer. The "Great Plague" that devastated London in 1665 probably was typhus.

plane comes from the Latin adjective *planus*, "flat," and has been used in English anatomy since the 16th century to designate various flat surfaces, real and imagined, in reference to the body. Among the most widely used of the imagined anatomic planes, referring to the body as a whole or any part thereof, are the **transverse** plane (Latin *transversus*, "lying crosswise"), the **frontal** plane (Latin *frons, frontis*, "facade"), and the **sagittal** plane (Latin *sagitta*, "arrow"). The last is so called because it is the plane within which an arrow would lie if it penetrated the body squarely from front to back, or vice versa, depending on the temerity or trepidity of the archer.

plantar is taken from the Latin *planta*, "the sole of the foot." The **plantaris muscle** makes up part of the calf of the leg, but when contracting it flexes the foot, i.e., turns the sole downward. The term **plantar wart** says nothing about the wart except that it is situated on the bottom of the foot.

-plasia is a suffix derived from the Greek *plassein*, "to mold," denoting an evolving development or formation. Cells and the tissues they make up can undergo hyperplasia or hypoplasia. There is a distinction between "-plasia" and "-trophy," the latter from the Greek *trophē*, "growth." **Hyperplastic** cells are in a state of proliferation; their numbers increase but not necessarily their size. **Hypertrophic** cells are in a state of growth; they enlarge but do not necessarily increase in number.

plasma is a direct borrowing of the Greek word for "anything formed," this being related to the Greek verb *plassein*, "to form or to mold." As noted by Professor H. A. Skinner, the ancients "believed that the vital principle or spirit of the body was a diffuse principle able to pervade any structure or tissue and adapt itself to any condition." It was in the 19th century that "plasma" was given as a name for the fluid content of blood (as opposed to its cellular elements). This was a logical extension of the idea that this "plastic" fluid substance pervaded all tissues of the body and, in a way, took their form.

plasmapheresis is the separation, customarily by centrifugation, of cellular elements in blood from the liquid plasma in which they are suspended (plasma + Greek *aphairein*, "to separate, to take away from"). Thereby the components can be used for the specific purposes to which they are individually suited; also, noxious substances in plasma can be removed without loss of the cellular elements. In the latter case plasmapheresis is a descendent of the ancient practice of bloodletting, but without sacrifice of the blood cells.

platelets are, as the diminutive ending suggests, "little plates," and this seems an apt name for the smallest of the formed elements in blood. When first identified in the mid-19th century, they were called **globulins** because they were thought to resemble little globes or spheres. However, this conflicted with the use of the same name, given about the same time, to the proteinaceous substance thought to be a product of the **globules** or cells of the blood. Later, the minute formed elements in blood were called, in German, *Blutplättchen*, and this was translated literally into English as "blood platelets," thus solving the problem.

platy- is a combining form taken from the Greek *platys*, "flat, wide, or broad."

platyhelminthes is a phylum of flatworms (platy- + Greek *helmins*, "worm"). Several of these, such as the trematodes or flukes and the cestodes or tapeworms, are parasitic to man.

platysma is the name given to a thin, flat muscle that lies just beneath the skin of the ante-rior neck and inserts in the lower jaw and the tissues around the mouth. (*see* **platy**)

pleio-, pleo- are variants of a combining form taken from the Greek *pleion*, "more."

pleiotropy in genetics means the capacity of a gene to manifest itself in different ways (Greek *pleion* "more" + *tropos*, "a turning").

pleomorphic describes whatever appears in more differing shapes than are normal (pleo- + Greek *morphē*, "form"). An example would be the varying size and configuration of parenchymal cells in certain liver diseases.

plethoric describes the florid countenance of a person whose skin, particularly that of the face and neck, is suffused with an excess of blood. **Plethora** offers an example of a disease having been demoted, through the ages, to the status of a symptom. To ancient Greek physicians, *plēthorē* meant an excess of "humors," notably blood. In modern medicine there is a disease characterized by an overabundance of blood, and it does confer on the patient a plethoric countenance, but it is called **polycythemia**. Today, "plethoric" is used to describe anyone who is red-faced for any reason. By extension, "plethora" has come to be commonly used as a word for any excess or surfeit; unfortunately, it is also sometimes mistakenly used as a substitute for "many" or "much," which it is not.

plethysmograph is an instrument designed to give an indication of the volume of blood flowing into a part by registering variations in the size of the part. As blood flows in the part swells. The name combines the Greek **plethysmos**, "increase," + *graphein*, "to write."

pleura is the plural of the Greek word for "the rib" and also refers to the side or body wall containing the ribs. Even ancient writers began to limit the term to the lining of the chest cavity. The combining form, "pleuro-," refers to whatever is related to the membrane lining the chest cavity or that covering the external surface of the lungs.

pleuritis was used by the ancient Greeks to denote any disease in the chest wall; now the word refers specifically to inflammation and has been Anglicized, through the French, to **pleurisy**.

pleurodynia is pain in the chest wall, especially that aggravated by breathing (pleur- + Greek *odynō*, "pain").

plexor is the proper name of the little rubber-headed hammer that doctors use to test neuro muscular reflexes. The name comes from the Greek *plēxis*, "a blow."

plexus originated in the Indo-European *plēk*, "to weave together," which gave rise to the Latin *plexus*, "plaited or braided." This is also related to the Greek verb *plekein*, "to twist or weave." In Anglo-Saxon the root word gave rise to *fleax*, which became "flax" as a name for the plant yielding a fiber that can be woven into cloth, specifically linen. A related Anglo-Saxon word, *fealden*, has become "to fold." In anatomy a plexus is an intricate network of fine nerve fibers or vascular channels. An example is the **solar plexus** (more properly designated the "celiac plexus"), the largest of the three sympathetic nerve plexuses situated in front of the lumbar vertebrae, so called because its processes radiate like the rays of the sun (Latin *sol*, "sun").

plica is the Latin word for "a fold" and is used to designate any structure having the appearance of a fold or ridge. The plicae **conniventes** (meaning with edges inclined toward each other, from the Latin verb *connivere*, "to wink") are the permanent transverse folds of mucosa and submucosa that characterize the lining of the small intestine. (Incidentally, the English verb "connive" is related; it is to do something "with a wink.") The plica **semilunaris** (Latin for "half-moon") is a curved fold connecting the palatoglossal and palatopharyngeal arches and forming the upper boundary of the supratonsillar fossa.

-ploid, -ploidy are suffixes denoting degrees of multiplication of chromosome sets in a karyotype, the number being indicated by the prefix. Thus, **euploidy** (Greek *eu*, "well or proper") is having a balanced set of chromosomes in a number appropriate to the species; **haploid** (Greek *haploos*, "single") means having only one member of each pair of homologous chromosomes; **diploid** (Greek *diploos*, "folded double or made two-fold") means having two sets of homologous chromosomes, as normally found in somatic cells of higher organisms; and **triploid** (Greek *treis*, "three") means having three sets of haploid chromosomes. The suffix "-ploid" is a back formation from the Greek *diploos*.

Trisomy is a condition wherein there is an additional (third) chromosome in at least one otherwise diploid set; the commonest example in humans is trisomy-21 (indicating an anomalous addition to the 21st pair of chromosomes) that is expressed as Down's syndrome.

plumbism is lead poisoning. The Latin for lead is *plumbum*, whence the chemical symbol "Pb." The Romans used this malleable metal to construct water pipes. Two causes related to lead water pipes have been postulated for the decline and fall of the Roman Empire. One is that Roman plumbers pauperized the populace by their ever-increasing charges for fixing the pipes, and the other is that citizens of Rome became afflicted with lead poisoning, a common symptom of which is mental impairment.

pneumat- (*see* **pneumo-**)

pneumo- is a combining form taken from the Greek *pneuma*, "wind, air, or breath." The Greek *pneumōn* is the lung. The list of medical terms incorporating "pneumo-" in reference to the lung, breathing, or air is expansive. When the combining form is **pneumat-**, the reference usually is to gas or air, as in "pneumatic," **pneumatosis** (an abnormal infiltration of air or other gas within a body tissue), and **pneumaturia** (+ Greek *ouron*, "urine"), the urinating of air, startling symptom pathognomonic of a fistula between the bowel and the urinary bladder.

pneumoconiosis is a term for any one of a number of diseases resulting from irritant particles in inspired air (pneumo- + Greek *konis*, "dust").

pneumonia is both a Greek and English word for "disease of the lungs"; to us it means specifically an inflammatory, usually infectious, disease. **Pneumococcus** is a species of bacteria that often causes pneumonia.

p.o. is an abbreviation of the Latin *per os*, literally "by way of the mouth."

podagra is a direct borrowing of the Greek word that originally denoted "a trap or snare for the feet." Later it came to mean "a seizure of pain in the foot," such as one might experience if one's foot were caught in a trap. The term is a combination of the Greek *podos*, "foot," + *agra*, "a seizure." Early on, podagra was identified with gout. Today, it refers to gouty arthritis as it specifically affects the big toe.

podalic version is an obstetric maneuver whereby the about-to-be-born fetus is turned so that the feet present first. "Podalic" is an adjective taken from the Greek *podus,* "foot," and "version" relates to the Latin *vertere,* "to turn."

podiatry is an invented combination of the Greek *pous, podus,* "foot," + *iatreia,* "a healing." A **podiatrist** is a specially trained therapist whose practice is limited to alleviation of various ailments of the foot. Formerly, such practitioners were known as "chiropodists," but **chiropody** was a confusing term, combining as it does the Greek *cheir,* "hand," + *podus,* "foot" (the idea being that the hand is used to manipulate the foot). What had been known as the National Association of Chiropodists officially changed its name, in 1958, to the American Podiatric Medical Association.

-poiesis is a combining form, usually a suffix, and a direct borrowing of the Greek *poiesis,* "a creation." Related English words are poem, poet, and poetry. An example of medical usage is **erythropoiesis** (+ Greek *erythros,* "red"), the generation of red blood cells, as in the bone marrow. Erythropoietin is a recently described principle that stimulates the creation of erythrocytes.

poikilocytosis (*see* **cyto-**)

poison came through the Old French *pocion* from the Latin *potio,* "a drink," from which we also derive **potion**. To the Romans *potio* also meant a magical draught. "Poison" acquired its meaning as a noxious potion in the 13th century. The Latin *potio* also gives "potable," meaning fit to drink.

polarity refers to the presence of an axial gradient, as in transmission of an impulse along a nerve tract, in a magnetic or electrical field, or along a conduit, such as a duct or a segment of the gut. The term is taken from the Greek *polos* (Latin *polus*) meaning, literally, "a pole," but more specifically an axis along or around which something moves. The related Greek verb is *pelein,* "to be in motion." An axis usually has extremities, and this idea is evident in "polar."

poliomyelitis is an acute viral disease characterized by inflammation of the central nervous system, particularly the anterior horn cells of the spinal cord and brainstem. Inasmuch as these are cells having to do with motor function, the aftermath of the disease can be a disabling paralysis. Because youngsters are particularly susceptible, the disease was once called "infantile paralysis." Older clinicians still remember the devastating onslaught of poliomyelitis in the summer and early fall of each year. Among the true triumphs of modern medicine has been the virtual obliteration of the disease by the universal use of effective vaccines. "Poliomyelitis" is a combination of the Greek *polios,* "gray," + *myelos,* "marrow," referring to the focus of the disease in the gray matter of the spinal cord.

pollex is the Latin name for the thumb and the big toe. In anatomy the reference is restricted to the thumb. The name is derived from the Latin *pollere,* "to be strong." In a contest of strength, the thumb wins over the other digits.

poly- is a combining form, usually a prefix, taken from the Greek *polys,* "many." When used in medical terms, "poly-" usually means "too many" or "more than normal." All medical terms incorporating "poly-" are too many to list, and only a few are cited here.

polyarteritis is not to be confused with **panarteritis**.

polycythemia is having too many red blood cells (poly- + Greek *kytos,* "cell," + *haima,* "blood"). This condition often is secondary to hypoxia of chronic pulmonary disease, but when it occurs as a primary manifestation of myeloproliferative disease it is called "polycythemia vera" (the feminine of the Latin *verus,* "true"). (*see* **plethora**)

polydactyly means having more than the normal allotment of fingers or toes (poly- + Greek *daktylos,* "finger").

polydipsia is excessive craving for water (poly- + Greek *dipsia,* "thirst"), whereas **polyuria** (+ Greek *ouron,* "urine") is the passage of an excessive volume of urine. Both are symptoms of diabetes.

polyp is a strange word, coming as it does from the Greek *polys,* "many" + *pous,* "foot." The allusion to many feet presumably relates to an observation that globular excrescences from the skin or mucous membranes can have an irregular, rootlike attachment. Actually, most such excrescences have a single, well-defined pedicle, but nevertheless the name "polyp" has become firmly attached. Another point: "polyp" often carries the connotation of a benign growth. This is not always true. A polyp can be cancerous, and not all benign growths are polypoid. "Polyp" should be used only as a descriptive term; it does not qualify as a diagnosis.

polyphlebitis (*see* **panarteritis***)*

polyuria (*see* **polydipsia**)

pons is the Latin word for "a bridge." The anatomic pons is that portion of the central nervous system "bridging" the mesencephalon and the medulla oblongata beneath the cerebellum. **Pontine** refers to that which may pertain to the pons, such as central pontine myelinolysis, a rarely observed lesion associated with severe malnutrition.

popliteal comes from the Latin *poples*, "the hollow of the knee," and refers to the concavity at the back of the knee. It has been suggested that *poples*, in turn, may have originated in a contracted combination of the Latin *post*, "behind," + *plicare*, "to fold," thus the "fold behind" the knee.

pore can be traced to the Greek *poros*, "a way through." Although the ancients could examine the skin only with the eye, aided at best by a primitive lens, they clearly recognized the presence of pores or passageways through which sweat was excreted.

porphyria designates a group of metabolic diseases, some of them hereditary, characterized clinically by neurologic and cutaneous manifestations and chemically by an excessive production of porphyrins, **pyrrole** derivatives that are ubiquitous in protoplasm. The terms are taken from the Greek *porphyra*, "purple," and the Greek *pyrros*, "red" (from *pyr*, "fire") because of the colors assumed by these compounds in certain chemical reactions.

porta is Latin for "gate" and is related to the verb *portare*, "to carry or convey." The porta hepatis is the fissure on the underside of the liver, a "gateway" into which enter the portal vein and hepatic artery and from which departs the bile duct.

positive and **negative** serve a number of useful functions in biomedical usage. "Positive" comes through the Old French *positif* from the Latin *positivus* "formally laid down," related to the verb *ponere*, "to place." "Negative" can be traced to the Late Latin *negatitivus*, related to the verb *negare*, "to deny, to say no." Both "positive" and "negative" have acquired, meanwhile, various meanings and connotations; in general, "positive" conveys a sense of "affirmative, certain, upward-and-onward," while "negative" conveys the opposite. However, one does well to consider how these terms are interpreted by different people under varying circumstances. Doctors are inclined to report test results that are "normal" or unrevealing of any defect as "negative." What is reported as "positive" affirms the occurrence of a suspected defect or lesion. Many years ago a thoughtful patient of mine, who happened to be the head of a large engineering laboratory, gently remonstrated when I told him his tests were "negative." He said, "Perhaps you should know that in my laboratory a 'negative' test is one that has produced an undesired result or that has gone wrong." I understood what he was telling me, and from that day on I banished "negative" from my vocabulary when talking to patients. Rather, I say a test result unrevealing of any defect is "in the normal range" or is "favorable." Also illustrating how these terms can be misunderstood is an amusing story—doubtless apocryphal—told of August Paul von Wassermann (1866-1925), the Berlin bacteriologist who devised a widely used complement-fixation test for syphilis that came to bear his name. While perfecting his procedure, Wassermann ran a test on a sample of blood provided by a physician-friend; the result required a telegraphed report: "Positive." The anxious response: "Are you positive?" Wassermann's wired reply: "Not me. You."

post- is a combining form taken from the Latin preposition and adverb *post*, "behind, backward, later, or afterward." It has been attached as a prefix to a host of medical terms to indicate a subsequent or following relation in space or time. Often the prefix is separated by a hyphen from the word it is intended to modify, but in recent usage the hyphen tends to be omitted. Sadly, "post" is extravagantly employed in the medical vernacular as a substitute for "after," as in "postsurgery" when what is meant is simply "after operation."

post hoc ergo propter hoc is a succinct statement of a well known but often ignored fallacy of reasoning. It translates literally as "after that, therefore because of that," but it sounds more forceful in the original Latin. The fallacy is pertinent to medicine, and its pitfall is to be carefully avoided by doctor and patient alike. The truth, as everyone knows but does not always remember, is that simply because two events occur in sequence does not necessarily mean the first is the cause and the second is the result. If a patient is given a dose of penicillin for a bad cold on Tuesday and then reports that he feels better on Wednesday, one cannot rightly assume that penicillin cured the cold. Medical practice is replete with similar examples of fallacious reasoning wherein *post* is confused with *propter*.

posthumous is understood to mean "after death," but the word itself is the result of a mistake. The original classical Latin *postumus* means "last or coming after." Some now-forgotten scribe, preoccupied with the idea of interment, must have thought the "-*umus*" represented the Latin *humus*, "ground or soil," and chose to amend the spelling as *posthumus* to look more like "after burial." When adopted into English, an "o" was slipped in near the end to make the word look like an adjective.

postmortem as an adjective in reference to time means, of course, "after death" (post + Latin *mors, mortis*, "death"). As a noun it is used as an alternative to "necropsy," the idea of examination being unvoiced but understood.

postpartum refers to a limited period after childbirth (post- + Latin *partus*, "born"), usually about 6 weeks.

postprandial is an oddly mixed-up word wherein "post-" is hooked onto the Latin *prandium*, "a late breakfast or lunch," which itself is derived from a combination of the Greek *pro-*, "before," + *endios*, "midday." Literally, then, "postprandial" translates as "after the time before midday." Nowadays, "postprandial" refers to the time after any meal.

potassium is a contrived, Latinized term for potash, the substance extracted from plant ash mixed with water in earthenware pots. The Arabic name for potash was *kali* or *qali*, which reminds us of **alkali**. Kali was a plant from which potash was derived. The Arabic *kali* was, in turn, Latinized to *kalium*, hence the initial "K" was taken as the chemical symbol for potassium. Recognition of potassium as a biomedical electrolyte of major importance led to the use of hypokalemia ("too little") and hyperkalemia ("too much") to designate abnormal potassium content in blood. (*see* **alkali**)

potion (*see* **poison**)

poultice comes through the French from the Latin *pulta* and the Greek *poltos*, both meaning "porridge." Originally, the idea was that of exerting heat on an afflicted part of the body by applying a warm, moist cloth on which had been smeared a boiled mixture of bread, cake, or herbs. Later, mildly irritating substances were incorporated and so applied. Oldsters may recall the mustard plaster of bygone days. The concept was that supposed "bad humors" would be thus "drawn out" from the affected part. This was a mistaken notion, yet the effect of a counterirritant was probably to allay a more deep-seated ache or pain. Moreover, counterirritation tends to increase local blood supply and might thereby enhance healing. Countless jars and tubes of mentholated products are still sold today for this purpose and, what's more, they often work. Incidentally, "poultice" bears no relation to "poultry," which comes from the Latin *pullus*, "a chicken."

pox is a variant spelling of the plural of "pock." The term seldom occurs in the singular except as in "pock-mark." "Pock" seems to have come from the Norman French *poque*, "pouch"; its diminutive, *poquet*, then, was "a little pocket" in the skin. In bygone times a great variety of pustular eruptions in both man and beast were called "pox." The smallpox was so called not only because the pustules, though many, were small, but also because the disease, as bad as it was, seemed the lesser of two evils. The "great pox" was syphilis. A still lesser eruption was degraded as "chicken pox."

pre- is a slightly shortened version of the Latin *prae*, "before, in front of, by reason of." "Pre-" usually appears as a **prefix** (pre- + Latin *figere*, "to fasten"). The number of medical terms incorporating "pre-" is almost endless. Some are near borrowings of actual Latin words; some are contrived. Some are obviously concoctions though perfectly serviceable, such as "precancerous."

precarious can describe the condition of a patient who may well be in need of prayer. The Latin *precarius* means "obtained by prayer" or "dependent on another's will," hence uncertain or risky. The adjective is derived from the Latin *precari*, "to pray for." The sense of uncertainty was epitomized by the phrase, popular during World War II, that described a crippled airplane as "coming in on a wing and a prayer."

precipitate relates to the Latin verb *precipitare*, "to throw down," which combines *prae* + *caput*, "head," in the sense of "headlong" or "headfirst." Used as a verb it means to suddenly or prematurely cause an event; as a noun it refers to a solid "thrown down" from a fluid solution.

predilection often is misspelled and mispronounced as if it were "predeliction." This error is avoided if one remembers the word comes from a combination of "pre-" + Latin *dilectus*, "selection." A disease that has a predilection for certain persons is one that tends to preselect its victims.

pregnant refers to a woman's state before giving birth (pre- + Latin *[g]natus*, "birth"); **prenatal** is used to describe circumstances preceding delivery. Both words share the same origin.

Premarin looks like it might begin with the prefix "pre-," but it does not; it is Wyeth-Ayerst's registered proprietary name for its brand of conjugated estrogen, originally isolated in *pregnant mare*'s u*rine*.

prenatal (*see* **pregnant**)

preparation in reference to a medicinal agent or to a preoperative procedure is a near borrowing of the Latin *praeparatus*, "to be ready in advance," this being a combination of *prae* + *paratus*, "ready."

presbyopia is a condition of faltering vision, especially for near objects, in the elderly. The term combines the Greek *presbys*, "an elder," + *ōps*, "the eye." **Presbycusis** (+ Greek *akousis*, "hearing") is diminished auditory acuity that comes with advancing age.

prescription is something written beforehand, i.e., preceding its preparation and use in treatment. The Latin *praescriptus* combines *prae* + *scribere*, "to write." In his *Devil's Dictionary*, Ambrose Bierce defines "prescription" a bit differently: "A physician's guess at what will best prolong the situation with least harm to the patient."

prevalence is the number of cases of a particular disease existing at a given time in a given place relative to the general population. The term relates to the Latin *praevalere*, "to be stronger, to exert greater influence," this being a combination of *prae* + *valere*, "to be strong." The origin of the term is more readily understood in the adjective "prevalent" and the intrasensitive verb "prevail."

priapism is a persistent, abnormal erection of the penis, such as occurs in the absence of sexual desire. It can be the consequence of certain spinal cord injuries or can be associated with a bladder calculus or sickle-cell anemia. Priapus was the mythologic god of procreation whose nude statues made abundantly evident his chief attribute. It is said that statues of Priapus were placed in vineyards or cultivated fields as scarecrows.

primum non nocere is a time-honored maxim essential to sound medical practice. Literally translated from the Latin it means "first of all do no harm." The principle dates back to Hippocrates, who is quoted as saying, "As to disease, make a habit of two things: to help, or at least do no harm." I vividly recall my own introduction to this fundamental precept. It came as the concluding remark in our medical school course on dermatology. Our professor was an earnest, diminutive, bald-pated Viennese. For 8 weeks he had been catechizing us on the various salves and ointments for what to me, as a junior medical student, was a bewildering array of rashes and eruptions. His final admonition, as he carefully lifted his pince-nez, was, "Boyce! [which is Viennese for "boys"—the three girls in our class were ignored]—vhatefer you do, for Gott's zake, don't make it any vorse!"

prion is a name coined by Dr. Stanley B. Prusiner (*Science.* 1982;216:136) for small proteinaceous particles, such as found in the disease scrapie, that appear to be self-replicating and infectious yet contain no nucleic acids or genome (as distinct from viruses or viroids). The name was extracted from "proteinaceous infection," with transposition of "o" and "i."

p.r.n. are the initials of the Latin *pro re nata*, "according as the circumstances arise," and when included in instructions for treatment mean "to be used as needed."

pro- is a combining form, usually a prefix, borrowed from the *pro* of both Greek and Latin, a preposition meaning "before, in front of, in behalf of, in place of, or the same as." In anatomy a **process** is a projection of a structure, the term being derived from the Latin *processus*, "a going forward," which combines *pro-* + *cedere*, "to go." A **procedure** is an action that must "go before" a desired result.

probe comes from the Latin *probare*, "to test or try." As surgical instruments in the form of slender, malleable rods with blunt ends, probes were used by the ancients, as they are now, to explore wounds, ducts, fistulas, and cavities. A **probang** is a slender, flexible rod (originally made from whalebone) to the end of which is affixed a small sponge. It was devised as a means of applying topical medication to inner recesses of the body and also to aid in removal of foreign bodies from the esophagus or larynx. The name was originally "provang," taken from the French *eprouver*, "to probe or test."

procaine was given as a name for a substance used in local anesthesia "in place of" or in preference to cocaine (with the misconception that "-caine" denoted an anesthetic property).

procidentia refers to a prolapse of the uterus; this Latin word combines *pro-* + *cadere*, "to fall," and therefore means "a falling forward."

proctalgia in the vernacular is literally "a pain in the arse" (procto- + Greek *algos*, "pain"). **Proctalgia fugax** (Latin *fugax*, "swiftly passing") is a fleeting anorectal pain due to muscular tension that, strangely, affects mostly men and strikes mainly during the night.

procto- is taken from the Greek *proktos*, "the anus or hinder parts," but is used only as a combining form. For nouns, we rely on the Latin-derived "anus" and "rectum."

proctology is the art and science of dealing with anorectal problems (procto- + Greek *logos*, "a treatise").

proctoscopy is the procedure by which the inner recesses of the anus and rectum can be inspected (procto- + Greek *skopein*, "to view").

prodrome signifies an early stage of a disease that "runs before" the period when the characteristic symptoms are fully evident (pro- + Greek *dromos*, "a running"). (*see* **syndrome**)

progeria is a rare condition of premature degeneration wherein young children acquire the appearance of wizened age (pro-, in the sense of "in advance of," + Greek *geraios*, "old").

progestin is the name given to a class of hormones capable of preparing the endometrium to receive the fertilized ovum; the term combines "pro-" in the dual sense of "before" and "in behalf of " with a derivative of the Latin *gestare*, "to bear." The active principle originally extracted from the corpora lutea of sows was called "progestin" by A. W. Corner and W. M. Allen (*Am J Physiol.* 1929;88:326). Later, this was refined as **progesterone**, to indicate both its action and its steroid structure.

prognathism is an abnormal protrusion of the mandible in relation to the maxilla (pro- + Greek *gnathos*, "the lower jaw").

prognosis is a direct borrowing of the Greek word for "perceiving beforehand." The word was used by Hippocrates, as we use it now, to mean a foretelling of the course of a disease. The word combines "pro-" and the Greek *gnosis*, "a knowing."

prolapse is taken from the Latin *prolapsus sum*, "to slip forward" and usually used in reference to a malpositioned uterus or to an intussuscepted gut.

prone (*see* **supine**)

prophylaxis is a borrowing of the Greek word for "an advance guard" and an apt term for whatever measure can be taken to fend off disease. "Pro" was once heard as a nickname for "prophylactic" and was commonly used, before the advent of penicillin therapy, to denote the method of genital lavage once promulgated as a measure to prevent venereal disease. In the early days of World War II, military authorities established "pro stations" at convenient locations in large cities where errant soldiers and sailors could repair for succor of sorts following a night of dalliance.

proprioception is a concoction of the Latin *proprius*, "one's own" + *capere*, "to take," and was introduced in 1906 by Sir Charles Sherrington (1857-1952), a renowned English physiologist, to describe the capacity of an organism to sense stimuli arising in its own body. By the faculty of proprioception we can tell whether our legs are crossed or outstretched, even with our eyes closed. **Nociception** (Latin *nocivus*, "harmful," + *capere*, "to receive, as an experience") is the faculty of perceiving stimuli arising in injured parts.

proptosis is a direct borrowing of the Greek word for "a fall forward." It combines "pro-" + *piptein*, "to fall." Most often it refers to an abnormal bulging of the eyeball.

prospective (*see* **retro-**)

prostaglandins are incredibly active autocoid derivatives of arachidonic acid. From their name one would think they were exclusively related to the prostate gland. Not so. Their naming was a misapprehension. Their activity was first noted in a chance observation that myometrium contracted or relaxed when exposed to semen. Understandably, it was thought the principle resided in prostatic secretion; actually it was mostly in that of the seminal vesicles. Later, substances originally called "prostaglandins" were found to exist and exert influence in almost all body tissues and fluids.

prostate is the name of the male gland that embraces the neck of the urinary bladder and the proximal urethra. Its naming followed a tortuous path. A Greek *prostatēs* (pro- + *histemi*, "to stand") was "one who stands before, as a leader of the first rank." To the Greek anatomist Herophilus, the *prostatai adēnoeidēs* was "that which stands before the glands," the glands being the testicles.

prosthesis is a direct borrowing of the Greek word for "an addition." Today, we use the term more in the sense of a substitution whereby parts lost to disease or injury are replaced by artificial devices, particularly for the purpose of restoring function. A set of false teeth is a dental prosthesis. **Enthesis**, a concoction of the Greek *en-*, "in," + *thesis*, "a placing or arranging," refers to the insertion or "putting in" of nonliving material to repair a defect or deformity of the body. Placing a metal plate to fill a hole in the skull is an example of an enthesis.

prot-, proto- is a combining form taken from the Greek *prōtos*, "first, foremost, or earliest." The prefix is useful in specifying whatever is "first-formed, primitive, or original." A **prototype**, in biology, is an ancestral form or species; in bioengineering, it is an original model as first conceived.

protamine is a term contrived in the late 19th century to designate certain elemental protein substances of low molecular weight (prot- + **amine**, an organic compound containing nitrogen, as a derivative of *ammonia*).

protean is always pronounced in three syllables and describes a capacity to assume different appearances. The word comes from Proteus, the name of a Greek sea god who had the peculiar ability to change his shape or appearance at will. A protean disease is one that can appear in various guises. Syphilis, so varied in its manifestations, is a good example of a protean disease. There was a time when it was said, "If one knows syphilis, one knows medicine." *Proteus* also is the name of a genus of bacteria that grow in culture as colonies of varying shapes.

protein is a term introduced in 1838 by a Dutch chemist, Gerard Johann Mulder (1802-1880), to designate what he thought to be the essential constituent of all organic bodies. He took the term from the Greek *proteios*, "the chief rank or first place."

protocol is used in medical circles to designate a particular scheme for a diagnostic, therapeutic, or experimental procedure. For example, an endoscopic protocol is an orderly outline of the planned examination and the observations to be made thereby. A protocol for chemotherapy is an agreed upon schedule, in orderly sequence, of the drugs and their dosages to be used in treating patients requiring such chemical agents. The word comes from the Late Greek *protokollon*, which was the first page or front leaf attached to a manuscript and which contained an outline of its contents. *Protokollon* combines *protos* + *kolla*, "glue," hence "something stuck on at the beginning."

protopathic describes primitive or primordial sensory perception, such as deep pain, firm pressure, heat, and cold (proto- + Greek *pathos*, "feeling"). Finer discrimination such as sharply localized pain or light touch is **epicritic** (Greek *epi-*, "upon," + *krinein*, "to decide").

protoplasm was introduced in 1839 by Johannes Evangelista Purkinje (1787-1869), a Czech anatomist from Breslau, as a term for the formative substance of embryos (proto- + Greek *plasma*, "the thing formed"). Shortly thereafter the term was extended by Hugo von Mohl (1805-1872), a professor of botany at Tübingen in Germany, to describe the mucilaginous substance contained within cell membranes of plants and animals. Previously, this substance had been known by the prosaic German *Schleim*, "slime or mucus."

protozoa is a term introduced in the early 19th century to more properly designate the single-celled, presumably primordial "animalcules" that had been described by van Leeuwenhoek in 1675 (proto- + Greek *zōon*, "a living animal").

proud flesh is an old, colloquial term for burgeoning granulation tissue, as seen at the edges of open, partially healed, skin wounds. In this case "proud" is used in the sense of "swollen," as if by pride. Old farmers sometimes spoke of "proud grain," that became unseasonably swollen beyond the normal stage of growth.

proximal is taken from the Latin adjective *proximus*, "nearest, next following, adjoining." With reference to position, proximal is opposed to **distal**, which is taken from the Latin verb *distare*, "to stand apart, to be distant from." Whenever such relative terms are used, there must be a point of reference. In most cases this is obvious. Everyone understands that in the finger a proximal phalanx is the bone nearest the hand. But in some cases the relation is not always clear unless stated. For example, in the aboral sequence of intestinal segments, the lower portion of the rectum is distal with reference to the colon but proximal with reference to the anus. The point of reference should be made clear in any ambiguous situation.

pruritus is from the Latin *prurire*, "to itch." The term has nothing to do with inflammation, and its ending must be spelled "-itus," never "itis." Communication with patients is made clearer if we use the simple "itch" in preference to the pompous "pruritus." **Itch** is a perfectly good Anglo-Saxon word that descended from the Old English *gyctha*, the initial "g" having fallen by the wayside. **Prurigo** is a generic term for an itchy skin eruption characterized by scattered vesicles that eventually become crusted and scaly. A prurient thought occurs in a mind itching with lewd or lascivious ideas.

psammoma is a combination of the Greek *psammos*, "sand," + *-ōma*, designating a tumor. Psammoma bodies are minute foci of calcification sometimes seen in various neoplasms, particularly those of the prostate gland.

pseudo- is a combining form taken from the Greek *pseudōs*, "false." When incorporated in medical terms, "pseudo-" is used in the sense of "mistaken" or "not of the true type" or sometimes "similar, but not quite." "Pseudo-" has been affixed to the names of a number of diseases to indicate a condition that can mimic a prototype or, sometimes, simply differ from it. For example, pseudohypoparathyroidism is a condition that resembles hypoparathyroidism except that the defect is a failure of response to parathyroid hormone rather than a deficiency in its secretion. Now we also have pseudo-pseudohypoparathyroidism which resembles the one-pseudo condition except that serum levels of calcium and phosphorus are in the normal range. Can "pseudo-pseudo-pseudohypoparathyroidism" be far behind?

pseudocyesis is a delusion of pregnancy (pseudo- + Greek *kyēsis*, "conception"). (Oddly, the Greek *kyēsis* is rarely, if ever, used is any other reference to pregnancy.)

pseudocyst is a real enough cavity, but it does not contain all the histologic components of its parent structure in its wall (pseud- + Greek *kystis*, "a bag or bladder").

pseudomembranous describes something that looks like a membrane, such as a sheet of exudate, but really isn't (pseudo- + Latin *membrana*, "a skin").

Pseudomonas (*see* **monad**)

psittacosis is a viral disease of birds, first

observed in parrots, that is transmissible to man, in whom it can result in illness ranging from a mild "flulike" indisposition to a febrile, sometimes lethal pneumonia. The term comes from the Greek *psittakos*, "a parrot." To the Greeks the parrot was an exotic bird, but they had a name for it nevertheless. Because the disease occurs in a variety of birds, probably **ornithosis** (Greek *ornis*, "bird") is the preferable general term.

psoas comes from the Greek *psoa*, usually used in the plural, *hai psoai*, "the loins." The psoas muscles are included in those of the loins. **Loin**, a term used more often by meat-cutters than by surgeons, refers to the muscular structures of the back from the lowermost rib margin to the pelvis, and it comes, through the Old French *loigne*, from the Latin *lumbus*, which to the Romans meant the same but also included the genital organs.

psoriasis is a direct borrowing of the Greek word denoting "an itchy or scaly condition" and is related to *psora*, "a cutaneous disease, particularly the itch or the mange." Ancient writers applied the term to a variety of pruritic, scaly diseases. By the end of the 18th century these diseases were more or less sorted out, and "psoriasis" was restricted to the chronically recurring, papulosquamous dermatosis we recognize today.

psyche is our word for the human faculty for thought, judgment, and emotion. To the Greeks *psychē* was "the spirit or soul of man" and also "the seat of the will, desires, and passions." (As in other terms originating from Greek words that end with the letter "eta," the final "e" is always pronounced as "ee.") The concept is felicitously defined in the Greek myth concerning Psyche, a mortal who aroused the jealousy and ire of Aphrodite, not only because of her surpassing beauty but also because she was beloved by Aphrodite's handsome son Eros. Seeking rapprochement with Aphrodite, Psyche was required to perform three nearly impossible tasks in which she almost failed because of her human character, but was then saved by the intervention of kindly gods. Eventually, Psyche was taken into the celestial realm by a benevolent Zeus and reunited with her beloved Eros. The allegory is that of a human soul gaining immortality.

The Greek name for the butterfly also is *psychē*, the allusion being to the transformation of the plodding caterpillar into the transcendent glory of the butterfly.

psychedelic is a word of more recent currency and incorporates the Greek *delos*, "visible." A psychedelic drug is one that evokes vivid mental images, particularly those that delight but sometimes those that depress.

psychiatry is that branch of medicine dealing with the diagnosis and treatment of mental disorders (psych- + Greek *iatreia*, "healing"). The term first appeared in medical writings about the mid-19th century.

psychoanalysis (*see* **analysis**)

psychology is that branch of science dealing with mental sensation and behavior. The term combines "psycho-" and the Greek *logos*, "a treatise"; however, no such word was known to ancient classical writers. Its first appearance was as the neo-Latin *psychologia* in the 16th century.

psychosis is a term borrowed directly from the Late Greek *psychōsis*, but to the Greeks this meant "animation, the spirit of life." When in the latter 19th century the term was first introduced in psychopathology, it was used to refer to mental derangement for which there was no known organic cause. Now with the advance in knowledge that such derangement can be attributed to definable biochemical aberration, this meaning will have to be revised. In medicine there is a curious distinction between "psychosis" and "psychoneurosis." A psychosis is a profound mental aberration whereby the afflicted person has lost all touch with reality, whereas a **psychoneurosis** is a behavioral disorder suggesting a functional nervous disturbance of mental origin.

psychosomatic describes whatever has an integral mind-body relationship (psycho- + Greek *sōma*, "the body"). Somewhat surprisingly, this is a relatively recent concept, gaining currency in the 1940s. Previously, the functions of the mind and body had been thought of as distinct. (*see* **soma**)

pterygoid combines the Greek *pteryx*, "wing," + *eidos*, "like," and describes whatever resembles a wing. The pterygoid processes are paired, winglike extensions of the sphenoid bone at the base of the skull. A **pterygium** is a sort of winglike, triangular membrane that sometimes emerges as an abnormal extension of the conjunctiva from the inner canthus of the eye. The usual cause is prolonged exposure of the eye to wind and weather.

ptomaine now has little, if any, medical significance, but one still hears occasional reference to any acute illness thought to be caused by ingestion of spoiled food as "ptomaine poisoning." An Italian chemist Francesco Selmi (1817-1881) is said to have invented the word *ptomana*, "from a corpse" (harking back to the Greek *ptōma*, "corpse"), to describe certain poisonous substances he extracted from cadavers. (The *Oxford English Dictionary* castigates Selmi for not using three syllables to construct a more proper "ptomatine.") The term was later used to refer to various products of organic decomposition.

ptosis is a direct borrowing of the Greek word for "a falling," and is related to the verb *piptein*, "to fall down." Although not used as a medical term by ancient writers, "ptosis" later was applied to drooping of the eyelid consequent to impairment of the third cranial (oculomotor) nerve. About the turn of the present century it was fashionable to attribute various obscure abdominal complaints to a downward displacement of the viscera. Gravity was blamed for a myriad of ills. There ensued a flurry of high-sounding but meaningless diagnoses, such as "gastroptosis," "nephroptosis," or—if one wasn't quite sure just which organ drooped—"visceroptosis." Fortunately, the organs were as difficult to pin down as the diagnosis, so little harm was done.

ptyalin comes from the Greek *ptyalon*, "saliva," this being related to the imitative verb *ptyein*, "to spit." Ptyalin, an enzyme occurring in saliva, converts starch into maltose and dextrose. The longer one chews a morsel of bread, the sweeter it tastes because of the action of ptyalin.

puberty is a term taken from the Latin *pubertas*, "coming to the age of manhood [or womanhood]." **Pubescent** can mean either covered with short hairs or soft down or, figuratively, having reached the age of puberty.

pubis is taken from the Latin *pubes*, which as an adjective means "grown-up, adult," and as a noun designates the growth of hair that comes to adorn the genital area of adults. In anatomy the term shifted in meaning from the hair-covered area to the underlying bone.

pudenda are what the Victorians primly called "the private parts." In the singular of the Latin neuter noun, **pudendum**, reference is particularly and collectively to the external genitalia of women, i.e., the mons veneris, the labia majora and minora, and the vestibule of the vagina. The word is related to the Latin *pudere*, "to be ashamed." The more familiar word "impudent" means "brazen or lacking in shame." Willard R. Espy tells us, "According to the Roman historian Livy, Pudicitia, personification of the chastity or modesty of women, was worshipped in a small shrine in the Roman Bovarium until at least 296 B.C., but the cult degenerated along with the simple Roman virtues, and spiders wove their webs in her altars."

puerperal is but a slight shortening of the Latin *puerperalis*, "pertaining to childbirth." The word is derived by a combination of *puer*, "child," + *parere*, "to bear or to bring forth." **Puerperal fever**, once an often fatal illness afflicting the mother shortly after delivery (and commonly known all too well as "childbed fever"), was recognized by Hippocrates. In 1660 the condition was described and named *febris puerperum* by Thomas Willis (1621-1675), the famous English physician and anatomist. But it was not until 1843 that Oliver Wendell Holmes (1809-1894), a proper Bostonian physician, and 1847 that Ignaz Semmelweiss (1818-1865), a Viennese obstetrician, proclaimed their conviction that puerperal fever was, indeed, an infectious disease spread by untidy, unwashed doctors. Needless to say, this was an affront to the profession and aroused bitter controversy on both sides of the Atlantic. When doctors and midwives were finally persuaded to employ antiseptic procedures as they attended women in labor, the malady became nearly extinct.

puke is a venerable English word for the act of vomiting. In *As You Like It*, Shakespeare describes the infant "mewling and puking in the nurse's arms." Probably it is an imitative word, akin to "spit." Nowadays, youngsters speak of "barfing," also imitative.

pulmonary comes from the Latin *pulmo* (genitive *pulmonis*), "the lung." Some authorities hold that this is derived, by a transposition of letters, from the Greek *pleumon*, a variant of *pneumon*, "the lung." In any case, the pulmonary vessels puzzled ancient anatomists. Lacking knowledge of the circulation of blood, they were perplexed by the structure of the vessels connecting the lung to the right and left sides of the heart. Thus, the pulmonary artery and vein were once known, respectively, as "the vein-like artery" and the "artery-like vein."

pulse comes from the Latin *pulsus*, "a pushing, beating, or striking," this being related to the verb *pello, pellere, pulsum* of similar meaning. The ancients connected the pulsation in peripheral arteries with the beating of the heart and came within a whisker of discovering the true nature of circulating blood. It was an ignorance of the capillary connection between arteries and veins that stumped them.

punctate comes from the Latin *punctum*, "a point or spot," this being related to the verb *pingere*, "to prick, sting, or stab." The **punctum lacrimale** is the pinpoint opening at the inner canthus of the eye, which leads to the tear duct that drains into the nasal cavity. This, of course, is why we often blow our nose when we weep. A **puncture** is the result of pricking or stabbing and may be more specifically designated as, for example, a venipuncture. A **pungent** odor is sharp or biting.

punk is a colloquial word commonly used to describe a state of feeling vaguely unwell or "out of sorts." Often, a patient will complain, "I'm feeling just punk." As a noun "punk" came to be applied to a callow, worthless youth inclined to hooliganism. Originally, "punk" was a name for touchwood or tinderwood, that soft, crumbly, partially decayed portion of a log that was useless except as tinder. It was fairly easily ignited and would smolder. When compressed into sticks and lit, punk was, in bygone times, an essential Fourth-of-July tool for every child intent on celebrating the national holiday by setting off fireworks. "Punk" probably had its origin in an Algonquin Indian word for friable, decayed wood.

puny can describe whatever is small, weak, and

feeble and comes from the Old French *puisne*, itself a combination of *puis*, "afterward," + *ne*, "born." *Puisne* was a legal term referring to one who was "born later," hence inferior in rank. This was important when inheritance was governed by the law of primogeniture (Latin *primogenitus*, "first born") which held that the eldest son got all and those "born later" got nothing.

pupil as the name for the aperture in the iris of the eye is derived from the Latin *pupa*, "a doll." Presumably, this came from the early observation that when one peers closely into the eye of another, one sees a minute image of himself. The Greeks, in similar fashion, used the word *korē* for "maiden or doll" and also for "the pupil of the eye." From the Greek word we obtain **anisocoria** (Greek *a-*, "not" + *iso*, "equal"), a condition wherein the pupils of the paired eyes are of different diameters.

purgative is taken from the Latin *purgatio*, "a cleansing," this being related to the verb *purgare*, "to clear away, to cleanse, to purify." The idea of cleansing the body by use of enemas or cathartics is as old as time itself. Incidentally, to "expurgate" a piece of literature is to remove from it whatever may be considered offensive or objectionable. The book you are reading has yet to appear in an expurgated edition.

purine was concocted in 1881 by Emil Fischer (1852-1919), a German chemist, by compressing the Latin *purus*, "clean, pure," + the German *Urin*, denoting a relation to uric acid. The synthetic heterocyclic compound $C_5H_4N_4$ is the prototype of uric acid compounds known as "purines." Perhaps because the prototype is not found free in nature it was perceived as "pure."

purpura is the Latin word for "purple" and may be related, in turn, to the Greek *porphyra*, the name of a mollusk or shellfish from which a purple dye was extracted. In medieval times patients afflicted with febrile illnesses marked by extensive subcutaneous hemorrhages were said to suffer from "purple fever." Later, it was recognized that similar hemorrhages occurred in the absence of fever, and such conditions were called simply "purpura." Purpura is distinguished from **petechiae** by the confluence of hemorrhagic spots and by their being observed at a stage when fresh blood has been degraded to a purple color. An **ecchymosis** usually is a larger, focal extravasation of blood in the skin.

pus comes from the Greek *pyon*, "corrupt matter, specifically that which exudes from sores." The Sanskrit root *pu-* meant "fetid or stinking." From this came the Latin *puter*, "rotten," and our word "putrid." Can it be that the colloquial exclamation "pee-yew!" represents a legacy from the Vedas of India two-and-a-half millennia ago?

pustule is a little pus-laden pimple (Latin *pustula*, "blister").

putamen is Latin for "whatever falls off with paring, such as a shell or husk." The related Latin verb is *putare*, "to trim or to prune." In anatomy the putamen is the outer part of the lenticular nucleus of the brain, so called because of its fancied resemblance to a husk or shell. The original sense of the Latin *putare* was "to make clean, as by pruning or trimming." Later, *putare* was extended to the sense of "making clear," hence "to think or reckon." From this sense we have derived a number of commonly used words, such as putative, compute, impute, and repute.

putrefaction is an enzymatic decomposition, especially of proteins and usually by bacteria, resulting in fetid products, such as hydrogen sulfide, mercaptans, and ammonia (Latin *putris*, "rotten," + *facere*, "to make").

pyelo- is a combining form taken from the Greek *pyelos*, "a pan or basin," to which the Latin *pelvis* is related. In modern anatomy "pyelo-" has been limited in reference to the pelvis of the kidney and has been incorporated in numerous terms pertaining thereto, e.g., **pyelography** (+ Greek *graphein*, "to write"), **pyelonephritis** (+ Greek *nephros*, "kidney"), and **pyelolithotomy** (+ Greek *lithos*, "stone," + *tomē*, "a cutting [for]"). It is necessary to distinguish between "pyelo-" and "pyle-"; the latter, from the Greek *pylē*, "gate," which refers to the portal vein.

pyemia is a contrived term combining the Greek *pyon* + *haima*, "blood," meaning, literally, "pus in blood." In modern medicine this has been superseded by the more precise "leukocytosis" (an excess of white blood cells), "septicemia" (bacterial toxins in the blood), and

"bacteremia" (bacteria in the blood).

pyknic is taken from the Greek *pyknos*, "close, compact, solid, or dense." A person of a pyknic habitus has a short, stocky build. A **pyknotic** nucleus of a cell is contracted by condensation of its chromatin into a dense clump, usually as a sign of impending mitosis or of degeneration.

pyle- is a combining form taken from the Greek *pylē*, "gate," to designate whatever pertains to the portal vein. Thus, **pylethrombosis** (+ Greek *thrombos*, "a clot") refers to the formation of a blood clot in the portal vein. **Pylephlebitis** is inflammation of the portal vein and looks like it might be related to *pyon*, "pus," but it is not. This term combines the Greek *pylē*, "gate" (a reference to the entry of the portal vein into the liver) + *phlebos*, "vein." Also, "pylephlebitis" (in which the "-le-" is pronounced as a separate syllable) is not to be confused with "pyelophlebitis," an inflammation of the renal pelvis.

pylorus is a near borrowing of the Greek word for "gatekeeper," this being related to *pylē*, "gateway." The Greeks used *pyloros* to designate the lower end of the stomach, whereas Latin authors tended to restrict the term to the narrow opening into the duodenum, as we do now.

pyorrhea can be taken to mean, literally, "a flow of pus" (pyo- + Greek *rhoia*, "a flowing") but currently the term tends to be restricted to purulent exudate issuing from infected tooth sockets.

pyretic denotes whatever pertains to an elevation in body temperature (Greek *pyretos*, "fever," from *pyr*, "fire") and, as a noun, is a substance that induces fever. An **antipyretic** is whatever quells fever. **Pyrexia** is a learned term for abnormally high body temperature due to any cause and is taken from the Greek *pyrexis*, "feverishness," related to *pyr*, "fire."

pyrogenic describes whatever may stimulate or cause fever (pyro- + Greek *gennaō*, "I produce").

pyrosis is a direct borrowing of the Greek word meaning "on fire" or "a burning." Transferred to the medical lexicon, "pyrosis" is restricted to the sensation of retrosternal distress that most sensible people would call "heartburn." It is not a febrile condition.

pyrrole (*see* **porphyria**)

pyuria is pus in the urine (pyo- + Greek *ouron*).

**Q fever** is the only disease whose name is qualified by a single letter. It is a self-limited, acute, febrile disease with constitutional manifestations, but its symptoms tend to focus on the respiratory tract. It occurs throughout most of the world but seems more prevalent where cattle and sheep are raised. Its odd name is shrouded in obscurity. Most writers interpret the "Q" as standing for "query" because the cause of the disease was unknown for so long. It is now recognized as an infection by *Coxiella burnetti*, a rickettsial organism named for Herald Rae Cox, an American bacteriologist, and for Macfarlane Burnet, an Australian microbiologist.

q. is used as an abbreviation for the Latin *quisque* (masculine), *quaque* (feminine), and *quodque* (neuter) meaning "each or every" and appears in a variety of shorthand prescription instructions. Many say we should discard all arcane Latin abbreviations and spell out instructions or notations in plain English. This is a worthy idea, but shorthand has been handy so long that it is unlikely we will give it up. There is no harm in using shorthand if everyone concerned knows what is meant thereby.

q.d. stands for "every day"; however, in classical Latin only a single initial would be required for *quotidie*, a single word for "daily."

q.h.s. is a quick way of writing "every bedtime" (Latin *hora somni*, "the hour of sleep").

q.i.d. stands for the Latin *quater in die*, "four times each day."

q.n.s. sometimes appears in laboratory reports to mean "quantity not sufficient," i.e., an inadequate specimen by which to perform a given test.

q.o.d. are initials that mix Latin and English, intended to mean "every other day."

Sometimes an Arabic numeral is inserted, as in "q. 4 h.," indicating "every 4 hours."

q.s. stands for *quantum satis* or *sufficit*, "quantity sufficient," as when completing a prescription with "q.s. 120 mL," meaning to add enough vehicle to make a total volume of 120 milliliters.

quack is a pejorative name for an unqualified practitioner of medicine and owes its origin to the sound of the word (and perhaps to that of a duck). "Croak" in Dutch is *kwakken*, which means "a loud, boisterous sound" or "a trifling utterance." According to one explanation, this form was long ago combined in Dutch as *kwakzalver*, meaning one who purveyed all sorts of salves and other remedies, all generously laced with humbug. This became "quacksalver" in English, later shortened simply to "quack."

quadrant is a near borrowing of the Latin *quadrans*, "a fourth part, a quarter." Thus, in surface anatomy, the right upper abdominal quadrant, for example, is the area extending from the midline laterally to the right flank, bounded above by the right costal margin and below by the level of the umbilicus. **Quadrate** (Latin *quadratus*, "squared") describes whatever is shaped like a square, as is, more or less, the quadrate lobe of the liver.

quarantine is a period of isolation of an individual decreed to control the spread of potentially contagious disease in the community. The duration might vary according to the known incubation period of the given disease or other circumstances. In the old days the period was a flat 40 days, hence the derivation of the term from the Latin *quadraginta*, "forty." Why forty? Probably because it was known empirically that the incubation period of most infectious diseases would fall within the 40-day range.

quartan (*see* **periodic**; *also* **tertian**)

queasy is a word some patients use to describe a feeling of nausea, especially that of relatively mild degree that may not culminate in vomiting. The word is of uncertain origin. Some writers have attributed it to the Old Norse *kveisa*, "a boil," which is related to the Norwegian *kveis*, "a hangover," i.e., a pronounced uneasiness following a debauch.

Others have related "queasy" to the Middle English *coisy*, which meant "tender or unsettled."

quellung is the German word for "swelling" and was applied to the reaction observed when pneumococci are mixed with a specifically immune serum. The organisms agglutinate, but there also is a swelling in the outer membrane of the cocci. The reaction and its naming are attributed to Fred Neufeld (1861-1945), a German bacteriologist.

quick is used to describe the keenly sensitive surface underlying the fingernails or toenails and is derived from the Anglo-Saxon *cwic*, "living," therefore reactive (*see* **whitlow**). Signs of life in a fetus nestled in a mother's womb are sometimes described as "quickening." The word also is used to distinguish the living when recited in the Apostle's or Nicene Creed: "... thence he [Christ] will judge the quick and the dead." The sense of reaction is evident when "quick" is incorporated in such names as "quicklime" (calcium oxide, which the Romans called *calx vita*) and "quicksilver" (elemental mercury).

quinine comes from a Peruvian Indian word *kina*, "bark of a tree," that was Latinized to *quina*. A particular bark came from what the Andean Indians called "the fever tree," now properly classified as *Cinchona calisaya* (*see* **cinchona**). The active principle in the extract from this bark was isolated and named "quinine" in 1820. When 18-year-old William (later Sir William) Perkin, an English chemist, unwittingly founded the coal-tar industry in 1856, he was actually seeking a synthetic source of quinine so as to relieve Europe of dependence on the cinchona bark, then available only in faraway South America and the East Indies. Perkin failed to form quinine, but he reaped rewards of serendipity on a grand scale. **Quinidine**, an alkaloid of conchona with quite different properties, was recognized in 1833 and so named because of its isomeric relation to quinine (a sort of "quinoidine"). A more detailed background is given in Saul Jarcho's *Quinine's Predecessor: Francesco Torti and the Early History of Cinchona* (Baltimore, Md: Johns Hopkins University Press; 1993).

quinsy is an almost archaic term for peritonsillar abscess. It originated as the Greek *kya[n]gchē*, "a bad sore throat," this being a combination of *kyōn*, "a dog," + *a[n]gchonē*, "a choking or throttling (whence "anguish"). The allusion might have been either to the pain and soreness one would suffer were a dog to chew on one's neck or, perhaps, to a sore throat "as mean as a dog." From *kyna[n]gchēa* shift in spelling led to the Medieval Latin *quinancia*, to the Middle English *quinesye*, and finally to "quinsy."

quotidian means "of daily occurrence," as a quotidian fever recurs and peaks every day (Latin *quotidie*, "daily").

Rabies is the Latin word for "rage or madness." This disease of warm-blooded animals, incidentally transmitted to man by a bite or other contact with an infected beast, was known to the ancients. Its dramatic neurologic manifestations led to its being called rabies. In medieval times the disease was known as **hydrophobia** (Greek *hydōr*, "water," + *phobos*, "fear") because its victims shied away from water because of the painful throat spasm induced by attempting to drink. In the 17th century the term "rabies" was revived, and the victims of the disease, both human and animal, were described as being **rabid**.

racemose is taken from the Latin *racemus*, "a cluster or bunch, especially of grapes." In anatomy the term is applied to whatever has the appearance of a bunch of grapes on a stalk, such as a cluster of glands attached to a ductal system.

rachitis (*see* **rickets**)

rad (*see* **radiology**)

radiation comes from the Latin *radius* (related to the Greek *rhabdos*, "a rod"), first a word for a stick or wand, then for the spoke of a wheel and, by allusion, for a ray of light or whatever emanated from a central source.

radical is used in science, particularly in mathematics and chemistry, to denote something essential or fundamental on which other forms can be constructed. Thus, sulfate ($-SO_4$) is a simple bivalent chemical radical from which, by combination with other elements or molecules, more complex compounds can be formed. When used in anatomy as a noun, the term is spelled **radicle**, in referring to the smallest extension of a nerve or vessel that is likened to "a little root." This scientific usage is much closer to the origin of the word, which is the diminutive of the Latin *radix*, "root," than the present-day vernacular use of "radical" would suggest. Yet there is a connection. In 18th century England certain political reformers came to be known as "radicals" because when in contention they insisted on getting to the root of a matter and advocated revamping the social structure from the ground up. Political "conservatives," on the other hand, were content with little or no change at all. In this regard there is a peculiar usage in medicine of the adjectives "radical" and "conservative" when referring to therapy. Radical therapy employs measures that are bold and unrestrained, if not audacious, "leaving no holds unbarred." The advocate of conservative therapy is content with more conventional, less disruptive measures, or, in the extreme, to "leaving well enough alone." For conditions wherein there may be a choice between medical and surgical treatment, the former tends to be considered as conservative and the latter as radical. Obviously, these are comparative terms, and their implication depends on who is using which and from what viewpoint.

radicle (*see* **radical**)

radiology as a name for the science that evolved from the discovery of X-rays in 1895 by Wilhelm Konrad Röntgen (1845-1923), a German physicist, had to be contrived by hybridizing the Latin *radius*, "a rod or ray," + the Greek *logos*, "a treatise." As a tribute to the discoverer, who was awarded a Nobel Prize in 1901, the science also has been known as **roentgenology**. A **roentgen** (usually symbolized by "R") is an international unit of X- or gamma radiation. The distinctly different **rad**, an acronym for "*rad*iation *a*bsorbed *d*ose," is a unit by which absorption of ionizing radiation, by any substance or tissue, is measured. Of increasing current use is the **gray**, the absorption at the point of focus of 1 joule of radiation energy in 1 kilogram of tissue, and equivalent to 100 rads. The term "gray" memorializes Louis Harold Gray (1905-1965), a British radiologist.

radium is the name given to a metallic elemental source of X-irradiation that was discovered in 1898 by Pierre and Marie Curie, the husband-and-wife French physicists. Their surname is commemorated in the **curie**, a term for the quantity of radionuclide in which the number of disintegrations is 3.7 x 10^{10} per second.

radius is the name of the smaller bone in the forearm and was so called because it was thought to resemble the spoke of a wheel. At least that is what it looked like to Celsus, the 1st century Roman writer who introduced the term to anatomy. The spoke of a wheel in Latin is *radius*. The **radial nerve** is so called because of its proximity to the radius, not because of its shape or distribution.

radon is a gaseous radioactive element with a suitably short half-life that has been used in implantable capsules as a source of radiotherapy.

rale is a French term adapted from the verb *râler*, "to make a rattling sound in one's throat, to grumble." This, in turn, appears to have been taken from the Vulgar Latin *ragulare*, "to bray." With slightly altered spelling, in English we use "rail" as a verb meaning "to condemn with harsh or abusive language." In medicine "râle" was first used as a term for the "death rattle" of mucus accumulating in the throat of a dying person. Laënnec, the French physician who invented the stethoscope in 1816, applied the term to certain adventitious crackling sounds he heard when he applied his new device to the chests of patients with various congestive cardiopulmonary diseases. **Rhonchus** is a near borrowing of the Greek *rhonchos*, "a snoring sound," obviously an imitative word. In physical diagnosis the term denotes the crackling or gurgling sounds emanating from the respiratory tract in which excess mucus or pus has accumulated in the larger passages. Rhonchi are louder and coarser than rales and tend to clear on coughing.

ramus is Latin for "a branch or bough." In anatomy a ramus is a small structure emanating like a branch from a larger structure, be it bone, nerve, or vessel. If there are many such branches, they are *rami* (the Latin masculine plural).

ranula is the diminutive of the Latin *rana*, "a frog," and has been given as the name of a cystic tumor, actually a mucocele, that can occur beneath the tongue when the submaxillary or sublingual salivary glands are obstructed. There are three possible explanations for the use of the term: (*a*) "ranine" is an archaic adjective referring to the tip of the tongue as "the frog of the mouth"; (*b*) a swelling in the floor of the mouth may be fancied to resemble the throat of a croaking frog; or (*c*) such a swelling may cause hoarseness, i.e., "a frog in the throat."

raphe is a near borrowing of the Greek *rhaphē*, "a seam," as joins two pieces of cloth when sewn together with a needle. The median line extending from the anus to the pudenda is known as the **perineal raphe**. From the same Greek source comes **-rhapy**, the suffix used in naming surgical procedures wherein seams are sewn (e.g., "herniorrhaphy").

rash comes from the Latin verb *rado, radere, rasi*, "to scrape or to scratch." An erythematous eruption in the skin has the appearance of having been scraped or scratched. Also, some rashes itch and thereby prompt scratching. "Rash" came into English from the French *raser*, meaning "to shave or slice thin." A rasher of bacon is a thin slice, and the connection with "razor" is obvious.

RAST is an acronym conveniently denoting a *ra*dio *allergo sorbent technique* as used to measure specific IgE antibodies in serum. It is a means of detecting sensitivity to various allergens.

reagin designates an antibody or whatever behaves like an antibody in complement fixation reactions. The term is modeled on **reagent** and is derived by combining the Latin *re-*, used as in "react," + *agere*, "to drive, act, or perform."

recalcitrant (*see* **refractory**)

receptor comes from the Latin *recipere*, "to receive." A receptor nerve ending is the sensory terminal that receives and registers a stimulus from its environment. Paul Ehrlich (1854-1915), the pioneer German immunologist, postulated the presence in cell membranes of special receptor sites where substances might attach, be recognized and received, then induce a particular activity. The basic validity of Ehrlich's "side-chain" or "receptor" theory has been borne out in modern immunology.

recrudescence comes from the Latin *recrudescere*, "to become raw or sore again." To the Romans this meant the reopening of a wound that had appeared to heal. Later, the meaning was extended to the recurrence of any symptom or disease, and now we may speak of the recrudescence of a rash or even of a fever.

rectum is derived from the Latin *rectus*, "straight." Aristotle referred to the most distal segment of the bowel as "the straight passage" from the lower colon to the anus. This reference puzzles most students of human anatomy because they find the lumen of the angulated rectum to be anything but straight. A possible explanation for the early and persistent use of the term is that the ancients derived most of what they learned of anatomy from the dissection of lower animals, and the most distal segment of the bowel is more nearly straight in many quadrupeds than in humans.

recuperate comes from the Latin *recupare*, "to regain, to get back, to recover." The Reverend W. W. Skeat, in his 19th century etymologic dictionary, explains that *recuperare* may have originally meant "to make good again," from the Sabine *cuprus*, "good or worthy," as related to the Latin verb *cupere*, "to desire." Another explanation is that *recupare* might be a transliterated combination of *re-*, "again," + *capere*, "to grasp or to gain."

recurrent is taken from the Latin *recurrere*, "to run back or to return." The recurrent laryngeal nerve is a branch of the vagus (10th cranial) nerve that runs down the neck then turns back up to invest the larynx. Otherwise, in medicine as generally, "recurrent" is used to describe anything that "comes back again." (*see* **periodic**)

reflex is derived from the Latin *reflectere*, "to bend back or to turn around," from which, obviously, we obtain "reflection." René Descartes (1596-1650), the celebrated French savant, may have been the first to perceive reflex arcs wherein sensations induced impulses, conducted automatically along nerve pathways, that were then "thrown back" to initiate a responsive action.

reflux is taken from the Latin *refluere*, "to flow back" (*see* **flux**). Fluid flowing in a retrograde direction from the stomach into the esophagus is an example of reflux, as is the motion of fluid and electrolytes from the internal environment into the gut lumen and back

again, through epithelial cell membranes. A term of related meaning is **regurgitation**, from a combination of the Latin *re-*, "back," + *gurgitare*, "to flood." This implies a somewhat more forceful action than "reflux." The retrograde flooding of blood from the left ventricle of the heart, during systole, through an incompetent bicuspid valve into the left atrium is known as "mitral regurgitation."

refraction comes from the Latin *refractus*, the past participle of *refringere*, "to break down (or up)." The original scientific application of the term was to describe the "breaking up," by a glass prism, of a beam of white light into its component colors of different wavelengths. The term was then applied to the deviation of light passing obliquely from one medium to another of different density, e.g., from air to water. Defective vision, notably hyperopia or myopia, can result from refractory errors, hence "refraction" came to be a term for the measurement of visual acuity.

refractory is a term adapted from the Latin *refractus* (*see* **refraction**). In physiology a muscle in its refractory phase is so "broken down" as to be incapable of responding to a contractile stimulus. In clinical medicine a refractory condition is one so utterly disordered that it resists treatment. An **intractable** condition is similarly resistant, but more in the sense of being obstinate. In this vein a patient or a symptom that defies treatment is said to be **recalcitrant**. This term is taken from the Latin *recalcitrare*, "to kick back." This relates to *calcaneum*, the Latin word for "the heel."

regimen is often confused with "regime," and vice versa. Both words have their origin in the Indo-European *reg*, whose dual meanings, "to move in a straight line," and "to rule" gave rise to the Latin *regio* and *rex*, and *regis*, respectively. A regime is a mode or system of government. A regimen, in medicine, is a regulated course of diet, exercise, or therapy designed to attain a favorable result.

regurgitation (*see* **reflux**)

relapse is a near borrowing of the Latin *relapsus*, the past participle of *relabi*, "to slide back or to sink down." In medicine a relapse is marked by a return of symptoms or signs of disease that had once appeared to subside. A **remission** (Latin *remissio*, "a release or abatement") is the period during which a disease appears to subside. The implication is one of uncertainty. A remission may lead to a cure or to a relapse.

REM is an acronym for "*rapid eye movement*," a phase of sleep during which brain waves are of low voltage but rapid and autonomic functions, such as the heartbeat and breathing, are irregular. This also is a phase of sleep associated with dreaming and with muscle twitching, of which rapid eye movement is a manifestation.

remedy designates anything that is known by repeated and convincing demonstration to cure or palliate a disease or disorder. The word comes from the Latin *remedium*, "that which heals again." The prefix "re-" is essential to the meaning in that a true remedy must have been proved to work, again and again. An experimental, unproved, or uncertain method of treatment cannot properly be called a remedy.

remission (*see* **relapse**)

renal is an adjective derived from the Latin *renes*, "the kidneys" (*see* **kidney**). We do not use a Latin-derived noun in modern English for this pair of organs, though *reins* (among other spellings) is an archaic English and Old French word for the kidneys or the lower back. None of this has anything to do with the reins by which a horse is controlled; this word comes from the Latin *retinere*, "to hold back."

research is obviously a compound of "re-" + "search" and is related to the French *recherche*, "a search, quest, or pursuit." If research is essentially an inquiry or a quest, why the "re-"? Why not just "search"? The explanation is found in translating the prefix "re-" as "back." We have to "search back" to find something new. We think of researchers as looking ahead, and they do. But they take their view from a vantage point previously established. As the Roman Didacus Stella put it, *"Pigmaei gigantum humeris impositi plusquam ipsi gigantes vident"* ("A dwarf sitting on the shoulders of a giant may see farther than the giant himself"). Even an investigator, in an etymologic sense, is not walking an untrodden path; he is looking for footprints. (*see* **vestige**)

resection is a near borrowing of the Latin *resec-* *tio*, "a trimming or a pruning." In surgery, the meaning of "resection" hews closely to the original Latin in being a "cutting away" of whatever is unwanted for the purpose of removal. Gastric resection is the surgical removal of all or part of the stomach. A related term is **extirpate** (Latin *ex-*, "out," + *stirpes*, "stem or stalk"), and another is **eradication** (Latin *e(x)-*, "out," + *radix*, "root"). These terms are aptly applied to the thorough removal of lesions, including their very stalks or roots.

respiration comes from the Latin *respirare*, "to breathe." The Latin *spirare* also is "to breathe," among its more figurative meanings. Why the "re-"? The Romans used *respirare* especially as "to catch one's breath" or "to breathe forcefully, as after combat or other exertion," i.e., "to breathe again." Also, "respiration" conveys the sense of breathing repetitively, which, experience teaches, is a good way to breathe. It is interesting to note that in the course of physical examination when an English-speaking patient is instructed, "Please breathe," nothing much happens; when a Spanish-speaking person is instructed, *"Respire por favor,"* the patient always takes in a deep breath. In biomedical usage "internal respiration" denotes the exchange of gaseous constituents between a cell and its environment.

restaurant is not a medical term but it has an origin that is health-related. In 18th-century Paris, certain places were established where a tasty and nourishing soup was concocted and purveyed, the soup being said to have a beneficial effect on the health of the partaker. The soup was purported to be a *restaurant*, the present participle of the French *restaurer*, "to restore or to refresh." Later, the name was transferred from the soup to the place where the restorative was made available. To go back further, the French word relates to the Greek *stauros*, "an upright stake in a palisade." To affix "re-" in "restore" conveys the idea of "fixing the fence."

retching means an involuntary and unproductive effort to vomit. It comes from the Anglo-Saxon *hraecan*, "to clear one's throat," whence we have the expression "to hawk up [phlegm]."

rete is Latin for "net." The name *rete mirabile*

("marvelous network") has been given to an elaborate vascular plexus found at the base of the brain in some animals and formerly believed to exist in man. At the base of the human brain there is a remarkable interconnection of arteries known as the "circle of Willis" (named after Thomas Willis, a 17th century English anatomist and physician), but this is not really a counterpart. If one defines *rete mirabile* as a capillary plexus interposed in an arterial channel, then the only example in man is the capillary tuft that makes up a renal glomerulus. The **rete testis** is the network of seminiferous tubules leading from the testis into the vas deferens.

reticulocyte is an immature erythrocyte, so called because its cytoplasm, when vitally stained, is seen to contain a fine, basophilic network. (*see* **reticulum**)

reticulum is the diminutive of the Latin *rete*; hence, "a little net." The term is used in histology to describe a fine network of connective or supporting tissues.

retina is a Latinized term, but no such word exists in classical Latin. According to Professor H. A. Skinner, Galen described the innermost layer of the eyeball using the Greek *amphiblēstron*, meaning "anything put on or thrown around," as a tunic, though the same word was also used for a fishnet. Galen used the term in the former sense when he described the eye, but translators read the Greek term in the latter sense and took it to be equivalent to the Latin *rete*. "Retina," although of confused origin, still serves adequately in modern anatomy.

retinaculum is the singular of the Latin neuter noun *retinacula*, used in the plural to mean "cable, rope, or tether." This relates to the Latin verb *retinere*, "to hold back." In anatomy a retinaculum can be a restraining ligament or a fibrous cord that restrains tendons. In surgery a retinaculum is a clawed instrument used to hold or pull back tissue from the field of operation, as a sort of small retractor. (*see* **tenaculum**)

retractor is related to the Latin adjective *retractus*, "withdrawn," from the verb *retrahere*, "to draw back." The ancients used the term, as we do, for an instrument designed to hold back structures that would obscure an operative field. The Latin *retrahere* also means "to

bring to light again," and that is what a retractor does in the hands of the surgeon.

retro- is a combining form borrowed from the Latin adverb *retro*, "backward, behind, or in the past." In anatomy "retro-" refers to space, as in **retrobulbar** (+ Latin *bulbus*, "onion"), meaning the space behind the eyeball that resembles, in shape, a medium-sized onion. In clinical investigation **retrospective** (+ Latin *spectare*, "to observe") studies are those that evaluate previous experience; **prospective** (Latin *pro*, "in front of") studies are those that are planned so as to evaluate forthcoming experience according to an antecedent protocol.

rh in biomedical terms is a sequence of Roman letters that often represent the aspirated Greek consonant rho (ρ), i.e., the pronunciation of "r" is followed by a slight puff of breath. Whenever you see a word that begins with the letters "rh," you can be almost sure the word is derived from the Greek.

Rh factor refers to one of the phenotypic blood groupings. "Rh" stands for "rhesus," the name of a macaque monkey, native to India, in whose red blood cells the factor was first recognized. It was later found that antibody to the "rhesus factor" agglutinated the erythrocytes of certain persons, who were then identified as being "Rh-positive." The initial letter of "Rh" when referring to the blood factor is customarily capitalized though the name of the monkey is not. Presumably, the monkey got its name from that of Rhesus, the mythic king of ancient Thrace, a realm northeast of Greece whose boundaries were indefinite and may have been thought to extend as far as the home of the monkey.

rhabdo- is a combining form taken from the Greek *rhabdos*, "a stick, rod, or wand," or from the Greek *rhabdōtos*, "striped." There is an obscure genus of rod-shaped microorganisms called *Rhabdomonas* (+ Greek *monas*, "unit," in this case taken to mean unicellular). More often, in medicine, "rhabdo-" is combined with "-myo-" to designate a reference to striated (striped) voluntary muscle, as opposed to "leiomyo-" (+ Greek *leios*, "smooth"), which refers to smooth or involuntary muscle. Thus, a **rhabdomyoma** is a tumor of striated muscle, whereas a **leiomyoma** is a tumor of smooth muscle origin.

rhagades is the plural of the Greek *rhagas*, "a rent or chink," this being related to the Greek verb *rhēgnymi*, "to break open or to burst forth." Originally, "rhagades" was used by the ancients to refer to chapping or excoriations in the skin of the scrotum, pudenda, or anus. Later, the term was extended to cracks or fissures occurring around any body orifice subject to movement, including the mouth.

-rhaphy (*see* **-pexy**)

rheumatism is derived from the Greek *rheuma*, "that which flows, as a stream or river." In ancient medical writings "rheuma" was used to describe any thin or watery discharge from a body surface or orifice. We still refer to a person with watery eyes as being "rheumy-eyed." In the 17th century *rheumatismos* was applied to an affection of the joints, presumably because various forms of arthritis are marked by effusion into the joint spaces. In modern medicine, an odd circumstance pertains. There is no disease entity medically recognized as "rheumatism," though laypersons often use the term to describe any sort of soreness or stiffness in their joints. Nevertheless, physicians skilled in musculoskeletal diseases and disorders have dubbed their specialty **rheumatology** (+ Greek *logos*, "a treatise") and themselves "rheumatologists." There is, of course, rheumatic fever, an acute febrile disease marked by polyarthritis and various immunopathic manifestations related to group-A streptococcal infection. There is also **rheumatoid** (+ Greek *eidos*, "like") arthritis, a term introduced in 1858 by Sir Alfred Garrod (1819-1907), a London physician, to distinguish that condition from acute rheumatic fever and gouty arthritis.

rhexis is a term, now seldom used, that denotes "a rupture." The word is a direct borrowing of the Greek term for a rent or a cleft and is related to the Greek *rhēgnymai*, "to break forth." **Angiorrhexis** (+ Greek *a[n]ggeion*, "a vessel") is rupture of a blood vessel.

rhin-, rhino- are variants of a combining form taken from *rhinos*, the genitive of the Greek *rhis*, "the nose." The rhinoceros (+ Greek *keras*, "horn"), as everyone knows, has a horny nose.

rhinencephalon is that part of the cerebral cortex associated with the sense of smell (rhin- + Greek *enkephalos*, "the brain").

rhinophyma is a form of rosacea characterized by a grotesque, knobby enlargement of the nose (rhino- + Greek *phyma*, "a swelling or tumor").

rhinoplasty is a cosmetic operation performed to improve the appearance of the nose (rhino- + Greek *plassein*, "to form or mold"). In the vernacular this is known as a "nose job."

rhinorrhea is a highfalutin way of characterizing a runny nose (rhino- + Greek *rhoia*, "a flowing").

rhizotomy is the surgical interruption of the sensory or posterior roots of spinal nerves and is performed for relief of otherwise intractable pain. The term combines the Greek *rhiza*, "a root," + *tomē*, "a cutting." The Greeks had a **rhizotomist** who practiced *rhizotomos*, but he was not a surgeon. He was a vagrant gatherer of roots and herbs for the preparation of agents used in medicine or in witchcraft (perhaps concurrently).

rhodopsin is the "visual purple," i.e., the purple-red protein substance in retinal rods that is bleached to "visual yellow" by light, thereby stimulating the sensory nerve endings in the retina. The term combines the Greek *rhodon*, "rose," + *opsis*, "vision."

rhomboid means "like a rhombus." The Greek *rhombos* was a sort of toy that could be spun around to make a whirring noise. A rhombus is an equilateral parallelogram. "Rhomboid" extends that definition to include an oblique, four-sided figure wherein adjoining sides may be unequal, but opposite sides and opposite angles are equal. The rhomboid muscles, major and minor, of the back (originating along the spinous processes and inserting on the scapula) were so named because of their shape.

rhonchus (*see* **rale**)

rib is probably derived from an obscure Teutonic root word for "strip, spar, lath, or rib." Most modern languages of Teutonic descent have similar words with such meaning, e.g., the German *die Rippe*. The classical Latin word for rib is *costa*. This yields **costal**, which designates whatever pertains to ribs, and the more common coast as the name for a strip of land that borders a sea.

riboflavin is a yellow-colored water-soluble vitamin naturally occurring in a variety of foodstuffs (ribo-, denoting its relation to nucleic acid + Latin *flavus,* "yellow"). When this vital factor was discovered in the 1930s, confusion arose by its being designated as vitamin G in the United States and as vitamin B_2 in Europe. It is now properly known by its name rather than by a letter. Deficiency of riboflavin leads to a syndrome that includes stomatitis, corneal vascularization, anemia, and retarded development.

ribose is a carbohydrate (an aldopentose) that characterizes the nucleic acid found in yeast. The term is derived from **arabinose,** also known as "gum sugar," a similar carbohydrate obtained by acid hydrolysis of certain vegetable gums, such as "gum arabic" (obviously a reference to its origin in Araby).

rickets is a disease of children, somewhat similar to osteomalacia in adults, wherein a dysplasia of the developing bone and cartilage results in spinal deformity with twisting and bending of the upper spine and long bones and a distortion of the skull. Because persons so afflicted with spinal deformity were impaired in posture and gait, "rickety" came to mean "shaky or tottering." The disease was recognized long before its cause was discovered to be a dietary deficiency of vitamin D or inadequate exposure to sunlight. A synonym is **rachitis** (which probably should be spelled "rhachitis"), taken from the Greek *rhachis,* "the spine," + "-itis." Rachitis, of course, is more a developmental deformity than an inflammation, as its name might suggest (remember, the Greek *-itis* was originally used to designate any condition). "Rickets" seems to be an Anglicized corruption of the Greek term. However, Professor H. A. Skinner makes a case for the origin of "rickets" in the Anglo-Saxon *wricken,* "to twist." Willard Espy, in *Thou Improper, Thou Uncommon Noun* (New York, NY: Clarkson N. Potter, Inc.; 1978) adds still another twist to the story. He points out that the 17th century gossip John Aubrey asserted:

> I will whilst 'tis in my mind insert this Remarque, viz., about 1620 one Ricketts of Newberye, a Practitioner in Physick, was excellent at the Curing of Children with swoln heads, and small legges: and the Disease being new, and without a name, He being so famous for the cure of it, they called the Disease of the Ricketts . . . and now 'tis good 'sport to see how they vex their Lexicons, and fetch it from the Greek.

As Espy says, "Those who vexed their lexicons had the right of it." But there is another, latter-day Dr. Ricketts whose name is properly in the medical lexicon, yet who has nothing to do with rickets. Howard Taylor Ricketts (1871-1910), an American pathologist, discovered in 1906 the cause and pathogenesis of Rocky Mountain spotted fever and other typhuslike diseases. The infecting microorganisms are now designated as members of the genus *Rickettsia* and the family Rickettsiaceae. In 1910 Dr. Ricketts died in Mexico City of typhus, the disease he helped to explain.

rifampin is a semisynthetic derivative of rifamycin B, one of a group of antibiotic substances produced by *Streptomyces mediterranei* and used to combat infection by staphylococci, meningococci, and mycobacteria (notably those causing tuberculosis and leprosy). The name is said by Elmer Bendiner (*Hospital Practice.* December 15, 1989:146) to have been given because the original organic source was found in a wooded area of northern Italy where, at the time, a camera crew was shooting the movie *Rififi.* This story, intriguing as it is, puts a strain on credulity. Rifampin, incidentally, happens to be a **zwitterion** (the second "i" is accented and pronounced as "eye") inasmuch as it is an ion possessed of both a positive and negative charge. *Zwitter* is German for "hybrid."

rigor is the Latin word for "stiffness or numbness" and also for "sternness or severity." This, in turn, is related to the Greek *rhigos,* "shivering or shuddering from cold or from horror." **Rigorous chills** are those attended not only by a sense of cold but by visible shaking. **Rigor mortis** (+ Latin *mors, mortis,* "death") is the stiffening of a corpse that ensues upon depletion of adenosine triphosphate in muscle fibers.

ringworm (*see* **tinea**)

risorius is "the laughing muscle," so called because when contracted it widens the mouth in a laughing posture. Its name is taken from the Latin *risus,* "laughter," the noun being derived from the verb *ridere,* "to laugh." **Risus sardonicus** is a pathologic grin due to spasm of the facial muscles, such as occurs in tetanus. It is so named because of the tradition that a poisonous herb found on the island of Sardinia caused a contorted grin on the face of any person in the throes of having been so poisoned. The adjective "sardonic" has come to refer to bitter or scornful derision.

robust describes whoever or whatever is strong and tough. The word is derived from the Latin *robustus*, "oaken." *Robus* is the Latin name for the oak. Anything robust is "sturdy as an oak." At one time a "corroborant" was a medicine intended to strengthen a patient. To corroborate is to support or reaffirm an assertion, thereby strengthening it.

rodent is derived from the Latin *rodere*, "to gnaw, to corrode." A rodent ulcer was at one time so called because it appeared to eat away at surrounding tissue, with no tendency to heal. This is now recognized as a form of skin cancer.

roentgen, roentgenology (*see* **radiology**)

rongeur is French for "a gnawer" and also "a rodent," being related to the verb *ronger*, "to nibble or eat away at." It is also the name given to a surgical forceps designed to gouge out unwanted fragments of bone at operation.

rosacea is an affliction wherein the skin, especially of the face, becomes a swollen, glowing red due to capillary dilatation. The term is a near borrowing of the Latin *rosaceus*, "made of roses." At one time a more odious term was "brandy face," reflecting a frequent association of the condition with uninhibited imbibition of alcoholic beverages.

rostrum is the Latin word for "a beak" and also "the pointed bow of a boat." In anatomy the term is used to describe certain beaklike prominences, such as the sphenoidal rostrum, the protuberant ridge on the inferior surface of the sphenoid bone that articulates with a depression between the wings of the vomer. In more common usage, a rostrum is a speaker's platform, so called because the dais in the Roman Forum was decorated with the beaklike prows of captured enemy ships or with the figure of a sharply beaked volant eagle.

rouleaux is the plural of the French *rouleau*, "a roll." The term was first used for a cylindrical stack of coins and later, because of the resemblance, for the manner in which agglutinated, disc-like red blood cells were observed to gather in stacked clumps.

rubella is the feminine form of the Latin adjective *rubellus*, "a reddish color." Beginning in the 16th century, a form of measles was called "rubella" because of its characteristic red rash. This is now known as "German measles," having been recognized as an entity by German physicians in the mid-18th century. It is also sometimes called "3-day measles" because of the typical duration of the rash.

rubeola has been adopted as a quasi-scientific name for ordinary measles, wherein the rash usually lasts about seven days. Both **rubella** and rubeola affect mainly children in populations where most adults are immune, and in children both diseases are relatively benign. Rubella is now more feared because of its teratogenic effect on women who contract the disease early in pregnancy. There is no etymologic difference between the terms "rubella" and "rubeola," but they serve a useful purpose in distinguishing the two similar yet distinct contagious diseases.

rugae literally means "many wrinkles" and is a direct borrowing from the Latin. The rugal folds of the stomach lining give a distinctly wrinkled appearance. The surface of the cerebrum can be described as being rugous. The singular of the feminine Latin noun is *ruga*. From the same Latin source comes the adjective "corrugated," as it refers to the alternating ridges and grooves of a sheet of cardboard or metal. Creating a rugous surface is one of nature's ways of increasing surface area within a limited expanse.

rumination is the act of chewing cud (i.e., food that has been once swallowed, then regurgitated into the mouth for further chewing). The process is normal for certain animals (cattle, sheep, goats, deer, and giraffes) but a distinctly odd and unusual symptom in man. Rumination as a symptom is to be distinguished from simple regurgitation and vomiting. The term is taken from the Latin *ruminare*, which is related to the noun *rumen*, "the gullet." Extended figuratively, "to ruminate" is also "to think over again, to meditate." An archaic synonym for "rumination" is **merycism** (Greek *merykismos*, "chewing cud") taken from *meryx*, the name of a ruminating fish.

rupture comes from the Latin *ruptus*, "a break or rent," this being the past participle of the verb *rumpere*, "to break down, break open, or burst through." "Rupture" is a common and serviceable word for hernia; both are of classical origin, the difference being that lay persons tend to use "rupture" whereas doctors prefer "hernia."

℞ is the symbol used in pharmacy for the Latin *recipe*, this being the imperative of the verb *recipere*, which in this context means "to take." Physicians traditionally write this symbol at the head of a prescription to say, in effect, "Take thou this!" But there is more to it than that. The letter "R" alone could stand for recipe. What about the mark that crosses the tail of the "R" to make "℞"? This is said to be significant of the astrological sign of Jupiter, ♃. At one time it was believed that to precede a formula with Jupiter's sign, as a sort of invocation, would assure a favorable result. Moreover, according to astrologers, the period during the ascendancy of the planet Jupiter was thought to be a good time to gather herbs and concoct medicines.

Sabot is French for "a boot or shoe." In medical parlance a *coeur sabot* is a boot-shaped heart and refers to the anteroposterior radiographic silhouette in cases of left ventricular hypertrophy, wherein the cardiac apex extends up and to the left, suggesting the toe of a boot.

sac is an abbreviation of the Latin *saccus*, "a bag or pouch," this being related to the Greek *sakkos*, "a coarse cloth made of hair." Usually, this was goat's hair, and when fashioned into a pouch, the cloth could be used for straining a fluid, such as wine. Numerous pouchlike structures in embryology and anatomy are referred to as "sacs." The diminutive **sacculus** is used to designate small pouches, such as the alveolar saccules of the lung.

sacchar- is a combining form taken from the Latin *saccharum* and the Greek *sakcharon*, both meaning "sugar." The Greek term is not native but seems to have come from an Oriental source. However, the need for the double-"c" signifies the sequence of the Greek letters kappa (κ) and chi (χ). **Saccharin** is a synthetic coal-tar derivative that is intensely sweet and is used as a noncaloric substitute for sugar. *Saccharo-myces* (+ Greek *mykēs*, "fungus") is the genus constituting yeasts that cause fermentation of sugars and other carbohydrates.

sacrum is derived from the Latin *sacer*, "holy or consecrated." The large, heavy bone at the base of the spine was called *os sacrum* by the Romans and *hieron osteon* by the Greeks, both meaning "sacred bone." Why sacred? One explanation often given is that the ancients observed that, because of its bulk, the sacrum appeared to be the last of the bones of an interred corpse to decay; hence this bone might be the nidus around which a body would be reassembled in the afterlife. Another explanation is that the Greek *hieron* could also mean "a temple," and that within the concavity of the large bone at the base of the spine lay the sacred organs of procreation. Finally, the shape of the bone may have resembled a vessel used in sacrifice, or the bone may have been used in some sacred rite.

sadism (*see* **masochism**)

sagittal (*see* **plane**)

salicylate designates a salt of salicylic acid, a compound once obtained from salacin, a bitter glycoside found, among other sources, in the bark of the willow tree. The Latin name for the willow is *salix*. The medicinal effect of decoctions from willow bark had been known for centuries. The antipyretic property of salacin was at one time presumed to be rationalized by the observation that willow trees grow in damp or marshy places where "agues (fevers) tend to abound." What came to be the best known salicylate, acetylsalicylic acid (trade-named **Aspirin**) was introduced to medical use in 1899 as a near-sovereign remedy for all that ached or was febrile. The salicylates are now subsumed in a class of agents called **NSAIDs**, an acronym (sometimes pronounced "en-seds") standing for "nonsteroidal, anti-inflammatory drugs, the "nonsteroidal" modifier thought to be necessary to distinguish such agents from hormonally active steroid substances related to the adrenal cortex.

saline can pertain to anything related to salts, but in medicine the term usually is restricted to a solution of sodium chloride. Physiologic saline is an aqueous solution of NaCl in a concentration isotonic with body fluids.

saliva is the Latin word for "spittle," commonly shortened to "spit," the mucoserous product of exocrine glands adjacent to the oral cavity. "Spit," of course, is an imitative word of which there are cognates in a number of languages. The Latin *saliva* would seem to be related, by transliteration, to the Greek *sialon*, having the same meaning. A **sialagogue** (Greek *sialon*, "saliva," + *agogos*, "leading,") is whatever stimulates the flow of saliva.

sallow describes a sickly, dusky yellow complexion, due to hypoxia of the skin, characteristic of various debilitating conditions. The word is of Old English origin and is related to the

French *sale*, "dirty." Reference to "sallow cheeks" is to their color and not to be confused with shallow or hollow cheeks.

salpinx is an almost direct borrowing of the Greek word for "a trumpet." It was only natural that the term would be applied to anatomic structures of a tubular configuration with a flared, bell-shaped end. There are two. The better known is the uterine or Fallopian tube, whose flared end embraces the ovary (much as the bell of a trumpet embraces a mute or sordino). Inflammation of the Fallopian tube is called **salpingitis** (a sort of "hot trumpet"). The second is the auditory or Eustachian tube that connects the pharynx with the tympanic cavity or middle ear. We no longer call this tube a "salpinx," but the term is preserved in the name of the **salpingopharyngeal** muscle, also called the levator palati. This muscle serves in two helpful ways. It widens and elevates the pharynx as one swallows a bolus of food, and it helps to open the pharyngeal orifice of the Eustachian tube when it is temporarily blocked. The latter action gives relief of ear discomfort when one descends from high altitudes.

salts owe their collective name to the Latin *sal*, "salt." However, it was not until the 18th century that salts were recognized as compounds formed by an interaction of acids and bases. In 1787 a committee of French chemists, including the famed Antoine Lavoisier (1743-1794), proposed a nomenclature for salts according to the acids and bases from which they are derived. This is the system we use today.

Salvarsan was once the trade name for arsphenamine, a trivalent arsenical compound, discovered in 1909 by Paul Ehrlich (1854-1915), the famed German bacteriologist. "Salvarsan" is a concoction combining the Latin *salvare*, "to preserve," + an abbreviation of the Latin *sanitas*, "health" (the "-ar" also conveniently suggests a reference to arsenic). Ehrlich called the compound "#606" because it was the result of his 606th experiment to find a drug specifically lethal to the spirochete of syphilis. Such an agent designed to seek out and destroy a pathogenic invader while sparing healthy cells of the host was hailed as a magic bullet.

Arsphenamine was long ago superseded by penicillin as a treatment for syphilis, but Ehrlich's aim ushered in a lasting era of definitive chemotherapy, and his heroic effort deserves to be remembered.

salve is derived from the Anglo-Saxon *sealf*, "a healing ointment," probably at first a clarified butter. The German word is *Salbe*, which relates to the Gothic *salbōn*, "to anoint." The sense of healing brings to mind the Latin *salvere*, "to be in good health." Incidentally, a "salver" is a small dish on which delicacies are served. This harks back to the dark days of yore when a small portion of a meal intended for persons of high rank was placed on a dish and eaten first by an expendable servant known as a **salver**. If the salver survived and showed no ill effect, the food was deemed safe and could be served to the company at large. The title of the servant to whom others owed their salvation was later transferred to the dish.

sanatorium (*see* **sanitarium**)

sanguineous means "bloody" and comes from the Latin *sanguis*, "blood." But many people forget the "e" in "sanguineous." The "e" must be there for both the correct spelling and the correct pronunciation. According to ancient humoral pathology, anyone with a preponderance of blood was thought to be of an optimistic temperament, hence our use of **sanguine** as an adjective meaning cheerful or full of hope.

sanitarium is one way of spelling and pronouncing the name of an institution for the care of invalid patients or for medically supervised recuperation. Another spelling is **sanatorium**. The former relates to the Latin *sanitas*, "a state of health," and the latter relates to the Latin *sanatorius*, "conducive to health." Both spellings and pronunciations are acceptable, and most would say the similar words mean much the same thing. A few would favor the fine point that a sanatorium is less a hospital and more a spa. There is no place for a hybrid such as "sanitorium."

saphenous is a term applied to but one anatomic structure and that is the saphenous vein, the longest vein in the body, extending in the leg from the foot to the groin. The origin of the term is confusing and somewhat contradictory. The spelling suggests a derivation from the Greek *saphēneia*, "clearness," in the intellectual sense of "the true picture." Yet this is anything but a true picture of the vein in question. A better explanation is that the name originated in the Arabic *al safin*, "the hidden" (which the vein is, in the tissues of the leg). The Arabic term was then mistakenly given a classical Greek spelling by some benighted scribe.

sapid refers to whatever gives a sensation of taste or flavor. Sapid substances are those that can be perceived by their characteristic taste or smell. The word is derived from the Latin *sapere*, "to have taste, smell, or flavor." To the Romans the meaning extended to embrace sensibility generally, and the Latin *sapiens* means "sensible, wise, judicious, and discriminating." Man distinguishes (and flatters) himself by referring to his own species as *Homo* (Latin for "person or being") *sapiens*.

saprophyte designates any vegetable organism, such as a bacterium or fungus, that takes its sustenance from dead or decaying organic matter. The term combines the Greek *sapros*, "rotten," + *phyton*, "plant." An example is the *Clostridium* genus of anaerobic gram-positive bacilli. Another example is the *Sarcina* genus of gram-positive cocci that tend to form cubical, packetlike clusters of eight cells; the name is taken from the Latin *sarcina*, "a luggage pack," such as that borne by soldiers.

sarcoma is from the Greek root *sarko*, "flesh," + *-ōma*, "tumor." A sarcoma is a malignant growth arising in tissues of mesenchymal origin; hence, most sarcomas are "fleshy tumors." **Sarcoid** (+ Greek *eidos*, "like") refers to whatever is "fleshy," but more specifically the term designates a disease characterized by the formation of exuberant granulomas found in lymph nodes, liver, spleen, and other tissues. From the same Greek root comes sarcasm, an utterance intended to "cut the flesh," and sarcophagus, a box or container intended to "swallow the flesh," i.e., a coffin.

sartorius is the name for a long, thin muscle that extends from the anterior superior spine of the ilium to the medial side of the proximal end of the tibia. By contracting it helps bring the thigh into the cross-legged position assumed by a tailor as he sits at his work. The name of the muscle is taken from the Latin *sartor*, "a tailor."

sassafras is an aromatic substance obtained from the bark of the root of the laurel tree, *Sassafras albidum*. Nowadays, sassafras is used as a flavoring agent in beverages and candy, but formerly it was regarded as a medicinal herb, whence comes its name. "Sassafras" may be a Spanish corruption of the Latin *saxifraga*, this being derived from a combination of *saxum*, "a rock," + *fragilis*, "brittle," from *frangere*, "to break into pieces." *Saxifraga* is the name given to a genus of small, flowering herbs that tend to grow in the crevices of rock, thus giving the appearance of having split the stone. The presumed explanation for "sassafras" is that a decoction of the root was supposed to exert a diuretic effect thought helpful in dislodging calculi in the urinary bladder. The name means "stone crusher." More up-to-date is the use of **saxifragy** to designate the effect of **lithotripsy** (Greek *lithos*, "stone," + *tribein*, "to rub or grind") as a means of pulverizing kidney stones or gallstones by ultrasonic shock wave or laser beam.

saturnine describes a person of a sluggish, gloomy, cold, and taciturn temperament. The mythologic Saturn was a Roman deity, identified with the Greek Kronos (Time), husband of Rhea, who devoured all of his children except Jupiter (Air), Neptune (Water), and Pluto (the Grave)—these Time cannot consume. Astrologers asserted that those born under the sign of Saturn are by nature cold, sluggish, and baleful. In alchemy Saturn became identified with lead, a heavy, sluggish metal. In the astronomy of the day, Saturn was given as the name for what was thought to be the outermost planet, farthest from the sun, that "moved slowly in its sullen orbit." In 18th century Europe and England there occurred an epidemic of what was called "saturnine gout." Remarkably, this affected only imbibers of port and Madeira, the so-called fortified wines that were imported from Iberia (Spain and Portugal); those who swilled common gin were spared. Fortified wines were those to which brandy was added; the brandy was distilled in apparatus equipped with lead tubing. Much later, another outbreak of "saturnine gout" was noted in the southern United States, where the local "moonshine" was contaminated with lead. It is now recognized that lead blocks the urinary excretion of uric acid and thus provokes attacks of gouty arthritis in susceptible tipplers.

satyriasis is an excessive venereal impulse in men, the counterpart of **nymphomania** in women. Just as female nymphs seductively cavorted in the mythologic sylvan glades, so male satyrs sought to satisfy what they perceived as a demand for their services. The satyrs, usually depicted in Roman sculpture as hybrids combining the head and torso of men with the lower body of goats, were companions of Bacchus, the god of wine, and were much given to revelry and lasciviousness.

saxifragy (*see* **sassafras**)

scabies is the Latin word for "the itch" and is related to the verb *scabere*, "to scratch," and probably to the Greek verb *skaptein*, "to dig." To the Romans, scabies originally meant any itchy, mangy disease of the skin. A common cause of such a condition, the itch mite, was described in the 12th century and is now known as *Sarcoptes scabiei* (the name of the genus being a combination of the Greek *sarx*, "the flesh," + *koptein*, "to smite or cut"). "Scabies" now specifically denotes the skin lesions produced by this mite. **Scab** comes from the Anglo-Saxon *scaeb*, "the crust on a sore." Because crusted sores in the skin often are the consequence of excoriation, doubtless there is a relation to the Latin *scabies*.

scala is Latin for "a ladder or flight of steps." The Romans always used the plural *scalae*. The **scala tympani** (Latin *tympanum*, "drum") and the **scala vestibuli** (Latin *vestibulum*, "entrance or forecourt"), parts of the cochlea, were so named because of their fancied resemblance to a circular staircase. Figuratively, any scheme of graded measurement is commonly known as a scale.

scald comes through the Italian *scaldare*, "to heat," as a shortened form of the Latin *excaldare*, "to wash in hot water," this being a combination of *ex-*, "out," + *caldus*, "hot."

scalenus is a near borrowing of the Greek *skalēnos*, "uneven or irregular." *Trigōnon skalēnon* was a triangle with uneven sides. The three (sometimes four) scalene muscles extend on either side from the cervical vertebrae to the first and second ribs. As a group they are of irregular triangular shape. The **scalenus anticus** syndrome involves pain in the shoulder, arm, and neck resulting from compression of nerves and vessels between a cervical rib and a tight anterior scalenus muscle.

scalp is the integument, usually covered by hair, that by cutting can be peeled from the top of the head to reveal the skull below. The term originated in the Old Norse *skalpr*, "a sheath or a husk." The sense is that of a covering that can be removed or cut away, a sense appreciated at one time by American Indians. The idea of separation or cutting away is evident in related words, such as cult, culture, and sculpture.

scalpel is a slight abbreviation of the Latin *scalpellum*, "a small knife," this being the diminutive of *scalprum*, "a chisel or a knife," and related to the Latin verb *scalpere*, "to carve." The instrument the surgeon uses to cut is simply a small, sharp knife, but it takes on a special aura when summoned by the surgeon: "Scalpel!" This is a signal that the operation is to begin.

scan (*see* **scintigraphy**)

scaphoid is an adjective derived from the Greek *skaphē*, "anything scooped out, as a trough, a bowl, or a small boat." The root verb is *skaptein*, "to dig." From this same source comes the Latin *scapha* and the English "skiff," both words for a light, open boat. One of the carpal bones is called "scaphoid" because it has a hollowed surface (to fit the head of an adjacent bone). A thin person, when supine, appears to have a boat-shaped belly that is referred to as a **scaphoid abdomen**.

scapula was always used by the Romans as the Latin plural *scapulae*, "the shoulder blades" and also "the shoulders or upper part of the back." The term probably relates to the Greek *skaptein*, "to dig," because the broad, flat shape of the shoulder blade suggests a sort of trowel or spade.

scar is derived from the Old French *escare* by aphesis (the dropping of an unstressed initial vowel) from the Late Latin *eschara*. One can call the visible trace of a healed wound either an **eschar** or "scar." Both mean the same, but plain English favors the latter. The Greek *eschara* means "the fire-place," doubtless a common source of many Hellenic scars.

scarlatina (*see* **rubella**)

scato- (*see* **copro**)

schisto-, schizo- are combining forms taken from the Greek *skhizein*, "to split or cleave." It is important to remember that the "sch-" in "schisto-" or "schizo-" represents in sequence the Greek letters sigma and chi (*not* the German "sch-") and always should be pronounced as "sk," not "sh." Also, the "z" in "schizo-" often is mistakenly given the non-Hellenic (or German) "ts" pronunciation rather than the proper "z" sound.

schistocytosis is a condition wherein fragments of cleaved erythrocytes are observed in the blood, as in hemolytic anemia (schisto- + Greek *kytos*, " cell").

schistosomiasis is an infection by trematodes or blood flukes of the genus *Schistosoma* (schisto- + Greek *sōma*, "body"). The male of this fluke has a deep cleft, the gynecophoric (female-carrying) canal, extending the length of his body; here the slender female is held during copulation.

schizophrenia is a term introduced in 1911 by Paul Eugen Bleuler (1857-1939), a Swiss psychiatrist, to characterize a form of dementia praecox in which the afflicted person seems to exhibit a "split personality" (schizo- + Greek *phrēn*, "the mind").

sciatic is derived from a Latinized corruption of the Greek *ischiadikos*, "subject to trouble in the hips or loins," this being taken from *ischion*, "the hip joint." The long thick, sciatic nerve (also known as the nervus ischiadicus) extends from the sacrum down the back of the thigh. **Sciatica** is a common term for pain anywhere along the course of the sciatic nerve.

scintigraphy is the two-dimensional pattern registered by gamma-rays emitted by a radioisotope, thus revealing its varying concentrations in a specific tissue, such as liver, brain, kidney, or thyroid gland. The term combines the Latin *scintilla*, "a spark," + the Greek *graphein*, "to write." These images formerly were called simply "scans," short for "scintiscans," but now that can be confusing because there are other types of unrelated scans, such as ultrasonographic scans and

CT scans. **Scan**, incidentally, is a verb converted to a noun, taken from the Latin *scandere*, "to climb or ascend." "To scan" is to observe from bottom-to-top or, in the case of a poem or paragraph, from top-to-bottom.

scirrhous is an adjective taken from the Greek *skiros* or *skirros*, "hard." The Greek word was used also for gypsum or stucco. Galen is said to have used the Latin *scirrhosus* for an indurated, fixed, painful tumor or swelling, but he distinguished this from *cancer*. Today, "scirrhous" describes any lesion of a hard, tough consistency.

scler-, sclero- are variants of a combining form derived from the Greek *sklēros*, "hard or tough." **Sclerosis** is a term used in pathology to describe a degenerative process marked by hardening.

sclera is the name for the tough, fibrous, outermost tunic of the eyeball. (*see* **scler-**)

scleredema is an indurated turgidity of subcutaneous tissues (scler- + Greek *oidēma*, "swelling").

scleroderma is a systemic disease of connective tissue that can result in hardening or stiffening not only of the skin (sclero- + Greek *derma*, "skin") but also of the viscera. When the disease is widespread it is called **progressive systemic sclerosis**.

sclerotherapy is the injection of irritant solutions to induce scarring and obliteration of varicose veins, as in hemorrhoids and in the esophagus (sclero- + Greek *therapeia*, "treatment or care").

scolex is the headlike portion by which a parasitic worm attaches to its host, but to the Greeks *skōlēx* was the whole worm.

scoliosis is an almost direct borrowing of the Greek *skoliōsis*, "a bending or a curvature." The term appears in Hippocratic writings to denote any sort of curvature, but now it is restricted to a lateral curvature of the spine.

-scope is a combining form, usually a suffix, taken from the Greek *skopein*, which, it is commonly held, means "to see or to view." But more than that it means observing for a purpose. To the ancient Greeks *skopein* meant "to look out for, to examine, to monitor." As it turns out these are the very functions of most instruments whose names end in "-scope," even the **stethoscope** (Greek *stethos*, "the chest"), the use of which is to examine or monitor the contents of the chest.

scopolamine is a naturally occurring antimuscarinic alkaloid paired with atropine in extracts of belladonna, originally obtained from a plant known as "deadly nightshade." In therapeutic doses (presumably lower than the doses employed in ancient times as a means of poisoning), scopolamine can induce drowsiness, euphoria, and amnesia; hence, the drug was long used as a preanesthetic medication, particularly in obstetrics, to produce a purported "twilight sleep." The name of the drug is taken from that of Giovanni Scopoli (1723-1788), an Italian naturalist for whom Linnaeus named a genus of plants that yield the alkaloid. Scopolamine also is identified as the levorotary form of **hyoscine**, so named because of its occurrence in plants of the genus *Hyoscyamus* (from the Greek *hys*, "pig," + *kyamos*, "bean"). The English had another name for the bean, "henbane," because of its adverse effect on pecking chickens.

scorbutus is a Medieval Latin term for scurvy. As such, it is said to have been taken from the Teutonic word *schaarbuyck*, this being a combination of *schaar*, "torn or ruptured," + *buyck*, "belly." This seems a bit farfetched inasmuch as neither rupture nor even swelling of the belly is a symptom of scurvy, now recognized as a manifestation of vitamin C deficiency. Of course, it is possible that in earlier times scurvy may have been confused with other nutritional deficiencies, notably protein deprivation, of which swelling of the belly can be a prominent symptom, especially in children. Whatever cures scurvy is known as an **ascorbutic** agent, hence the name **ascorbic acid** for vitamin C. **Scurvy** is somewhat of a misnomer, too. It is an adjectival derivative of "scurf," a scaly exfoliation of the skin which is not a symptom of vitamin C deficiency as we know it today. Again, when scurvy was so named it may well have been mixed up with other scruffy expressions of malnutrition.

scotoma is derived from the Greek *skotos*, "darkness or gloom." The Greeks used the term *skotodinia* to denote dizziness, probably because severe giddiness often is accompanied by ephemeral loss of vision or "dark spots before the eyes." Today, scotoma refers to a focal area of diminished or suppressed acuity in the visual field. A variant is "scintillating scotoma," wherein there is a luminous appearance before the eyes, sometimes as a serrated wall-like outline. The latter is called **teichopsia** from a combination of the Greek *teichos*, "a city wall" of the type that is crenellated as a fortification, + *opsis*, "vision."

scrapie is a debilitating, invariably fatal disease of sheep manifested by a patchy loss of woolly coat and impaired gait. The name comes from the afflicted animal's compulsion to scrape itself because of itching. In Scotland "scrapie" also is known as "cuddy trot," in England as "the rubbers" or "the goggles," in France as *la tremblante* ("the trembles"), and in Germany as *die trabe Krankheit* ("the trotting sickness"), according to J. R. Grief (*Trans High Agric Soc Scotl.* 1940;52:71-90). Its importance lies in its being the animal counterpart of the human disease called **kuru**, the native name given to the condition that was first recognized among the Fore people indigenous to remote areas of New Guinea. Both scrapie and kuru are "slow-virus diseases," i.e., symptoms appear only long after infection has occurred.

scrofula is a now almost archaic term for tuberculous swelling of the cervical lymph glands. It is the diminutive of the Latin *scrofa*, "a breeding sow." Apparently, someone fancied that the puffy visage of a patient with cervical lymphadenopathy resembled that of a little pig.

scrotum as a name for the baglike male appendage that contains the testicles seems to be a transliterated variant of the Latin adjective *scorteus*, "of leather," the allusion being to a pouch made of animal hide.

scurvy (*see* **scorbutus**)

scutwork is a cant term used by medical students serving as clinical clerks or by neophyte doctors in training in referring to menial tasks foisted on them by their immediate superiors, as when ordered to perform lowly jobs no one else wants to do. The first part of the term probably was taken from the intransitive verb "to scuttle," meaning to scurry about, to run with quick, hurried steps.

sebum is a direct borrowing of the Latin word for "tallow, suet, or grease." Probably, it is related to the Latin *sus*, "hog." The derived adjective **sebaceous**, was applied to a fatty cyst or to an oil-producing gland in the skin. **Seborrhea** (+ Greek *rhoia*, "a flow") is excessive elaboration of oil by the skin.

secretin is the name contrived for the first recognized hormone, discovered in 1902 by the English physiologists W. M. Bayliss (1860-1924) and E. H. Starling (1866-1927). The term was taken from the Latin *secretus*, "that which is separated." Secretin is a potent stimulus to the flow of water and bicarbonate from the exocrine glands of the pancreas.

secretion is derived from *secretus*, the past participle of the Latin verb *secernere*, "to separate, one from another." In strict usage "secretion" denotes the elaboration of a substance that acts for a specific purpose within an organism (*see* **hormone**), whereas **excretion** denotes the elaboration or separation of a substance intended to be discharged from an organism.

section comes from the Latin *sectio, sectionis*, "a cutting off." To the Romans this often referred to the auctioning off of confiscated property. In anatomy a section is a slice of tissue cut away for gross or microscopic examination. In surgery, a section or a sectioning is a division of tissue. A **resection** is a division for the purpose of removal. A **cesarean section** is the surgical opening of the uterus for the extraction of a baby.

sedative is an adjective (sometimes used as a noun) taken from the Latin *sedare*, "to allay, to calm." In pharmacy a sedative drug is one that helps a patient to settle down by allaying excessive stimulation or excitement. From time immemorial, potions have been concocted to induce lethargy or sleep. Among the earliest of the relatively modern sedative agents were the bromides and chloral hydrate (trichloracetic aldehyde), introduced in the mid-19th century. The popular use of bromides (an effervescent concoction with the trade name Bromo-Seltzer was once commonly dispensed at soda fountains) led to the coining of "bromide" in reference to a trite remark uttered by a dull person. In the first half of the 20th century, various derivatives of barbituric acid were the most widely used sedative agents. In recent years it has been more fashionable to use **tranquilizers** (Latin *tranquillare*, "to calm or to make quiet") or **anxiolytics** (Latin *anxius*, "being troubled," + Greek *lysis*, "setting free [from]").

sediment comes from the Latin, *sedere*, "to sit," and refers to an insoluble substance that settles out or down from a fluid mixture. The sedimentation rate measures the extent to which erythrocytes settle out or down from a column of anticoagulated blood.

segment is an abbreviated form of the Latin *segmentum*, "a trimming." To the Romans this meant a flounce or brocade attached to a garment as a trimming. In anatomy, a segment is a defined portion of a larger structure.

sella turcica is Latin for "a Turkish saddle." The Latin *sella* means "chair or stool." Roman horsemen used no saddle but rode on a cover tied to the back of a horse and called it an *ephippium*, "that which is put on a horse." The saddles in which the Turks and Arabs rode had supports, front and rear, and it is from resemblance to such a saddle that the fossa in the sphenoid bone containing the pituitary gland is named. The anterior and posterior extensions of this fossa are called the **clinoid** processes, from the Greek *klinē*, "a couch or bed," + *eidos*, "like." They look a little like bedposts. (*see* **clinic**)

seltzer (*see* **effervescence**)

semen is a direct borrowing of the Latin word for "seed or germ" and designates the fluid that conveys the male spermatozoa. From the same Latin source comes the word **disseminate**, literally "to scatter seed," although the scattering may give rise to things as disparate as tumors and knowledge.

semester is taken from the Latin *semestris* or *semenstris*, these being composites of *sex*, "six," + *menstruus*, "monthly," thereby denoting a 6-month period or whatever occurs at a 6-month interval. The "sem-" in the word has nothing to do with "semi-," as in "semiannual," and it is only a coincidence that a 6-month period and a semiannual period are the same. A **trimester** is a 3-month period. Again, only by coincidence is this one third of the usual period of human gestation.

semi- is the Latin prefix denoting "half," and used as a combining form in words of Latin origin. It is equivalent to the Greek *hemi-*

which is used in words of Greek origin. "Semi-" has been attached to various biomedical terms to indicate half of something. The semicircular canals of the ear are so named because of their shape. Certain structures are described as semilunar because they are shaped like a half-moon. The semimembranous and semitendinous muscles of the thigh are composed almost half of connective tissue. Sometimes "semi-" is fallaciously used to mean "sort of" or "not quite," as in "semipositive" when referring to a borderline value obtained by a laboratory test. This is as ludicrous as would be "semipregnant."

semilunaris (*see* **plica**)

seminal describes whatever sews a seed (Latin *semen,* "germ or seed") from which a fruitful idea may sprout. A **seminar** is a gathering of thinkers where new and potentially productive ideas are examined. A **symposium** (Greek *syn-,* "together," + *posis,* "a drink") might also be a productive gathering, perhaps more convivial.

senile comes from the Latin adjective *senilis,* "aged or old." **Senescent** is taken from the Latin verb *senescere,* "to grow old." The Romans had an exalted view of advanced age, and their *senatus* was "a revered council of elders." Our own founding fathers doubtless held a similar view when they established the United States Senate, but there are times when reality would seem to fall short of noble intent.

senna is a cathartic substance obtained from the dried leaves or pods of the plant *Cassia acutifolia.* "Senna" comes from the Arabic *sana,* "acute," and refers to the sharply pointed leaves of the plant (as does the Latin *acutifolia*).

sensation as a biomedical term denotes the registration of an afferent nerve impulse in that portion of the brain, the **sensorium,** capable of such perception. This meaning is faithful to the origin of these terms in the Latin *sensus,* "the faculty of perceiving." In common usage "sensation" is often escalated to convey the idea of heightened, more intense excitement.

sepsis is a derivative of the Greek *sēpsis,* "putrefaction," though the meaning has changed. The Greek term was used by earlier writers to mean the culmination of inflammation in corruption and rottenness. Today, "sepsis" means a condition of illness marked by the noxious effect of toxic products of microbial infection.

septum is an almost direct borrowing of the Latin *saeptum,* "a dividing wall or enclosure." The related Latin verb is *saepire,* "to fence in." The Latin noun being neuter, the plural is "septa." The term is used in anatomy and pathology to denote various wall-like or dividing structures, such as the nasal septum and the interventricular septum of the heart. **Septate** describes whatever is divided.

sequestrum is the Latin word for "a thing surrendered or deposited for safekeeping." In skeletal pathology a sequestrum is a particle of dead bone that has become separated, by injury or disease, from adjacent healthy bone.

serendipity can account for a fortuitous discovery or diagnosis, not at all uncommon in biomedical research and practice. More than mere luck is implied by serendipity. The encounter is unexpected but is turned to advantage by a prepared mind. The word comes from Horace Walpole's 18th century version of *The Three Princes of Serendip.* Serendip is an old name for Ceylon, now Sri Lanka. The princes in their travels had a knack for making remarkable discoveries they were not seeking.

serosa (*see* **serum**)

serotonin is a chemical neurohumoral transmitter substance, widely distributed in a variety of tissues, that was first recognized as such and named by M. M. Rapport and coauthors (*J Biol Chem.* 1948;76:1243) because of its property of inducing vasoconstriction. The name combines derivatives of the Latin *serum,* here used in reference to blood + the Greek *tonus,* "a tightening." The active moiety of serotonin is 5-hydroxytryptamine, often abbreviated as 5HT. A limerick telling of some of the effects of excessive serotonin is attributed to the late Dr. William B. Bean:

> This man was addicted to moanin',
> Confusion, edema, and groanin',
>> Intestinal rushes,
>> Great tricolored blushes,
> And died from too much serotonin.

serpiginous is an adjective derived from the Latin *serpere,* "to creep, to crawl, or to spread slowly." An ulcer that spreads slowly is said to be serpiginous. Although the related Latin noun *serpens* means "a creeping thing, as a snake or serpent," the term "serpiginous" refers to the mode of spreading, not to the shape. A structure or lesion that appears shaped like a serpent is properly described as **serpentine**. Thus, an ulcer with a serpentine border can also, but in a different sense, be serpiginous.

serratus is the Latin word for "notched," taken from the Latin noun *serra*, "a saw." The serratus muscles of the back and thorax have interdigitating slips that resemble the notches on the cutting edge of a saw. Any finely notched border can be referred to as serrated. Incidentally, "sierra" is a Spanish way of describing the saw-tooth profile of a ridge of mountain tops.

serum is the Latin word for "whey." Milk, when it coagulates, as in the making of cheese, separates into solid clumps (curds) and a slightly turbid, watery liquid (whey). It was such a dish that Miss Muffet was eating when she took offense at the proximity of the spider who sat down beside her. "Whey" is of Anglo-Saxon origin. The Latin *serum* may be related to the Sanskrit *sara*, "flowing." The use of "serum" to designate the watery residue of clotted blood, as analogous to whey, dates back to the 17th century. Serum differs from plasma in that it lacks **fibrinogen**, which has been consumed in the clotting process. From the same Latin source comes **serous** to describe any watery fluid of the consistency of serum or a gland that might give rise to such fluid, as well as **serosa** as a term for a smooth membrane immersed in serumlike fluid.

sesamoid relates to the Greek *sēsamon*, "the sesame plant." The tendons of certain muscles, particularly those in the hands and feet, may be inlaid with bony nodules that were fancied to look like sesame seeds.

setaceous describes whatever is slender and firm, like a bristle (*see* **hair**). The word comes from the Latin *seta*, "a bristle." A **seton** is a thin, durable wick, usually of woven silk or linen, that can be inserted in a wound or sinus to promote drainage.

sex is a word of obscure origin. According to one explanation it is a shortening of the Latin *sexus* (not to be confused with the Latin *sex*, "six"), which is related to the Latin verb *secare*, "to cut or to divide." The word thus denotes a division of living beings into male and female. Another hypothesis has it that "sex" is related to the Latin *secus*, "otherwise." In Latin *secus muliebre* (the second word means "womanly") are females and *secus viriles* (the second word means "manly") are males. In any case, we can join with the French in exulting, *"Vive la différence!"*

shingles (*see* **herpes**)

shock generally means a violent impact, as by a heavy blow, or the disruption of function consequent to such a blow. More specifically, in medical usage, the term denotes a state of dire physiologic reaction to severe trauma, typically associated with vascular collapse and depression of vital processes. The word is a near borrowing of the French *choc*, "a harsh impact," related to the verb *choquer*, "to strike against."

sialagogue (*see* **saliva**)

sibilant describes the shrill, whistlelike breath sounds heard on stethoscopic examination of the chest in cases of partial bronchial obstruction. The term is taken from the Latin *sibilans*, "a hissing sound."

sicca describes a syndrome or complex associated with immunopathic degeneration of salivary and lacrimal glands resulting in excessive dryness of the mouth (*see* **xerostomia**) and the eyes. The condition is a prominent feature of Sjögren's syndrome, named for the Swedish physician Tage Sjögren (1859-1939), but it can also be observed in other collagen-vascular diseases. **Siccative** describes an agent, such as may be used in certain dermatological preparations, to lessen exudation and thus promote dryness. The terms are taken from the Latin *siccativus*, "drying." (*see* **desiccate**)

sick is a simple word that can be traced to the Old English *seoc* and is related to the German *siech*, the Dutch *ziek*, the Danish *syg*, and the Swedish *sjiek*, all being close in meaning. (Actually, *krank* is more often used by Germans when they refer to being unwell; *die Krankheit* means "an illness.") This derives from an Old German word meaning "to stumble or grow weak." *Krank*, which bears an obvious relation to our colloquial "cranky," is pronounced "krawnck," and some say it was corrupted to become the deprecatory "crock," regrettably used by unfeeling doctors in reference to complaining patients. "Sick" and "ill" are often used interchangeably, though to say "I've been ill" seems to have a more genteel ring than "I've been sick." This is odd insofar as ill has descended, unchanged, from the Old Norse word meaning "bad or evil." "Sick" is more often used in a sense of bodily or physical impairment due to disease, in contrast to "injured" as a consequence of trauma, whereas "ill" frequently is used subjectively, as in "ill-conceived" or "ill at ease."

siderosis is a condition marked by an accumulation of iron in the tissues of the body. The term is derived from the Greek *sideros*, "iron." Curiously, we use the Latin *ferrum* as a root for designating iron-containing compounds, but we use the Greek *sideros* for terms pertaining to abnormalities in iron metabolism. **Sideropenia** (+ Greek *penēs*, "poverty-stricken") is a deficiency of iron in the body. **Sideroblastic** (+ Greek *blastos*, "a bud or germinal form") anemia is characterized by the presence of abnormal, "ringed" sideroblasts in the bone marrow, signifying impaired utilization of iron and, hence, deficient red cells in the circulating blood.

sigmoid is taken from the Greek letter sigma (Σ), equivalent to "S," to which is added *-eidos*, "like." "Sigmoid" describes whatever is Σ-shaped or S-shaped. The best example is the sigmoid segment of the distal colon, which is typically coiled like the letter "S."

sine qua non is a Latin phrase meaning "without which nothing." Whatever is *sine qua non* is indispensable. A feature of a disease essential to its pathogenesis or diagnosis is a *sine qua non*. For example, gastric acid secretion is a *sine qua non* of peptic ulcer disease.

sinew (*see* **nerve**)

singultus is medicalese for **hiccup**. It is a Latin word meaning "a gasp or sob," especially occurring in series. *Singultus*, in turn, is related to the Latin adjective *singuli*, "one at a time."

sinister is the Latin word for "left," but its common English usage has come to mean "evil or corrupt." This pervasive association of "right" with right and "left" with wrong has been noted in the entry about the word **adroit**. In addition to the tyranny of the majority of right-handed persons exercised over the minority of left-handers, there is another explanation for the ill repute of "left." In Roman **augury** (an art of divination whereby future events presumably could be foretold by scanning the sky), the observer faced north; because on his right was the east with its auspicious connotation related to the dawn, whatever was on his left was deemed unfavored. The combining form **sinistro-** is used in anatomy to mean "on or toward the left."

sinus is a Latin word meaning "a concave or hollowed-out surface" and also "a pocket, purse, valley, or gulf." The related Latin verb is *sinuare*, "to wind, curve, or arch," from which we derive "sinuous" and "insinuate." In anatomy, "sinus" is used to designate subsidiary cavities that open into larger spaces, e.g., the nasal sinuses. In some instances the term has been extended to refer to widened channels, e.g., venous sinuses. The hybrid term **sinusoid** (+ Greek *eidos*, "like") is similarly used.

siriasis is injury resulting from ambient heat, especially in athletes, and includes sunstroke. The term is taken from the Greek *seiros*, "burning." **Sirius** is the proper name of the "dog star" which burns brightly in the summertime night sky. In the northern hemisphere calling the time of oppressive heat at midyear "the dog days of summer" relates to the common name for the star. Dr. R. E. Sinclair cautioned, "Be Serious about Siriasis" (*Postgrad Med.* 1985;77:261), and Dr. J. P. Knochel reflected on "Dog Days and Siriasis: How to Kill a Football Player" (*JAMA.* 1975;233:513).

Sister Mary Joseph node is a lump or nodule that becomes externally visible or palpable at the umbilicus. It is so called from the name of the nursing nun at Saint Mary's Hospital in Rochester, Minnesota, who often assisted Dr. William Mayo at operations. It was she who called attention to such a lump when preparing a patient's abdomen for laparotomy, and Dr. Mayo identified the nodule as a metastatic growth from peritoneal carcinomatosis. (For more information, see *Amer Surg.* 1996;62:328.)

sitophobia describes a symptom that can lead to devastating weight loss. The term comes from a combination of the Greek *sitos,* "food," + *phobein,* "to fear." Sitophobia differs from other phobias in that it does not signify a mental quirk but rather an avoidance or fear of eating because of severe abdominal pain induced by any attempt to eat. A typical setting for sitophobia is in cases wherein mesenteric arterial blood supply has been markedly impaired by atherosclerosis. A patient so afflicted may be ravenously hungry, yet refuses to eat so as to avoid pain. The result can be grave nutritional deficiency.

skeleton is derived from the Greek *skeletos,* "dried up, parched, withered." It has been said that the Greeks applied the term to a mummy or a withered corpse, not to the bony framework of the body. So far as the record indicates, it was during the 16th century that "skeleton" was given its modern meaning.

skin is an almost unchanged descendent of the Old Norse *skinn,* "that which one peels off." **Skinny** describes one whose appearance is more peel than plush.

skull is of Scandinavian descent and harks back to such Nordic words as *skál* and *skul,* which meant "bowl or shell." Some say the ultimate origin is in the Teutonic *skal,* "to cleave." The traditional Nordic toast *"Skoal!"* has been said to derive from the ancient word for the skull and the supposed custom of using the inverted dome of the skull to contain ceremonial potions. More likely the call for a toast comes from the Old Norse *skál,* meaning "bowl." Incidentally, the custom of touching glasses in response to a toast and before drinking can be traced back to the days when poisoning was a prevalent means of gaining an advantage. Fellow quaffers felt more at ease when they could exchange the contents of their cups.

slough comes from the Middle English *slughe,* "the cast off skin of a snake." In pathology the term refers to a mass of necrotic tissue that separates, as a result of injury or disease, from a living part or organ.

smegma is the Greek word for "a soap or wax used in cleaning or polishing." The Greek root verb is *smekhein,* "to rub or cleanse." The accretion of fatty discharge under the prepuce from sebaceous glands at the corona of the penis is known as smegma.

smell (*see* **olfactory**)

snake oil is a term for an unguent of dubious value, if not worthless, purveyed by mountebanks or charlatans as a purported remedy for almost any ill to which the flesh is heir. The term has nothing to do with snakes or serpents. In the backwoods of Pennsylvania there seeped from the ground a viscid substance of umber hue and unpleasant odor known as "rock oil" or, more classically, "petroleum." This vile substance appeared to have no useful purpose other than as a topical ointment, and in this manner "rock oil" was applied by the local Indians to their burns and scratches. White settlers observed this practice and certain unscrupulous operators, seeing a market among their gullible countrymen, began bottling the stuff and selling it as "Seneca Oil." By appropriating the name of a native tribe in the Allegheny region, they cast the allure of a mystical Indian remedy. Seneca was often mispronounced as "Sen-*ake*-a" and thus "Seneca Oil" became "snake oil."

sodium by its "-ium" ending is recognized as an elemental metal whose designation is derived from *soda,* the medieval Latin name for the compound now known to be sodium carbonate. *Soda* is said to be a back-formation from *sodanum,* the glasswort plant whose name can be traced to the Arabic *suda,* "a splitting headache," which a decoction of the glasswort was purported to cure. However, the Late Latin name for the mineral hydrated soda was *natron,* taken from the Arabic *natrun* which, in turn, seemed to be confused with the Greek *nitron,* "saltpeter." In any case, when the distinction between sodium and potassium became clear, it was Martin Heinrich Klaproth (1743-1817), a professor of chemistry at the University of Berlin, who suggested that sodium be given the classical Latin name *natrium;* hence, its elemental abbreviation as "Na." Sodium and potassium were first isolated in 1807 by Sir Humphry Davy (1778-1829), a pioneer of electrochemistry. Incidentally, Davy was a close friend of Samuel Taylor Coleridge and others among the Romantic poets.

Thomas Castle wrote, "It was impossible to doubt that if he had not shone as a [natural] philosopher, he would have become conspicuous as a poet." Davy was asked by his friend William Wordsworth, later poet laureate of England, to oversee publication of the second edition of *Lyrical Ballads*.

sodoku is the Japanese name for "rat-bite fever," a relapsing illness caused by the microorganism *Spirillum minus*, transmitted by the bite of an infected rat. The disease was originally described in Japan. The Japanese term is a modification of the Canton Chinese *shue*, "rat," + *tuk*, "poison."

solar plexus (*see* **plexus**)

solecism is not a medical term but is a word worth noting in any book on words and their usage. A solecism is a mistaken use of words or error in grammar, usually for want of knowing better. The inhabitants of the remote Greek colony of Soloi spoke what proper Athenians regarded as atrocious Greek and derided as being *soloikismos*, i.e., characteristic of those ignorant oafs of Soloi. It is hoped that in this book there are relatively few solecisms.

soleus is a masculinized form of the Latin *solea*, which means "the underside or flat of the foot," "a sandal" (conforming to the shape of the foot), and "the sole-fish" (similarly shaped). The soleus muscle in the calf of the leg was so named because of its fancied resemblance to the fish.

soma is a direct borrowing of the Greek *sōma*, originally "a corpse" but, later, "a body, dead or living." The Greeks used *sōma* particularly as opposed to *psychē*, "the soul." In like manner, whatever is described as **somatic** pertains to the body, especially in contrast to the mind. Only recently was there contrived **psychosomatic** to refer to the interplay between the corporeal substance and the mind. "Somatic" also distinguishes cells of bodily tissues, in contrast to cells of germinal descent. Also derived from *sōma* is the suffix -**some**, indicating "a body, in the sense of a particle," as contributing to the dark-staining **chromosome** (Greek *chrōma*, "color") and to **lysosome** (Greek *lysis*, "loosening"), a minute intracellular particle that can release substances exerting an enzymatic effect.

somatostatin is a remarkable polypeptide occurring naturally in a variety of tissues and now synthesized as a pharmacologic agent that inhibits the action of other polypeptide effector substances, including various hormones. Originally detected in 1968 as a hypothalamic peptide acting on the pituitary gland to inhibit the release of growth hormone, the substance was first called "growth hormone release-inhibiting factor (GHRIF)" or "somatotropin release-inhibiting factor (SRIF)." These cumbersome terms were then reduced to "somatostatin" by contriving a combination of the Greek *sōma*, "body," + *statikos*, "causing to stand (still)."

-**some** (*see* **soma**)

somnus is the Latin word for "sleep." In Roman mythology Somnus is the name given to the god of sleep, who, with his brother Mors (Death) and his father Nox (Night), lived at the western edge of the world, where the sun is seen to set. A **somnambulist** (+ Latin *ambulare*, "to walk") is one who walks in his sleep, and a **somniloquist** (+ Latin *loqui*, "to speak") is one who talks in his sleep. A **somnifacient** (+ Latin *facere*, "to make or bring about") is an agent that induces sleep, as employed for the benefit of one who suffers from **insomnia** (Latin -*in*, "lacking").

sonde (*see* **sound**)

soporific describes whatever induces sleep, be it a drug or a tiresome lecture. The term combines the Latin *sopor*, "a deep sleep or stupor," and "-fic," a suffix indicating "a making" and derived from the Latin *facere*.

sore as both noun and adjective can be traced to the Anglo-Saxon *sar*, "distressing, grievous, painful." This is also the origin of "sorry" but not of "sorrow" (which relates to the Old English *sorgful*, "a sense of care or anxiety").

sound is an English word that can have almost 50 different uses, many of them of different origins and several with medical implications. To be sound in body and mind (or, as some would say today, "to have it all together") relates to the Latin *sanus*, "healthy and rational." Heart sounds, as perceived by means of a stethoscope, relate to the Latin *sonus*, "a noise or tone." A sound or **sonde** used as a probing instrument takes its name from the French *sonder*, "to fathom or explore." In nautical parlance a sound is a weighted line dropped from a boat to measure the depth of the underlying water. This may have been derived from a sort of garbled contraction of the Latin *sub-*, "under," + *unda*, "a wave or billow."

spa is a term for a health resort featuring a mineral spring or, more broadly, to any fashionable hostelry in a naturally soothing setting. The word is taken from Spa, the name of a town in the province of Liege, Belgium, celebrated since the 16th century for its purportedly curative mineral springs.

spasm is a near borrowing of the Greek *spasmos*, "a convulsion." Hippocrates used this word in reference to an epileptic fit. The Greek root verb is *span*, "to draw or pull tight, or to wrench" (which, incidentally, explains why the British insist on calling a wrench, the tool, a "spanner"). Although the Greek word could mean either "to stretch out" or "to tense up," the medical use of the term is usually restricted to the latter sense.

species is a direct borrowing, but with altered meaning, of the Latin word for "view, image, or appearance." The Indo-European root is thought to be *spek-*, "to look keenly." In taxonomy those entities that have a similar appearance or structure are grouped together as species. An anatomic or pathologic **specimen** is looked at keenly as representative of whatever is being studied. To call corrective glasses "spectacles" or to refer to "the spectrum of diseases" hews closer to the meaning of the root words.

speculum is the Latin word for "mirror," in which to see a *species* (an image). In medical diagnosis a speculum is an instrument by which a passage or cavity of the body can be examined. The mirrored instrument that a dentist uses is a true speculum. Most speculums (or specula) used to examine the ear, nose, vagina, or anus are cylindrical or bivalved tubes that provide an image but do not use mirrors.

sperm is a slight contraction of the Greek *sperma*, "the seed or germ of anything." (*see* **insemination**)

spermatozoa are the male seeds of animals (+ Greek *zōon*, "a living animal").

spermicide is any agent that is destructive of sperm (+ -cide, a suffix derived from the

Latin *caedere*, "to strike down or to slay").

sphenoid is the name of a prominent bone at the base of the skull. The name is taken from the Greek *sphēn*, "a wedge," + *eidos*, "like." Galen described the bone as being "like a wedge thrust between the skull and the superior maxilla."

sphincter is a near borrowing of the Greek *sphinktēr*, "that which constricts," being related to the verb *sphingein*, "to bind tightly." In anatomy a sphincter is a muscle, usually ringlike, that constricts whatever it surrounds when it contracts. The mythical Sphinx was a monster that had the body of a lion and the head and breast of a woman. The Sphinx was wont to perch on a rock outside Thebes and there pose unanswerable riddles to passing travelers. A wrong answer or no answer at all elicited an asphyxiating embrace by the Sphinx. The Sphinx met its match when Oedipus passed by. The challenging riddle: "There is a thing on earth that has four, two, then three feet. Of all the creatures that creep on the earth or move in the air or in the sea, it alone changes its nature—when it moves on the largest number of its feet, the strength in its limbs is the smallest. What is this creature?" Quickly came Oedipus' answer: "*Man*, who as a helpless babe crawls on all fours, then stands erect on his own two feet as a man, but with age requires a cane or crutch, the third leg." In a fury of frustration, the Sphinx squeezed itself to death. The association of the Sphinx with insoluble puzzles apparently led to the naming of **sphingolipids**, unusual fatty substances abnormally stored in body tissues, as in Tay-Sachs disease. Johann Heinrich Wilhelm Thudichum (1829-1901), a German-born investigator working in a laboratory at London's Saint Thomas' Hospital on the chemistry of nervous tissue, is quoted as writing, in 1881: "A body remained insoluble (in ether) . . . and to which, in commemoration of the many enigmas which it presented to the inquirer, I have given the name 'sphingosine.'"

sphingo- is a combining form that indicates a relationship to sphingosine or sphingolipids (see **sphincter**). A more prosaic attribution is to the Greek *sphingein*, "to bind tightly."

sphygmomanometer was contrived by combining the Greek *sphygmos*, "the beating of the heart or the pulse," + "manometer," the origin of which is given elsewhere in this book. A sphygmomanometer measures not the frequency of the pulse but, as its name implies, the pressures created by the pulse, commonly called "blood pressure." The instrument, essentially as we know it today, was introduced in 1896 by Scipione Riva-Rocci (1863-1937), an Italian clinician.

spica is the name given to a bandage applied by figure-eight turns that overlap in a chrevron pattern, which might be thought to resemble the overlapping covering of an ear of grain. The name is taken from the Latin *spica*, "an ear of grain."

spine comes from the Latin *spina*, "a thorn or prickly bush." The Romans used this word for the backbone because the series of vertebrae has so many bony protuberances. It was fancied to resemble a thorny twig.

spirochete is a hybrid term wherein the Latin *spira*, "a coil, as of a serpent," is combined with the Greek *chaitē*, "long, flowing hair." The spirochete is an organism that resembles a coiled hair. In 1905 Fritz Schaudin (1871-1906), a German bacteriologist, discovered the causative organism of syphilis. It was found to be a spirochete (the type having been named earlier), which Schaudin named *Treponema* (Greek *trepein*, "to turn," + *nēma*, "a thread") *pallida* (Latin for "pale").

spit (*see* **expectorant**)

splanchnic comes from the Greek *splan[n]gikos*, "pertaining to the entrails." Thus, the splanchnic nerves and vessels serve the internal organs.

splayfoot is a physical deformity characterized by abnormally flat feet turned outward. "Splay" is a shortened form of "display" that, in turn, is taken from the Latin *displicare*, "to unfold."

spleen is an almost direct borrowing of the Greek *splēn* as the name for the parenchymatous organ situated high in the left hypochondrium and which serves in the regulation of cellular elements of the blood. The Latin name for the organ, *lien*, appears to be almost the Greek name, with the "sp" lopped off. Possibly they both relate to the Sanskrit *plihan*. An archaic Teutonic term for the spleen is *milt*, preserved in the German *Milz*.

This, in turn, seems to relate to the Icelandic *melta*, "to digest." The ancients had no concept of the function of the spleen. Because it is situated in close company with the stomach, they may have assumed that it in some way served in the digestive process.

spondylo- is a combining form taken from the Greek *spondylos*, "a vertebra" or "any round body, such as the weight that twirls a spindle." **Spondylitis** is an inflammation of a vertebra. **Spondylolisthesis** (+ Greek *olisthos*, "slippery") is a forward displacement of one vertebra over another, usually of the fifth lumbar vertebra that has slipped over the sacrum.

sporadic comes from the Greek *sporadikos*, "isolated," this being related to *sporas*, "scattered." A sporadic disease is one that occurs here and there in space or now and then in time, as opposed to a disease that is either endemic or epidemic in a given place or population. Incidentally, Sporades is the name given to two groups of Greek islands scattered about in the Aegean Sea. (*see* **periodic**)

spore is derived from the Greek *spora*, "the sewing of seed." Originally the term was applied to plant seeds and to offspring. In the mid-19th century, it was appreciated that certain bacteria or fungi could survive unfavorable conditions by developing certain resistant forms called "spores" that, like seeds, then gave rise to further generations of the organism.

sport (*see* **mutation**)

sprain may have come through the Old French *espreindre* or *espraindre*, "to wring out," from the Latin *exprimere*, "to express or squeeze out." By the same token, **strain** comes through the Middle French *estreindre* or estraindre, "to wring hard," from the Latin *stringere*, "to draw tight." In medicine there is a particular distinction between "strain" and "sprain." A strain is an overextension of a muscle; a sprain is a partial rupture of the ligaments supporting a joint. Moreover, there is a distinction between **stress** (related to the Old French *estrece*, "straitness or oppression") and "strain" that is not always observed by otherwise careful speakers and writers. Stress is the potentially injurious action, whereas strain is the resulting injury. Twisting one's arm constitutes stress; it may or may not lead to a strain of the arm muscles. An odd and colloquial use of "strain" was by unschooled men as a name for gonorrheal urethritis, the painful penile discharge being wrongly attributed to a physical stress, such as that of heavy lifting.

sprue is a name for a condition marked by impaired intestinal absorption and consequent malnutrition. There are two types. **Tropical sprue** occurs in persons who live in or visit for an extended time certain areas of India, Southeast Asia, or the Caribbean islands, and who are subject to an enteric infection that has not yet been precisely defined. **Nontropical sprue** and **idiopathic steatorrhea** are now seldom used as synonyms for coeliac disease, particularly that occurring in adults. The term "sprue" was introduced in 1880 by Sir Patrick Manson (1844-1922), a widely traveled British physician, as an Anglicization of the Dutch *spruw* or *sprouw*, which meant "thrush," i.e., a patchy exudative inflammation of the oral and pharyngeal mucosa. Coeliac disease can be marked by redness of the tongue and mouth, but exudation is not a feature unless there is secondary infection. Persons afflicted with coeliac disease, because of their depleted state, may be subject to candidiasis. (*see* **moniliasis;** *also* **thrush**)

sputum is the substance of whatever is spit out. The word is a direct borrowing of the neuter past participle of the Latin *spuere*, "to spit."

squamous comes from the Latin *squama*, "the scale of a fish or serpent." The **squamal** portions of various bones of the skull (frontal, temporal, and occipital) are so called because of their thin, flat, platelike shape. The squamous cells of the outer layer of the skin (epidermis) are similarly named. They tend to occur in overlapping layers and thereby constitute a stratified squamous epithelium. **Desquamation** is the shedding, because of underlying dermal injury, of the outer layers of the skin. To the Romans *desquamare* meant "to scrape the scales off a fish."

squint (*see* **strabismus**)

stain is ordinarily thought of in the sense of adding color, yet the origin of the word suggests the opposite. "Stain" is an aphetic, Anglicized, back-formation from the Old French *desteindre*, "to take away the color,"

this being derived from a combination of the Latin *dis-*, "apart, away," + *tingere*, "to dye." Perhaps the idea is that by applying a stain one takes away the original color of an object, albeit by adding another color. A variety of stains have been developed for use in microscopy whereby particular features of tissues and cells can be more clearly discerned.

stapedius (*see* **stapes**)

stapes is a Late Latin term for "a stirrup." It cannot have been, and was not, a classical Latin word because the Romans rode their horses with neither saddles nor stirrups. The barbarians, however, were more clever. They used saddles from which they hung a looped rope by which a man could quickly mount a horse. This was known as a *stigrap*, from the Anglo-Saxon *stigan*, "to rise or mount," + *rap*, "rope." Later, supports for the rider's feet were hung from both sides of the saddle, and these became called *stapes*, by combining the Latin *stare*, "to stand," + *pes*, "foot," i.e., "a place for the foot to stand." One of the three small bones in the middle ear is shaped like a tiny stirrup and was given the Late Latin name (*see* **incus**). The genitive of stapes is *stapedis*, and the little muscle attached to the stapes is thereby called **stapedius**.

staphylococcus (*see* **coccus**)

starch comes from the Anglo-Saxon *stearc* or *starc*, "stiff or strong," and is related to the German *stark*, "strong." Starch is a substance long known to stiffen cloth. This property led to its naming centuries before starch was recognized as a polysaccharide of vegetable origin with the generic formula $(C_6H_{10}O_5)_n$.

starve has descended from the Old English *steorfa*, "death," which is related to the Old Norse *deyja*, "to die." So, the expression "starve to death" is, etymologically, a redundancy. "Starve" is an example of how a word, in its travel through time, can acquire a special and restricted meaning. Today, one can die from any number of causes, but one can starve only by being deprived of nourishment.

stasis is a direct borrowing of the Greek word for "the posture of standing," from the verb *histemi*, "to make stand still." In physiology, stasis is a stoppage in the flow of blood or other body fluid.

stat is a slight abbreviation of the Latin *statim*, "immediately, at once, on-the-spot." To issue an order such as "Intravenous fluids, stat!" is a mandate for prompt, imperative action.

status is a direct borrowing of the Latin word for "state or condition." In medicine the term is applied particularly to conditions that are sustained and prolonged, e.g., status asthmaticus.

status lymphaticus (*see* **lymph**)

steatopygous means just what it would have meant to the Greeks, "having a fat rump." The word combines the Greek *steat-*, from *stear*, "stiff fat or suet," + *pygē*, "the buttocks."

stellate comes from the Greek *stella*, "star," and means "star-shaped." Various anatomic structures with processes radiating from a central point or body are described as being stellate. The stellate (or cervicothoracic) ganglion is situated on the sympathetic trunk anterior to the lowest cervical or first thoracic vertebra.

stenosis comes from the Greek *stenos*, "narrow." Pyloric stenosis is a narrowing of the outlet from the stomach. Spinal stenosis causes impingement on the spinal cord within its vertebral canal. A stenotic vessel is one in which the lumen is narrowed but not completely closed.

stent is the name of a supporting device, such as a mold fashioned to hold a graft in place, or a stiff cylinder used either to support an **anastomosis** or to preserve a dilatation during the ensuing healing process. Tubular stents also can be implanted in blood vessels, the esophagus, or biliary ducts to keep open a stenotic lumen. But "stent" has nothing to do with "stenosis." Most authorities believe "stent" to be a colloquial (probably Scottish) version of "stint," meaning a limitation or restraint. Another explanation, perhaps only a coincidence, is that the term memorializes Charles Stent, a 19th century English dentist, who fabricated a plastic resinous substance that would set hard and provide a firm impression of the teeth from which a dental prosthesis could be made. The substance became known as Stent's mass and was readily adapted to other uses.

sterco- is a combining form taken from the Latin *stercus*, "dung." **Stercobilin** is a bile pigment found in feces. A **stercoral** ulcer results from erosion of the rectocolic mucosa by a hard, abrasive clump of feces.

stereo- is a combining form adapted from the Greek *stereos*, "solid," as a mass having three dimensions. For example, **cholesterol** (Greek *cholē*, "bile") was so named because it was first found in gallstones and appeared to be "solid bile."

stereognosis is the faculty of perceiving the shape and identifying an object by the sense of touch alone (stereo- + Greek *gnōsis*, "knowledge").

stereotype is used figuratively in medicine, as it is generally, to denote whatever conforms to an unvarying pattern. Thus, a stereotype of a given disease is predictable in terms of its pathogenesis, manifestation, and course, based on knowledge of a particular model. The term combines the Greek *stereo-* + *typos*, "impression," but the ancient Greeks never would have seen or heard the word because it was not conceived until the 18th century. Originally, the "-type" of "stereotype" was literally printers' type. In 1725 William Ged, a Scottish inventor, patented a process for casting a duplicate metal plate from a mold made up of movable type. Later, French typecasters perfected a means of using papiermache to receive the impression. The resulting "solid type" had the advantage of being durable and reproducible when compared to loose and movable type, thus it was better suited to use in high speed presses. Workers who made stereotypes began calling them "cliches," from the French verb *clicher*, "to click or clap," as that was the sound made when the mold was struck against near-molten lead to create a stereotype. It was not until the late 19th century that the nickname appeared as a metaphor for any expression reiterated so often as to become trite.

sterile is a near borrowing of the Latin *sterilis*, "unfruitful, barren, empty, or bare." The related Greek word of the same meaning is *steiros*. The original reference was to a female animal or to a woman who was unable to conceive and bear offspring. This usage persists for both the male and female of any species. In medicine the term has been adapted to mean totally free, or "barren," of infectious microorganisms, as surgical paraphernalia must necessarily be.

sternum is a Late Latin term taken from the Greek *sternon*, "the breast or chest." The term was used by some early writers for the chest generally, but this use was soon supplanted by that of "thorax," and "sternum" became the name of the bone in the middle of the anterior chest to which the ribs are attached. Often this is called the breastbone.

steroid describes a substance that resembles cholesterol chemically and contains in its structural formula a cyclopentanoperhy-drophenanthrene ring. Included in this group are certain hormones, bile acids, and cardiac glycosides. Steroid therapy refers usually to the use of **corticosteroid** hormones, such as cortisone or one of its many kin. The "corti-," of course, indicates an original source in the adrenal cortex.

sterol began as a sort of nickname for "cholesterol" and is now used as a collective term for unsaturated solid alcohols, of which cholesterol is the prototype.

stethoscope comes from the Greek *stethos*, "the breast or chest," combined with *skopein*, "to view or examine." A prototype of the instrument, little more than a simple rigid tube to conduct sound, was invented in 1816 by the French physician René Théophile Hyacinthe Laënnec (1781-1826), who also conceived the term "cirrhosis." The stethoscope was later developed as a binaural device by a New York doctor, George Philip Cammann (1804-1863). One might wonder why the name given to an instrument for listening carries the suffix "-scope," which usually is attached to the names of instruments intended for viewing. Perhaps the stethoscope should have been called a "stethophone." But there is more to the meaning of the Greek verb *skopein* and the Greek noun *skopos*. The former could mean viewing in the broader sense of observing or monitoring; the latter means "a watchman or a scout."

-sthenia is a combining form taken from the Greek *sthenos*, "strength, might, or prowess." To be **asthenic** is to lack strength. **Neurasthenia** is a condition marked by nervous exhaustion, less precisely defined as "weak nerves." A **hypersthenic** person is well-muscled to the point of being "muscle-bound," and heavy-set at that. There was a time when much significance was attached

to a person's **habitus** (Latin for "condition," from the verb *habere*, "to hold"), i.e., how the person "held" himself or herself. A person of the asthenic habitus was slender and frail; asthenic habitus denoted a person of normal proportions; a person of hypersthenic habitus was stocky or disproportionately thick.

stigma is a direct borrowing of the Greek word meaning "puncture by a pointed instrument," particularly a "brand mark." The latter is the sense in which "stigma" is used medically as a visible sign of a particular disease. A telangiectasis can be a stigma of cirrhosis.

stimulus is the Latin word for "a pointed stick used as a goad." To a Roman soldier a *stimulus* was a sharp, partially buried stake concealed in such a way as to injure an unwary enemy. Such a simple, nefarious device has been used as recently as the Vietnam War. The related Greek word is *stigma*. "Stimulus" came to be used in physiology in the 18th century when it was observed that pricking caused a frog's leg to twitch.

stoma is the Greek word for "the mouth." By extension, the term has been applied to various mouthlike openings in plants and animals. In medicine **stomatitis** is inflammation of the oral mucosa. A surgical stoma is an artificial opening in any viscus, created for the purpose of ingress or egress. These usually are specified as gastrostomy, enterostomy, or colostomy, according to their location. Occasionally, there is an unwitting confusion between "-stomy" and "-tomy" (Greek *tomē*, "a cutting"). A **gastrotomy** is simply an incision in the stomach wall, whereas a **gastrostomy** is a mouthlike opening fashioned between the stomach and the anterior abdominal wall to accommodate a feeding tube.

stomach was cited as a spoof of outrageously fanciful etymology by Willard R. Espy in his *Another Almanac of Words at Play* (New York, NY: Clarkson N. Potter, Inc.; 1980) when he informed: "Septimus Thaddeus O'Mach's great treatise on gastrointestinal anatomy led to the general use of the term 'the gastric organ of Septimus Thaddeus O'Mach.' O'Mach's contemporaries got fed up with such a mouthful, and it was digested down to 'the organ of S. T. O'Mach,' and finally just to 'stomach.'" There is, of course, not one morsel of truth in this gulp. The fact is that the term originated in the Greek *stomachus*, "the throat or gullet," this being related to *stoma*, "the mouth." In this sense the gullet was a passage that had a mouth. Through the ages, the assignment of the term "stomach" seems to have gradually descended the alimentary canal: first the throat, then the gullet or esophagus, later the opening into the *ventriculus* (medical Latin for "stomach"), and finally the saclike organ we now know as the stomach. **Stomachic** is a bygone term for a digestive tonic.

stool can be traced to the postulated Indo-European root word *stā*, "that which stands firm," which led to the Anglo-Saxon *stōl*, "a seat." When the universal custom of squatting when evacuating the bowel was made more comfortable by some sort of firm support, "to stool" became a euphemism for "to defecate." We still speak of "stooling pattern" when we describe a patient's bowel action. Later, "stool" became a relatively inoffensive word for the product of "stooling," viz., the fecal deposit itself.

strabismus is a visual defect in which the two eyes cannot coordinately focus because of an imbalance in their respective extraocular muscles. The term is taken from the Greek *strabizein*, "to squint." Persons with deviating or "crossed" eyes tend to squint in order to compensate for their imperfect focus. Indeed, **squint**, which in an older sense meant "to look askance or askew," is another word for strabismus. There are two forms of strabismus: one or both eyes deviate inward (**esotropia**, from the Greek *eso-*, "inward," + *tropē*, "turning"), and one or both eyes deviate outward (**exotropia**, from the Greek *ex-*, "out").

strain (*see* **sprain**)

stratum is the neuter past participle of the Latin verb *sternere*, "to spread out." The term has been incorporated in a number of anatomic terms for sheetlike structures, particularly those that occur in layers. The stratum corneum (Latin *cornu*, "horn") is the outermost layer of keratinized squamous cells in the skin. The stratum granulosum (Latin *granulum*, "a small grain or sed") of the ovary is the layer of cells lining the theca of an ovarian follicle.

streptococcus (*see* **coccus**)

stress (*see* **sprain**)

stria is the Latin word for "a groove," especially in architecture, where it means the flute of a column. A series of parallel flutes separated by elevated strips gives the appearance of stripes. **Striated** is used in anatomy to described structures that are striped, e.g., the striated fibers of voluntary muscle. The so-called stretch marks on the bellies of some women who have had children are known as striae.

stricture is an almost direct borrowing of the Latin *strictura*, the past participle of the verb *stringere*, "to draw tight or to compress." In pathology a stricture is an abnormal constraint or narrowing caused by a contracting scar, as in the urethra or the esophagus.

stridor is the Latin word for "a shrill sound or a harsh noise." In medicine "stridor" denotes such a respiratory sound produced by the strenuous effort to inhale through a spastic or constricted larynx and is a sign of respiratory distress. In times when diphtheria was rampant, stridor would send chills to the marrow of parents whose children were stricken with the disease. It meant the diphtheritic membrane in the throat was choking off breath.

stroke (*see* **apoplexy**)

stroma is a direct borrowing of the Greek *strōma*, "anything spread out for lying or sitting upon." This, of course, would be a sort of mat. It is in this sense that "stroma" was adopted in anatomy as a term for the matrix in which functional elements of a tissue are supported.

Strongyloides is the name for a genus of roundworms that infect both people and animals. The most notorious is *Strongyloides stercoralis* (Latin *stercus*, "dung"), which is transmitted by contact with feces expelled by an infected person. The parasites tend to resemble worms of another genus, ***Strongylus***, similarly infectious, mainly in animals. The names come from the Greek *strongylos*, "round."

strophanthin (*see* **ouabain**)

struma is the Latin term for "a glandular swelling in the neck" and is related to *strues*, "a pile or heap." (When we construe or misconstrue what someone has said, we build up a heap of belief from what we have heard.)

Both "struma" and "scrofula" are old terms for what is now recognized as cervical lymphadenopathy. We have abandoned "scrofula" but kept "struma," as in struma lymphomatosus, a swelling of the thyroid gland consequent to degeneration of its epithelial components, infiltration by lymphocytes, and proliferation of connective tissue. (*see* **goiter**)

Student spelled with a capital "S" is used to designate Student's *t* test, a measure of statistical significance. "Student" was the *nom de plume* of William S. Gossett (1876-1937), a British mathematician who published his exposition of statistical inference in 1908, while he was in the employ of Arthur Guinness & Sons, the brewers.

stupe is a direct borrowing of the Greek *stupē*, "the coarse fiber of flax or hemp." This was woven into cloth that, among its other uses, was soaked in hot water and applied as a therapeutic fomentation or poultice. Thus, a hot stupe is what we would otherwise call a "hot pack."

stye comes from the Anglo-Saxon *stīgend*, "a rising." A sty, which is a swollen, inflamed, sebaceous gland of the eyelid, is a "rising on the eye." A polysyllabic name for the same lesion is **hordeolum**, Latin for "a barleycorn."

styloid is derived from a combination of the Greek *stylos*, "a pillar or post," + *eidos*, "like." The Latin *stilus* was a pointed instrument used for writing. The styloid process is a long, slender projection of the temporal bone that serves as a point of attachment for several muscles of the throat and tongue.

styptic comes from the Greek *styptikos*, "an astringent," being related to the Greek verb *styphein*, "to contract or draw together." A styptic pencil, which can be applied to stop bleeding from minor cuts, contains a core of alum (a double sulfate of aluminum and potassium) that exerts an astringent effect on small blood vessels.

sub- is a prefix taken from the Latin preposition *sub*, "under, beneath, or to come after." Often it is used in the sense of "less than."

subacute is a word generally understood in medicine to indicate the duration of a symptom or disease that is longer than "acute" but shorter than "chronic." Strictly speaking,

a better word for an intermediate duration would seem to be "subchronic," but such a word enjoys no currency and probably never will.

subclinical is a term contrived to describe a disease that is present but not clinically manifest. An example would be impaired glucose tolerance signifying diabetes but in the absence of any symptom of the disease.

sublimate is an interesting word taken from the Latin *sublimis* (or a collateral form, *sublimus*), "high or lofty" in the sense of "lifted to a higher plane." In analyzing the Latin *sublimis* most authorities translate the prefix *sub-* as "up to" and relate *-limis* to *limen*, "threshold," but it would seem as likely to be related to the Latin *lima*, "a polishing or revision." In any case "sublimate" has two meanings, one as a noun and the other as a verb, pertinent to medicine. In chemistry a sublimate is a substance that can change from a solid to a vapor without intervening liquefication. In psychology to sublimate is to divert unacceptable, instinctive drives into personally or socially acceptable channels.

subliminal is used in psychology to describe whatever exists or operates below the threshold (Latin *limen*) of consciousness. In physiology a subliminal stimulus is of insufficient intensity to elicit the expected response. (*see* **liminal**)

subluxation is a partial (or "less than complete") dislocation of a bony articulation (sub- + Latin *luxare*, "to put out of joint"). Incidentally, the Latin *luxus* (hence "luxury") has an almost pejorative meaning of extravagance or splendor in excess. (*see* **luxation**)

substantia is a Latin word meaning "the essence of anything, that of which it is composed"; as such, substantia has been given as a name to various anatomic structures, particularly those of the brain.

substrate is whatever an enzyme acts on, as if the enzyme were placed atop an "underlayer" (sub- + Latin *stratum*, "a layer")

subtilis is Latin for "finely woven or of fine texture" and combines sub- + *tela*, "a web." By allusion to whatever was so finely woven as to be almost invisible comes the word "subtle." The microbe *Bacillus subtilis* may have been so named because it is a common contaminant of bacterial cultures, i.e., it often seems to be just lying around, almost invisibly.

subungual (*see* **ungual**)

succus is the Latin word for "sap or juice" and is related to the verb *sugere*, "to suck." The succus entericus is the digestive juice elaborated by the mucosa of the small intestine. **Succinic** acid was so named because it was originally detected in amber, a fossil resin called *succinum* by the Romans.

succussion describes the means of eliciting a splash heard or felt in the abdomen of a person whose fluid-filled stomach or bowel fails to empty normally. The term is taken from the Latin *succussus*, "a shaking or a jolt."

sudamen is a small white vesicle in the skin produced by sweat (*see* **sudor**) trapped in a swollen sweat gland. Such vesicles are about the size of millet seeds, and the eruption is sometimes called **miliaria**.

sudor is the Latin word for "sweat." **Sudoriferous** (+ Latin *ferre*, "to bring forth") glands in the skin are those that produce sweat. They can also be called **sudoriparous** (+ Latin *parere*, "to produce") glands.

sulcus is the Latin word for a furrow made by a plow or the rutted track of a wheel. The related Greek word is *holkos*, "track or trail." An almost endless number of grooves, depressions, and wrinkles in anatomic structures have been called a sulcus or, in the Latin plural, **sulci**.

super-, supra- are combining forms, used in English as prefixes. They have been taken from the Latin preposition *super*, "over, above, more than," and the Latin adverb *supra*, "over, above, beyond." As a general rule "super-" is used with nouns and participles whereas "supra-" is affixed to adjectives, but the rule is by no means inflexible.

supine is a near borrowing of the Latin adjective *supinus*, "face up, turned upward." This is almost, but not quite, the opposite of the Latin *pronus*, "leaning, stooping, or bent forward." The supine position is that in which the body is lying on the back with the face up. In the **prone** position the body lies face and belly down, with the back turned up. This distinction is unknown or forgotten by the careless speaker who says, "He was lying prone on his back," an impossible posture. The terms also are used to describe positions

of the arms: supine is with palms up, prone is with palms down. Thus, a **supinator** muscle turns the arm so that the palms are up, whereas a **pronator** muscle turns the arm in the opposite direction. The supinators are stronger muscles, thereby enabling a right-handed person to more effectively tighten a screw. The fact that most persons are right-handed has determined the angle of the threads on screws and bolts. By the same token, a left-handed person is better at loosening a screw. Derivatives of the Latin *supinus* and *pronus* are also used figuratively. Whoever takes an affront supinely takes it "lying down." Whoever or whatever leans toward something is said to be prone to it.

supplement (*see* **complement**)

suppository is derived from the Latin *suppositus*, the past participle of *supponere*, "to put something under or next to something else." In pharmacy a suppository is a fusible or easily melted form of medication that can be inserted in a body orifice, usually the vagina or rectum, there to exert its intended effect.

supra- (*see* **super-**)

supratentorial (*see* **tentorium**)

sura is the Latin term for the calf of the leg. The **sural** nerve, a cutaneous branch of the medial popliteal (tibial) nerve, descends between the two heads of the gastrocnemius muscle and serves the skin overlying the calf of the leg and the lateral aspect of the foot.

surgery is an example of a word whose path from Greek to English has been so tortuous as to obscure its origin. It began with the Greek *cheirourgia*, "working with the hands, the practice of a handcraft or art." This was taken into Latin as *chirurgia* and thence into Old French as *surgerie*, finally becoming the English "surgery." The original Greek word combines *cheir*, "the hand," + *ergon*, "work, a person's employment," and the reference in all derived languages is to manual procedures. To the British, the noun "surgery" also means the place where treatment is given, i.e., the room where the doctor performs his manual procedures. Cognitive activity presumably takes place in the consultation room (Latin *consultario*, "thoughtful deliberation or consideration"). An old English spelling of "surgeon" is **chirurgeon**, and a former medical school in Philadelphia was known as the Medico-Chirurgical College.

suspensory is from the Latin *suspendere*, "to hang up or to support," this being derived from the Latin *sub-*, "under," + *pendere*, "to hang down." A support is placed above or below whatever hangs down to keep it up. The term is applied to various anatomic supporting structures, particularly ligaments, as well as to certain bandages and appliances. Women's breasts are supported by a brassiere (from the French *bras*, "the arm," + *-iere*, a suffix denoting "something connected with"). Some men wear suspenders to keep their pants up.

sustentaculum is another anatomic term used to denote a supporting structure and is taken from the Latin *sustinere*, "to hold up." An example is the projection on the calcaneus that serves to support the talus.

suture is a near borrowing of the Latin *sutura*, "a sewn seam," this being derived from the Latin verb *suere*, "to sew, stitch, or tack together."

sycosis is not to be confused, either in pronunciation or meaning, with "psychosis." The "y" in sycosis is pronounced as a short "i", as in "bit." Sycosis is an inflammation of the hair follicles, especially of the beard, whereby the surface of the skin becomes rough and irregular. The word comes from the Greek *sykon*, "a fig," a fruit that has a puckered skin.

sym-, syn- are variants of a prefix representing the Greek preposition *syn*, "together with, invested or endowed with, or in connection with." Other variants are "sy-" (as in system) and "syl-" (as in syllable or syllogism). "Sym-" and "syn-" must be the most useful prefixes in the language of medicine; they are attached to more words than any other. Only a few examples can be given.

symbiosis is literally "living together," as of two or more organisms (sym- + Greek *bios*, "life"), but with the important provision of harmony or, at least, of no harm to each other. (Incidentally, "harmony" and "harm" are of wholly unrelated Greek and Anglo-Saxon origins.) The earliest English use of "symbiosis," in the 17th century, was in a social sense. The term was introduced in biology, in the 19th century, to denote a friendly relation between host and parasite.

sympathetic as originally used in physiology was a name proposed for the whole of the autonomic or involuntary nervous system (sym- + Greek *pathos*, "feeling or suffering"), and only later was restricted to that portion characterized by adrenergic neuroeffector transmission, the cholinergic component being given the name **parasympathetic** (Greek *para*, "beside"). Presumably because the autonomic tracts serve the viscera, the idea came into being that the "sympathies" of the organs were thereby aroused. **Sympathomimetic** (+ Greek *mimetikos*, "imitative") became the term of reference for drugs that mimic the effect of adrenergic stimulation (adrenalin was the prototype).

sympathy (*see* **empathy**)

symphysis is a direct borrowing of the Greek word for "growing together" and is applied in anatomy to a fixed union of bones, such as that at the pubic symphysis.

symposium (*see* **seminal**)

symptom comes from the Greek *symptōma*, "anything that has befallen one, by chance or mischance" or, literally, "that which falls together with," the Greek verb being *piptein*, "to fall."

synapse as a term for the connection between processes of two nerve cells was introduced in 1897 by Sir Charles Sherrington (1857-1952), the English physiologist, with the acknowledged help of classical scholars of his acquaintance. The Greek source is *synaptein*, "to join together," this being related to the Greek verb *haptein*, "to fasten."

syncope is an almost direct borrowing of the Greek *sy[n]gkopē*, literally "a cutting to pieces" but also used by the Greeks for "a fainting spell or swoon," the allusion apparently being to a "cutting off" of consciousness in a person so afflicted. From its Greek derivation we are reminded the word is pronounced in three syllables.

syncytium is a multinucleated mass of protoplasm resulting from an agglomeration of cells (syn- + Greek *kytos*, "cell").

syndrome denotes a group of symptoms that "run together" in the course of a given condition. Sometimes "syndrome" is used rather than "disease" when the full picture of a condition as a true entity has not yet been defined. **Prodrome** comes almost directly from the Greek *prodromos*, "a running ahead," which combines the Greek *pro-*, "before or ahead of," + *drōmos*. In medicine a prodrome is a set of symptoms or signs that precedes or "runs ahead" of the full manifestation of a disease. "Prodrome" is usually pronounced in two syllables, whereas often one hears "syndrome" sounded in three ("syn-drō-mē"). The three-syllable pronunciation would seem to be in deference to the origin in the Greek *syndromē*, but prodrome is also derived from a Greek word. This is a tempest in a teapot. To insist on different pronunciations of such similar words seems pedantic, and only two syllables will suffice for either of the two words.

synechia is a near borrowing of the Greek *synecheia*, "a continuity," related to the Greek verb *synechein*, "to hold or keep together." In medicine today the term is restricted to an adhesion of the lens of the eye to the cornea or to the iris.

synovia is a term contrived by Paracelsus in 1520. He combined "syn-" + Greek *ōon*, "an egg," to come up with a term for various fluids in the body that resemble the seromucoid white of an egg. The term has persisted but now is restricted to that slippery fluid found in joint spaces, and sometimes it is used to refer to the membranes that line the joint spaces, as in **synovitis**.

syphilis became astonishingly widespread in Europe during the decade following 1495, the year in which Charles VIII of France and his motley army occupied the Kingdom of Naples. Rumor had it that the cunning Neapolitans deliberately dispatched prostitutes to infect Charles's troops, who were more than susceptible to dalliance. When the army disbanded, the mercenary soldiers returned to their homelands, where the scourge rapidly became rife. Charles blamed his troubles on "the Neapolitan disease," while the English and Germans called it "the French disease." In France it was "the Spanish pox." In Russia it was "the Polish disease," in Persia it was "the Turkish disease," and so on, each nationality reproaching another. The Spanish tried to contend that the disease was imported from the newly discovered West Indies, but it is likely that syphilis was well entrenched in Europe in a less virulent form long before the Age of Discovery. In retrospect

the emergence of the scourge of syphilis in the 1490s seems not unlike that of AIDS in the 1980s. The term "syphilis" is said to have been coined by Girolamo Fracastoro (1478-1553), a Veronese physician and poet who in 1530 published *Syphilis sive morbus gallicus*. In this poem Fracastoro concocted a myth wherein the protagonist was a swineherd named Syphilus, who was scourged with a disfiguring, debilitating disease because he defied the sun god. The fellow's name may have been taken from the Greek *sypheos*, "a hog sty." A rare form of tertiary syphilis involving the stomach is called **linitis plastica**, from the Greek *linon*, "flaxen thread," (which also gives "linen"), and *plastikos*, "form." The allusion is to the thickened, stiff, stomach wall composed of densely packed fibrous connective tissue. Another obviously descriptive name is "leather-bottle stomach." The same condition can be the result of intense desmoplasia induced by certain forms of poorly differentiated adenocarcinoma in the stomach. (*see* **lues**; *also* **tabes**)

syringe comes from the Greek *syri[n]gx*, "a shepherd's pipe" such as that played by Pan, the deity of flocks and herds, who also gained a reputation of being a lusty lad. In ancient Greek lore the musical instrument was named for the nymph Syrinx, who was both chaste and, on one fateful occasion, chased. The chaser was the panting Pan. Syrinx took refuge in the River Ladon, where, to escape "a fate worse than death," she prayed to be turned into a clump of reeds. When finally Pan sought to embrace the nymph, he was dismayed that he was clutching only a handful of reeds. Letting out a great sigh, he found that his breath elicited a pleasant tone from the hollow reeds. And so it was, if you can believe it, that the shepherd's pipe was invented. Actually, the Greek *syri[n]gx* could be any cylindrical container or conduit, and so became, in English, "syringe."

syringomyelia refers to abnormal, fluid-filled cavities in the spinal cord consequent to a developmental defect or in association with a degenerative process. The term was contrived by linking the Greek *syri[n]gx* (*see* **syringe**) + *myelos*, "marrow," i.e., of the spine, as ancient anatomists conceived the spinal cord to be.

systole is the period of contraction of the heart muscle that impels the circulation of blood. The term is a direct borrowing of the Greek *systolē*, "a drawing together or a contraction," the root verb being *systellein*, "to draw together or to pull in, as in shortening a sail."

In the 16th century the noun was used for the contraction of heart muscle. In "systole" tribute is paid to its Greek origin by always pronouncing the final letter as a long "e", as in "be."

syzygy (*see* **zygote**)

Tabagism is any condition resulting from the excessive or harmful use of tobacco. The term is taken from *tobaco*, the Spanish name for the weed, which the Spaniards in turn took from the Cariban Indian name for the pipe in which the weed was smoked.

tabes is the Latin word for "decay," related to the verb *tabere*, "to waste away." Originally, the term was applied to any wasting disease. In 1836 the term "tabes dorsalis" was suggested as a name for the disease otherwise known as "locomotor ataxia," in the belief that the condition was due to a wastage of the dorsal or posterior columns of the spinal cord. It was not until 1876 that the cause of the disease was identified as syphilis. Later, "tabes" became used as an alternative term for syphilis in its advanced stages.

tabloid was originally a contrived term officially registered in 1884 at Stationers' Hall in London by Messrs. Burroughs, Wellcome & Company as a trademark for their innovation of a small, compressed medicinal tablet. **Tablet** is taken from the Old French *tablete*, "a small table." The "-oid" in "tabloid" comes from the Greek *eidos*, "like, but not the same as." In the early 1900s, "tabloid" came into wider use as the name for an undersized, condensed newspaper, the contents of which were easily consumed.

tachy- is a combining form, usually a prefix, taken from the Greek *tachys*, "quick, swift, or fast."

tachycardia is an abnormally rapid heartbeat (tachy- + Greek *kardia*, "the heart"), customarily applied to rates in excess of 100 per minute.

tachyphylaxis is a rapid dissipation of the effect of an active substance by its frequently repeated administration (tachy- + Greek *phylaxis*, "a guarding"). For example, tyramine acts directly as a sympathomimetic agent by displacing norepinephrine from binding sites at certain nerve endings; the released norepinephrine then is available to act at receptor sites on effector cells. But the amount of norepinephrine liable to displacement is limited and can be depleted by repeated administration of tyramine.

tachypnea is abnormally rapid breathing (tachy- + Greek *pnoia*, "a drawn breath").

tactile refers to perception in the sense of touch. The word is a near borrowing of the Latin *tactilus*, "tangible," from *tactus*, the past participle of *tangere*, "to touch." To be sensitive is to exhibit tact; to be tactless is to be insensitive or inconsiderate of the feelings of others.

taenia is Latin for "a ribbon or tape" and is related to the Greek *tainia*, "a band, such as worn around the head in token of victory." In parasitology *Taenia* is a genus of tapeworms. *Taenia saginata* (Latin *sagina*, "a fattened animal") is found in beef, and *Taenia solium* is found in pork (here the *solium* refers to the ring of hooklets around the scolex of the worm and may have been taken from either the Latin *solium*, "a throne" or, more likely, from the Latin *sol*, "the sun's rays"). The taenia coli are the three prominent, tapelike, longitudinal bands of muscle in the wall of the colon.

talipes is the Latin word for "clubfoot" and is a combination of the Latin *talus*, "the ankle," + *ped*, "the foot." The deformity is such that, with the foot turned in sharply, the afflicted person appears to be walking on his or her ankle.

talus is the name of the second largest of the tarsal bones, supporting the tibia above and resting on the calcaneus below. It is also called the **astragalus**. Curiously, both terms once referred to dice, as used in games of chance. The Greek *astragalos* originally meant the upper cervical vertebrae. Soldiers of ancient Greece made their dice from the second cervical vertebrae of sheep, and the word came to be applied mainly to the dice. Roman soldiers made their dice (which in the Latin singular is *taxillus*) from the ankle bone or heel bone of the horse. *Taxillus* was later shortened to *talus* and given as a name for the ankle bone. Thus, both "talus" and "astragalus" came to be applied to the ankle bone—by chance, as it were.

tampon is the French word for "a plug or stopper" and is a sort of nasalized derivative of the French *tapoter*, "to tap," as to open a keg. In medicine a tampon is a gauze plug inserted in a body cavity to stop or to absorb a flow of fluid.

tamponade is the procedure of occluding a lumen, as by inflating a balloon in the esophagus or stomach, or applying pressure to a vessel in order to stop bleeding. Cardiac tamponade is a condition wherein constrictive pressure is exerted on the beating heart by an accumulation of fluid within the pericardial sac. The term is taken from the French *tamponner*, "to plug up."

tantalum is a rare metallic element often used, because it is malleable and resists corrosion, to fabricate prosthetic appliances, wire sutures, and implantable plates or mesh for covering bony or soft tissue defects. The name comes from that of Tantalus, a mythologic king of Lydia. Tantalus presumed on his friendship with the gods and was condemned to everlasting torment in the infernal regions; in other words, he was told to go to hell. Plagued by unrelieved hunger and thirst, he could not eat because fruits were held just beyond his reach, and he could not drink because water receded whenever he stooped to sip—thus, the verb "to tantalize." The derivation of the name for the metal seems a bit more strained. It was probably chosen because the element was considered to be beyond the reach of corrosive fluids.

tarsus is a Latinized form of the Greek *tarsos*, "a wicker frame or basket," or any broad, flat surface, such as the flat of the foot. In anatomy "tarsus" also is used in reference to the plate of connective tissue that serves as a framework for the eyelid.

tartar is a calcareous substance (calcium phosphate and carbonate together with organic matter) that becomes encrusted on teeth. It also is the substance (potassium bitartrate) that becomes encrusted in vats during the fermentation of grape juice as it becomes wine. Just as the process of fermentation harks back to time immemorial, so "tartar" is of ancient lineage. Some scholars have related the word to the Persian *durd* and the Arabic *durdi*, but more clearly it is derived from the Medieval Greek *tartaron* and the Late Latin *tartarum*, all referring to the dregs of winemaking. Tartaric acid is so called because it was first obtained from tartar accumulating in wine vats.

taste comes through the Old French *taster*, "to handle, feel, or taste," from the Latin *taxare*, "to appraise." Thus, a discriminating person does not have all of his taste in his mouth.

taurine is an amino acid first obtained from ox bile, its name being taken from the Latin *taurus*, "a bull." **Taurocholic** (+ Greek *cholē*, "bile") acid is the product of conjugation of taurine and cholic acid in the liver. This is one of the primary bile acids that, being **amphiphilic** (Greek *ampho*, "both," + *philos*, "affinity"), help solubilize lipid substances in an aqueous medium. The bile salts accomplish this by interspersing with aggregates of fatty acids and monoglycerides to form **micelles** (from a neo-Latin diminutive of *mica*, "a grain").

technique is a French word derived from the Greek *tekhnikos*, "belonging to the arts." A Greek *tektōn* was "a worker in wood or a carpenter," and the Sanskrit *taksh* meant "to cut wood." This sense is preserved in the scientific use of "technique" to designate a means of accomplishing a procedure, usually by deft use of the hands.

tectum, tegmen are terms taken from the Latin verb *tego, tegere, texi, tectum*, "to cover over, to shelter, or to hide." The mesencephalic tectum is the rooflike covering of the midbrain. The tegmen tympani is the roof of the middle-ear cavity. The Latin *tegmentum* means "a covering," and this term is applied to that part of the cerebral peduncle above the substantia niger. The skin covering the body is an **integument**.

teichopsia (*see* scotoma)

tel- is a combining form, usually a prefix, taken from the Greek *telos*, "the completion or fulfillment of anything" or, adverbially, "at the end, at last." In science the sense of "tel-" often is "at a distance."

tela is the Latin word for "web," particularly the warp, i.e., the threads that run lengthwise in the loom. The term has been applied to numerous weblike anatomic structures, often alternatively with "tunica," as a covering, or with "lamina," as a layer.

telangiectasia is a condition wherein the end

branches of arteries and capillaries are abnormally dilated (tel- + Greek *a[n]ggeion*, "vessel," + *ektasis*, "dilatation"); a **telangiectasis** is the spot where telangiectasia has occurred.

telemetry is the means whereby measurements are recorded at a distance from the subject (tel- + Greek *metron*, "a measure"), particularly when the signals are transmitted by radio waves.

telencephalon is sometimes called the end-brain and is made up of the cerebral cortex, the corpus striatum, and the rhinencephalon, all comprising the terminus of higher brain activity (tel- + Greek *enkephalon*, "the brain").

telophase is the completing or last of the four stages of mitosis (tel- + Greek *phasis*, "appearance").

temperature comes from the Latin *temperatio*, "a blending, a constitution," related to the Latin verb *temperare*, "to apportion or to regulate." These words can be traced further to the Latin *tempus*, "time," which was early recognized as being regularly apportioned in days, months, seasons, and years. We retain the idea of the Latin *temperatio* in **temperament** as the combined attributes or mental cast of an individual being. Presumably, the heat of the body was taken to be representative of temperament, hence the temperature. The first **thermometer** (Greek *thermē*, "heat," + *metron*, "a measure") was devised by Galileo in 1592, and shortly thereafter it was discovered that the human body, in health, maintains a relatively constant temperature and that abnormal deviations signal illness. For many years body temperature was one of the few objective measurements that could be made, and clinical thermometry became almost a science in itself. Occasionally one hears, "The patient is running a temperature." What is meant, of course, is that the patient is "running a fever."

temple is derived from the Latin *tempus*, which means both "time" and "the temple of the head," i.e., the area just behind and lateral to the forehead. To understand the connection one must go back to the Greek *temnein*, "to cut or to divide." Time was clearly divided into days and nights by the rising and setting of the sun, into months by phases of the moon, and into recurring seasons of the year. Most of these divisions of time were evident by observing the heavens. Ancient augurs would gaze at the sky, mark off a given sector, and study it for signs of things to come or other divine revelations. Such a precinct of the sky or an area of earth marked off for the observation of omens was known by the Greek word *temenos* and the Latin word *templum*. Some say the temple of the head was so called because, by observing the visible subcutaneous vessels and palpating their pulsations, one could divine the temperament of a person. Others have said that graying of hair at the temple was looked on as a sign of the ravages of time. But the Greek *temnein* also meant "to wound or maim in battle," and the sides of the head toward the front were early found to be the thinnest part of the skull and, therefore, the most vulnerable to a crippling or lethal blow. A well-aimed blow at the temple would surely cut off one's time on earth. Whatever the origin of the word, we still use **temporal** to refer to the bone, muscle, artery, vein, and nerve that occupy that region of the head.

tenaculum is an elongated hook used in anatomic or surgical dissection to seize and hold tissue. The term appropriates the Late Latin word for "a holder," and is related to the Latin verb *tenere*, "to grasp or hold tightly." A closely related term is **retinaculum**, an appropriation of the Latin word for "a rope or cable," used in anatomy to designate the structure that holds an organ or tissue in place. With various descriptive modifiers, a number of tendons, ligaments, and connective tissue bands are known by this name. Similar in sound but different in origin is **tentacle**, a flexible protrusion intended to explore its environment. "Tentacle" is taken from the Latin *tentare*, a variant of *temptare*, "to probe or to test." A tentative diagnosis is a sort of hypothesis subject by testing to proof or disproof.

tendon is derived from the Latin *tendere* and the Greek *teinein*, both meaning "to stretch." The Greek *tenon* is "a sinew or tendon." Both tendons and ligaments are tough, fibrous cords or bands; they differ in that tendons are the fibrous extensions by which muscles are attached to bones, whereas ligaments bind bone to bone, as at joints. The tendon by which the calf muscles are attached to the calcaneous or heel bone is called **Achilles tendon** because of the Greek legend, which is related under that entry.

tenesmus is a near borrowing of the Greek *tenesmos* (from the verb *teinein*, "to stretch"), which Hippocrates used for "straining at stool," and so do we.

tensor describes a muscle that stretches or tightens a part (Latin *tensus*, "drawn tight"), such as the tensor of the soft palate or the tensor tympani that makes taut the eardrum.

tentacle (*see* **tenaculum**)

tentorium is Latin for "tent," and the **tentorium cerebelli** is a broad infolding of the dura mater that is stretched over the cerebellum like a tent. Because this tentorium separates the "thinking" forebrain from the lower "vegetative" portions of the brain, disturbances attributed to psychologic aberration are sometimes referred to as **supratentorial**.

terato- is a combining form taken from the Greek *teras*, "a sign or portent" and also "a monster." The connection is that the ancient Greeks looked upon the appearance of a deformed creature, human or animal, as an omen by which the gods were seeking to deliver a message.

teratogen denotes any agent or factor identified as a cause of defects in the developing embryo (terato- + Greek *gennan*, "to produce").

teratology is the study of congenital defects (terato- + Greek *logos*, "a treatise").

teratoma is a true neoplasm composed of aberrant tissues, none of which is indigenous to the area where the tumor occurs. Such a malformation was so named (terato- + Greek *-ōma*, "tumor") because its components suggested parts of an implanted monster.

teres is the Latin word for "smooth and round or cylindrical" and is applied to various ligaments and muscles. The round ligament of the uterus is more formally known as the ligamentum teres uteri. The ligamentum teres hepatis is the smooth cylindrical anterior edge of the falciform ligament that helps suspend the liver in the upper abdomen.

tertian is a near borrowing of the Latin *tertianus*, "pertaining to the third," and **quartan** is taken from the Latin *quartanus*, "pertaining to the fourth." However, a "tertian fever," such as is typical of infection by the malarial parasite *Plasmodium vivax*, actually recurs every other day, and a "quartan fever," such as that caused by *Plasmodium malariae* with a life cycle of 72 hours, recurs every 3rd day. The seeming confusion is explained by the ancient custom of counting the day of occurrence as the first day; therefore, whatever is "tertian" recurs after an interval of only a single period. (*see* **periodic**)

test comes from the Latin *testa*, "a brick, tile, jug, or crock." An earthenware pot with a lid was a *testum*. Such ceramic utensils were commonly used by the ancients to assay ores and also by alchemists to conduct their experiments. Substances placed in pots and subjected to heat, to see what changes might occur, were said to be "tested." Today, many of the tests in a research or clinical laboratory are conducted in flasks, dishes, or tubes, and all of these utensils are usually made of glass.

testis is a direct borrowing of the Latin word for "witness." In ancient times testimony was validated by the swearer grasping the scrotum, presumably his own, but on occasion someone else's. In Genesis 24:9 the following is recorded: "And the servant put his hand under the thigh of Abraham his master, and sware to him concerning the matter."

tetanus is a near borrowing of the Greek *tetanos*, related to the verb *teinein*, "to stretch." Infection by the anaerobic bacillus *Clostridium tetani* results in elaboration of a potent neurotoxin that causes hyperreflexia and muscular contractions, manifest in severe cases by trismus ("lockjaw"), glottal spasm, respiratory paralysis, opisthotonus, and seizures.

tetany is a symptom complex that may include hyperreflexia, carpopedal spasm, muscle cramps, and laryngospasm with inspiratory stridor (*see* **tetanus**). Such symptoms can occur in any condition marked by severely diminished extracellular ionic calcium from any cause.

tetralogy is a series of four related things, the word being derived from the Greek *tetra*, "four," + *logos*, "a statement." A tetralog in ancient Athens was a series of four dramas, three tragic and one satiric, performed consecutively at the festival of Dionysus, the god of wine, whose Roman name was Bacchus. The term is applied, uniquely in medicine, to the tetralogy of Fallot, so called because it was described by Etienne-Louis Fallot (1850-1911), a French physician, and because it had four components: (*a*) stenosis of the pulmonary conus; (*b*) an interventricular septal defect; (*c*) dextroposition of the aorta that overrides the interventricular septum, and (*d*) right ventricular hypertrophy. Fallot's description in 1888 was preceded in 1771 by that of Edward Sandifort (1742-1814), a pathologist of Leiden.

thalamus is the Latin name for "an inner chamber," usually a bedroom occupied by the principal married couple in a house—what we would call a master bedroom. How or why Galen gave the name to that solid portion of the diencephalon, which we now know serves as a relay center for sensory impulses to the cerebral cortex, is a bit of a mystery. Perhaps he was alluding to its relation to the adjacent ventricles of the brain. Nevertheless, the name stuck.

thalassemia is a genetically determined hemolytic anemia that occurs predominantly in persons of Mediterranean stock. The name combines the Greek *thalassa*, "sea," + *haima*, "blood." The *thalassa* best known to the Greeks was the Mediterranean Sea.

theca is a near borrowing of the Greek *thēkē*, "a case to put anything in." The **theca folliculi** is a fibrous envelope containing an ovarian follicle.

thenar is the Greek word for "that part of the hand with which one strikes," i.e., the flat of the hand. The related Greek verb is *thenein*, "to strike." Originally, the term referred to the entire palm of the hand. Later, the thenar eminence was considered to be the area at the base of the thumb, and the hypothenar (or lesser) eminence was the area at the base of the little finger.

theobromine (*see* **theophylline**)

theophylline is one of three closely related xanthine alkaloids that occur in the leaves and berries of various plants widely distributed in tropical climes throughout the world. The other two are theobromine and caffeine. The alkaloids are best known for their stimulant and antisoporific effects. They also have been used as diuretic agents. The story is told that they were introduced into Western culture by the prior of a convent in Araby who was informed by native shepherds that goats nibbling on the berries of the coffee plant were observed to frolic and gambol through the night rather than to sleep. The prior asked that samples of the berries be brought to him so he might brew a beverage that would enable him to keep awake during the long, nocturnal, prayer vigils. Legend would have us believe that this was the first cup of coffee. The alkaloids are readily extracted from tea leaves and from coffee, coca, and cola beans. **Caffeine** comes from the French *café*, "coffee," + "-ine," denoting a derivative. "Theophylline" combines the Latinized *thea* (taken from the Amoy *t'e*, but *ch'a* in Mandarin Chinese), "tea," + the Greek *phyllon*, "leaf." **Theobromine** incorporates the Greek *broma*, "food." Some authorities relate the combining form "theo-" to the Greek *theos*, "a god," but a derivation from the word for tea seems more down-to-earth. "Theo-" is not to be confused with the combining form **thio-**, taken from the Greek *theion*, "sulfur." **Aminophylline** is so named because it is a complex of ethylene diamine and theophylline, the former being added to increase the solubility of the xanthine.

therapy is a near borrowing of the Greek *therapeia*, "a service, an attendance," the related Greek verb being *therapeuō*, "I wait upon." **Therapeutics** is that branch of medicine dealing specifically with the treatment of disease. One who calls himself a **therapist** owes his name to the Greek *therapōn*, "a servant," but is distinguished from a *doulos*, "a slave," in that a *therapōn* gave his services willingly, without bondage or coercion. Distinction between cure, remedy, and treatment is posited in those entries.

thermometer (*see* **temperature**)

thiamine was the first member of the vitamin group to be recognized and is often called vitamin B_1. **Beriberi**, the disease resulting from a dietary deficiency of thiamine, was not widely known until steam-powered rice mills were introduced in the 19th century. These marvels of technology so refined rice that the cereal was divested of its vitamin-containing husk. In 1882 the Japanese admiral Kanehiro Takaki (1849-1915) found that he could eliminate beriberi in his sailors by adding fish, meat, and vegetables to their regular diet of polished rice. More to the point, Christian Eijkman (1858-1930), a Dutch physician working in Java, demonstrated that feeding the discarded rice husks to victims of beriberi could cure their disease. For this discovery Eijkman was awarded a share of the Nobel Prize for medicine in 1929. Thiamine contains one sulfur atom in its pyrimidine-thiazole nucleus, hence its name from the Greek *theion*, "sulfur or brimstone," + -amine.

thigh as a name for the thick segment of the leg can be traced, through Germanic descent, from the Indo-European root word *teue*, "a swelling or enlargement."

thio- (*see* **theophylline**)

thirst can be traced to the Indo-European root word *ters*, "dry or arid." The Greek *tersomai* means "to become dry or parched." (However, the Latin *tersus* , the past participle of *tergere*, "to wipe," means "clean, neat, polished"; hence, a terse lecture is succinct and pithy—but also might be dry.) Meanwhile, the Gothic *thaurstei*, from the same Indo-European stem, led to the English "thirsty."

thorax is the Greek word for "a breastplate or cuirass." For added protection of the torso, a double-cuirass was fashioned from a breastplate and a backplate joined with clasps. By extension, the Greek thorax came to refer also to that part of the body thus encased, i.e., the chest.

thrombin is an enzyme that converts fibrinogen to fibrin, thereby promoting formation of a blood clot (Greek *thrombos*, "a clump").

thrombo- is a combining form taken from the Greek *thrombos*, "a curd or clump," to refer specifically to clotted blood.

thrombocyte is not in itself an actual cell (despite the derivation of its name from thrombo- + Greek *kytos*, "cell") but rather a fragment of a **megakaryocyte** (Greek *megas*, "large," + *karyon*, "kernel," + *kytos*, "cell"). The particle is better known as a "blood platelet," and its function is to facilitate the clotting of blood.

thrombocytopenia is a deficiency in blood platelets (thrombocyto- + Greek *penēs*, "poverty-stricken").

thromboplastin is a factor essential to the production of thrombin and thus to the promotion of blood clotting (thrombo- + Greek *plassein*, "to shape").

thrombus is an almost direct borrowing of the Greek *thrombos*, "a lump or a clump," but also "a curd of milk or a clot of blood." Now, in medicine, a thrombus is a clot that forms within a blood vessel or chamber of the heart; a clot that forms outside the cardiovascular lumen is simply a clot, not a thrombus.

thrush is a term, now almost obsolete, for oral infection by *Candida albicans*, also known as **moniliasis**. "Thrush" is of murky origin. Possibly it is related to the word "frush," by which farriers referred to the tender hind part of a horse's foot, just above the hoof, an area subject to infection and exudation. "Frush," in turn, is said to have been a slurring of the French *fourchette*, as applied to anything shaped like a small fork.

thumb is the name given to the stoutest digit of the hand and can be traced, through Germanic descent, to the Indo-European root word *teue*, "a swelling or an enlargement." To the Romans the thumb was *pollex*, related to the Latin verb *pollere*, "to be strong." The Latin term is used to describe certain muscles pertaining to the thumb, e.g., the flexor (also the extensor, adductor, and abductor) pollicis longus (and brevis).

thymus is a fleshy, bilobed, lymphoid gland situated in the anterior mediastinum. The name was given because of its fancied resemblance to a bunch of thyme (which, purists insist, is pronounced "time" because of its French antecedent). Thyme is a member of the mint family of shrubs, and its aromatic leaves are used for seasoning in cooking. The Greek name for the plant is *thymos*, seemingly related to the Greek *thyōma*, "that which is burnt as incense," which in the plural means "spices." Another Greek word, a homonym, is *thymos*, "the soul," and some people have said the thymus gland, being near the heart, was taken to be the seat of the soul, but the Greeks didn't hold such a view.

thyroid is a name first given to the largest cartilage in the larynx and later transferred to the gland that sits in front of the cartilage. The Greek *thyreos* originally was the word for a large stone placed in front of a door to keep it shut. Later, it was given as the name of a warrior's oblong shield, with a notch at the top for the chin. The notched thyroid cartilage resembles such a shield, hence *thyreos + eidos*, "like," became "thyroid." The thyroid gland looks only vaguely like a shield, but the name serves just as well.

tibia is the Latin word for both the shinbone and a sort of flute. No one is sure which bore the name first. It has been said that primitive flutelike musical instruments were once fashioned from the shinbones of animals.

tic is a little French word that means, as it does when used in English, "a twitching of the muscles." Probably, it originated as imitative of an abrupt, evanescent, muscular contraction.

tick is a name given to a blood-sucking parasitic arachnid of the family Ixodidae, notorious as a vector of various infectious diseases. The creature takes its common name from an old Teutonic word for "bug." A bed may or may not be infested with ticks, but the "tick" that encases a mattress or pillow traces its name rather to the Greek *thēkē*, "a covering."

tincture comes from the Latin *tinctus*, the past participle of *tingere*, "to dip or soak," as one would do in dyeing cloth. In medieval times extracts of various herbs were prepared in alcoholic solutions to which the dissolved substance often imparted a distinct color. The solutions were then used as dyes. In pharmacy an alcoholic solution of a drug is a tincture.

tinea is the Latin name for "a gnawing worm," such as the bookworm or book louse, an insect now classified in the order Corrodentia. The book louse is fond of chewing on paper. In figurative usage a "bookworm" is a person who, too, devours books. The name "tinea" was early given to the skin eruption commonly called **ringworm**. The latter term reflects the ringlike shape of the spreading eruption and, presumably, an early belief that the eruption was caused by a worm. It isn't. It is the result of infection by a fungus. Calling the disease "tinea" may have been a misunderstood translation of the Arabic *al-tin*, a name given to various eruptions of the scalp. In any event a variety

of tineas have been described: **tinea capitis** (Latin *caput*, "the head"), **tinea barbae** (Latin *barba*, the beard), and **tinea cruris** (Latin *crus*, "the leg"). The last form affects the crotch more often than the leg itself.

tinnitus is Latin for "a ringing or tinkling sound." The word obviously imitates the sound. In medicine tinnitus (never "tinnitis") is a ringing in the ears.

tissue can be traced, through French, to the Latin *texere*, "to weave." This came from the Greek *tekhnē*, "a skill or craft," which is related to the Indo-European root *tek, tegh*, "to twine or to build." The Old French word was *tistre*, and from its past participle *tissu* came "tissue." To early anatomists many prominent components of the body, such as skin, fascia, mesenteries, and muscle, resembled woven cloth. Later, the term "tissue" was extended to all aggregates of living or once-living material.

titer is a modification of the French *titre*, "a title or qualification," this being derived from the Latin *titulus*, "an inscription or label." By extension, a *titre* was also proof of the fineness of alloyed gold or silver. When it is important, as it is in knowing the content of a precious metal or of an alcoholic beverage, we insist on a statement of "proof." In chemical or biologic analysis, "titer" has become a term for the dilution of a substance at which a certain reaction is registered.

tongue is said to go back to the Indo-European root word *dnghu*, which referred to that active and useful muscular organ in the floor of the mouth. In early languages there was much confusion between "d," "t," and "l." Thus, the root word led to the archaic Latin *dingua*, which became the classical Latin *lingua*; it led, too, to the Anglo-Saxon *tunge*, which became the English "tongue" (the modern spelling probably is in imitation of the French *langue*). The Greek word for the tongue is *glossa*, from which is derived the adjective **glossal** and the combining form **glosso-**, as used in anatomy. This is another example of using a noun derived from one language as the name of a structure and an adjectival form from another language to describe what pertains to it.

tonic is a common name for a medicinal agent intended to restore or enhance vigor. (*see* **tonus**)

tonsil comes from the Latin plural *tonsillae*, by which the Romans referred to the small glands stuck in the back of the throat. The singular *tonsilla* meant "a pointed pole stuck in the ground, as a mooring stake." The connection between the apparently divergent uses of the singular and plural in Latin is not known. Possibly, it relates to the appearance of the glands as being moored to the adjacent pharyngeal folds, looked upon as "pillars" of the throat. It is mere coincidence that the Roman *tonsor* was a barber who cut hair and who later became a surgeon with a proclivity to cut out tonsils.

tonus is taken from the Greek *tonos*, which has a variety of meanings, such as "that which strains or tightens a thing, as a sinew, cord, or brace," "a stretching or tightening, as of the voice in pitching the sound uttered," and "the exertion of force or intensity." Hence, we speak of the tonus or tone of a muscle as its degree of vigor or tension and of the tone of voice as its degree of pitch, intensity, or stridency.

tooth can be traced far back to the Indo-European *ed*, "to eat." This led to the Sanskrit *danta*, from which came the Greek *odous*, *odonta* and the Latin *dens, dentis*, all meaning "the teeth." The Anglo-Saxon *toth* was "the eating tool" and became the English "tooth." The Latin *dens* provides **dental, dentist, dentistry**, and **dentifrice** (the last being a word for toothpaste and incorporating the Latin *fricare*, "to rub"). From the Greek stem *odont-* has been taken the combining form **-dontal**, as in **periodontal** (Greek *peri-*, "around"), in reference to the tissues around and supporting the teeth, and **orthodontics** (Greek *orthos*, "straight"), as the practice of straightening irregular or misaligned teeth.

tophus is a Latinized version of the Greek *tophos*, "a porous volcanic stone." In medicine a tophus is a chalklike deposit of urates in tissues, as seen in gout. Such deposits occur in and around joints, particularly that of the big toe, and in cartilage, particularly that of the ear. Such deposits were called "tophi" long before their content of urate was known.

torpor is a benumbed state in which the victim is deprived of the capacity for feeling or motion. The term (and the adjectival "tor-pid") is taken from the Latin *torpere*, "to be sluggish or numb."

torsade de pointes is a term used to describe a polymorphous ventricular tachycardia that occurs in a setting of prolonged QT intervals recorded electrocardiographically. Typically, the condition is a complication of antiarrhythmic drug therapy. Translated literally from the French, the term means "a twisting of the points."

torsion as a medical term refers to an abnormal twisting of a joint, its ligaments, or a mesentery and is taken from the Latin *tortus*, "twisted."

torso is a direct borrowing of the Italian word for "stump or stalk," this being derived from the Latin *thyrsus*, meaning the same, but more particularly the wand of Bacchus, the god of wine. The wand or staff was intertwined with vine tendrils and ivy and capped by a fir cone. With some imagination, this configuration can be likened to that of the main part of the body with its dangling extremities and topped by its head. **Trunk** is often used synonymously with "torso" as a term for the bulk of the body, shorn of its head and extremities. "Trunk" also can mean the main stalk of a tree and, in anatomy, the principal stem of an artery or nerve. The term is derived from the Latin *truncus*, "whatever is stripped of its branches or appendages." The related Latin verb is *truncare*, "to lop off." Hence, whatever is truncated is diminished by having a part or parts chopped off.

torticollis is a condition wherein, because of asymmetric spastic contraction of the cervical muscles, there is a distorted twisting of the neck resulting in an unnatural posture of the head. The term is a combined derivative of the Latin *tortus*, "twisted," + *collum*, "the neck." From *tortus* also comes tortuous, torture, and even tort, the last being a legal term for a wrongful act resulting in injury to another's person or property. *Collum* also gives "accolade," the bestowing of praise such as might be symbolized by placing a wreath around the neck, and *décolleté*, a French word for a garment cut low at the neck. **Wryneck**, the common term for torticollis, is also the name of an Old World bird capable of twisting its neck into unusual contortions. The "wry-" comes from the Old English *writhan*, "to twist," which also gives "to writhe."

torus is Latin for "a rounded protuberance or swelling" and has been appropriated to designate certain normal or abnormal bumps, e.g., the **torus palatinus**, a moundlike protuberance of bone sometimes seen at the midline of the hard palate. The diminutive **torulus** designates a small bump or elevation, e.g., the **toruli tactiles** in the skin of the palms and soles, richly supplied with sensory nerve endings. *Torula* formerly was a genus of budding yeasts, now known as *Cryptococci*.

tourniquet is a French word meaning "that which turns," such as a turnstile or swivel. The related French verb is *tourner*, "to turn." The original tourniquets were rather elaborate devices with variations of a screw-type mechanism for constricting a limb in order to stop the flow of blood. Now a simple length of cloth or rubber tubing tied around a digit, arm, or leg suffices. This is a rare, perhaps unique, example of something that has become simpler rather than more complex in its evolution. Being a French word, "tourniquet" probably should be pronounced with a final "-ay," but no red-blooded American would think of saying anything but "toor'-ni-ket."

toxin is a term introduced to medicine in 1888 by Ludwig Brieger (1849-1909), a Berlin physician, as a name for poisonous substances elaborated by pathogenic organisms. Among the first toxins so recognized were those evolved in decaying meat, but it was soon observed that similar substances were present at the site of bacterial infection in living tissues. **Endotoxins** (Greek *entos*, "within") are contained within bacterial cells and exert their effect only when the bacteria disintegrated, whereas **exotoxins** (Greek *exō*, "on the outside") are excreted by certain living bacterial cells. The term "toxin" was taken from the Latin *toxicum*, "poison." But the Greek *toxon* referred to a stringed bow used for shooting arrows, typically used by the Persians. Some archers took to tipping their arrows with poisonous substances, hence the Latin *toxicum*. An **antitoxin** (+ Greek *anti-*, "against,") is a substance that destroys a toxin or inhibits its effect. The

term was first used in reference to the substance that could be induced in the blood of animals, then administered as a serum to antagonize the toxin of diphtheria.

trabecula is the diminutive of the Latin *trabes*, "a beam or plank of wood," such as used in supporting structures. In anatomy **trabeculae** are strands of supporting connective tissue, particularly those that extend from the fibrous capsule of an organ into its substance.

trachea is taken from the Greek *traxus*, "rough." The explanation is that ancient anatomists thought that all prominent conduits of the body (other than the alimentary tract) served to conduct air. The Greek *artēria* (combining the Greek *aēr*, "air," + *tereō*, "I carry") was the windpipe. Because its wall contained prominent, corrugated, cartilaginous ridges, the windpipe was more specifically called *artēria traxeia* (or, in Latin, *arteria aspera*), "the rough artery," to distinguish it from the large afferent vessels of the heart, which were called *artēriai leiai*, "the smooth arteries." About A.D. 1500, the *artēria* was dropped, and the windpipe became known simply as the trachea.

trachoma is an inflammatory eye disease characterized by redness and swelling of the conjunctiva and cornea. The condition was well known to ancient writers as a contagious disease that sometimes led to blindness. It was given the Greek name *trachōma*, "a rough swelling," from the Greek *traxus*, "rough," + *-ōma*, "a swelling."

tract comes from the Latin *tractus*, "a drawing or dragging out, a trail." The related Latin verb is *trahere*, "to drag or to haul." Applied to anatomy, "tract" can refer to a pathway, such as that followed by a bundle of nerve fibers, or to a series of connected organs through which a common substance travels, such as the alimentary, biliary, or urinary tract.

tragus is a near borrowing of the Greek *tragos*, "a he-goat." One of the he-goat's characteristic features is a sort of beard that hangs from his neck. The little projection in front of the external orifice of the ear is called the tragus because in elderly men it often carries a little tuft of hairs. Also, not surprisingly, the Greek *tragos* and the Latin *tragus* were used to refer to the fetid odor of the armpits.

trait is an appropriation of the French word for "a drawn line or mark" and, figuratively, "a characteristic feature." A genetically transmitted trait is a phenotypic feature that can be traced in a line through a pedigree.

tranquilizer is a word only lately taken into medicine to designate certain psychotropic drugs, particularly the benzodiazepines, touted as having a soothing effect on the troubled body and mind (*see* **sedative**). The term is taken from the Latin *tranquillitas*, "stillness or calm." These drugs also are sometimes described as being **anxiolytic**, a mongrel term made up of the Latin *anxietas*, "a troubled state," + the Greek *lysis*, "a breaking up." So-called tranquilizing drugs act as sedatives. Barbiturates were formerly the most popular sedative agents but fell into disrepute because they were abused. Not surprisingly, the newer tranquilizers have been similarly abused and already are losing their charm. We can expect to see the emergence of yet another class of similar drugs, under a newly conceived rubric, that repeats the pattern—and so it goes.

trans- is a combining form taken directly from the Latin preposition *trans*, "across, over, or beyond." The related Latin verb is *transire*, "to pass or cross over, or to pass beyond."

transfusion is the process whereby a fluid, typically blood, is transferred from one body to another. The first transfusion in humans, attempted in the mid-17th century, was "direct," i.e., the donor of blood and the recipient lay side-by-side, their antecubital veins being connected by a tube. This was in accord with the meaning of the Latin *transfus-*, past participle stem of *transfundere*, "to pour from one vessel across to another." Later, when blood was first collected from the donor in a flask, then injected into a recipient, the procedure was known as "indirect transfusion." Today, this is the only way it's done, so there is no need to qualify the term.

translucent describes whatever transmits light (trans- + Latin *lucere*, "to shine") but not an image, as would whatever is **transparent** (+ Latin *parere*, "to be visible").

transplant as used in medicine is the grafting of a tissue from one place to another, much as the ancients grafted a bud from one plant to the stem of another (trans- + Latin *planta*, "a sprout or shoot"). An **autotransplant** (Greek *autos*, "self") occurs in the same individual, whereas a **heterotransplant** (Greek *heteros*, "different") involves tissue from one individual engrafted on another. A **homologous** (Greek *homologus*, "agreeing") transplant is between two individuals of the same species having the same or similar genetic composition. An **orthotopic** (Greek *orthos*, "straight," + *topos*, "a place") transplantation is the grafting of an organ in its customary position, whereas **heterotopic** transplantation puts the grafted organ in an unaccustomed place.

transposition means an anomalous configuration (trans-, in the sense of "cross-over"+ Latin *positus*, "placed"), as in transposition of the great vessels, a congenital anomaly wherein the aorta arises from the right ventricle of the heart and the pulmonary artery issues from the left ventricle.

transudate is a fluid that has been generated within a tissue, then passed through a membrane so that its resulting consistency is watery (trans- + Latin *sudare*, "to sweat") and relatively devoid of high molecular weight substances or formed cellular elements. This is in contrast to an **exudate** (Latin *exsudare*, "to sweat out or sweat profusely"), which is an outpouring of inflammatory products relatively rich in protein and cellular elements, principally leukocytes.

transverse in anatomy is descriptive of anything that lies crossways (trans- + Latin *versus*, "turned, so as to face").

trapezius comes from the Greek *trapeza*, "a table, especially a dining table or a money-changer's counter," this being a derived combination of *tetra*, "four," + *peza*, "foot" (presumably, a four-legged table or counter). In geometry a trapezoid is a four-sided plane figure of which two sides are parallel. "Trapezius" has been given as the name of one of the wrist bones and also of one of the muscles of the back because of their shape.

trauma is a direct borrowing of the Greek word for "a wound" and also for "damage or defeat." In medicine trauma refers to any physically or emotionally inflicted injury.

treadmill describes a device now commonly used to test cardiovascular function. The original treadmill was a wheel fitted with steps or treads that, when mounted, applied power to an axle, thence to a millstone for grinding grain. Now, in the test or exercise machine, the relation is reversed.

treatment comes from the French *traitement*, "a handling or a ministration" and also "a salary or stipend." The French noun *traite* means "a compact or agreement" and has been taken into English as "treaty." In medicine a treatment is a form of handling a problem according to the requirements of a given case. Furthermore, in this modern day, treatment implies an informed consent by the patient, a sort of treaty. In medical parlance treatment is closely akin to **management**, taken from the French *manège* (originally applied to horsemanship) that can be traced to the Latin *manus*, "hand," and thus "a handling."

trematode is the name of a class of flatworms that includes various flukes that are parasitic in man and animals. The name was taken from the Greek *trēmatōdes*, meaning "pierced or having holes." Apparently, the allusion was to the one or more prominent openings or suckers by which flukes attach to their hosts. The more common name **fluke** (from a Germanic root word meaning "flat") was originally attached to a flatfish, especially a flounder; the parasite, in its shape, appeared to be a miniature of a flatfish. A fluke can also be the flattened tail of a whale or a fish (or the flattened points of an anchor). To catch a fish by accidentally hooking its tail rather than its mouth became known as a "fluke," i.e., an unintentional but lucky event. This use was soon adapted in billiards to describe, with some disdain, an awkward yet successful shot. By extension, any chance gain, especially by a novice, has come to be put down as "a fluke."

tremor is the Latin adjective that describes "shaking, trembling, or shivering," and it was so used by ancient medical writers. "Tremor" is now an English noun. In physical diagnosis a tremor may be fine or coarse. An intention tremor is one that becomes evident or is intensified when a voluntary or purposeful movement is attempted. An unintentional tremor is one that persists when the tremulous part is otherwise at rest.

trench foot is a term for injury to the foot caused by prolonged exposure to moist cold. It came out of World War I when the common plight of soldiers was to be stuck in cold, damp trenches for days, weeks, and even months on end.

trephine is an instrument with a circular cutting blade or saw (sometimes called a "crown saw") for the purpose of incising and removing a disk of tissue, as from the skull or cornea. The finding of neatly cut holes in ancient skulls unearthed the world over suggests that operations for cranial decompression may have been among the earliest practices of surgery. Presumably the procedure was intended to allow the escape of evil spirits. Most authorities attribute "trephine" as a corruption of the now almost archaic *trepan*, taken from the Greek *trypanon*, "a carpenter's tool used as an auger or borer," related to the Greek *trypē*, "a hole." But Dr. John H. Dirckx points out that "trephine" was chosen by the 17th century inventor of the instrument, John Woodall, as an adaptation of the French *tres fines*, "three ends," descriptive of the three sharp prongs at the cutting edge of the original device.

Treponema is the name of a genus of microorganisms, including spirochetes, many of which are pathogenic for man and animals. The name was contrived by combining the Greek *trepein*, "to turn," + *nēma*, "thread." The most notorious is the species *Treponema pallidum* (Latin *pallidus*, "pale") that causes syphilis. Another species, *Treponema pertenue* (Latin *pertenuis*, "very thin or fine") causes yaws.

triad is taken from the Late Latin *tria*, a neuter form related to the Greek *treis*, "three." A triad is a group of three related things and, in medicine, is applied to a concatenation of three symptoms, signs, or other features that make up a syndrome or a disease entity. The prefix **tri-**, taken from the Latin *tres, tris, tria*, "three," is incorporated in a number of biomedical terms.

tribadism is the mutual friction of the genitals between women for the purpose of sexual arousal. The term is derived from the Greek *tribein*, "to rub, as one thing on another." The practice is a feature of **lesbianism**, so called because of the reputed character, in antiquity, of the female inhabitants of Lesbos, a Greek island in the northeast Aegean Sea. Generally acknowledged to be the foremost of early Greek poets was Sappho, a lady who was born and lived on the island of Lesbos. One of the longest and best known surviving fragments of her poetry is an invocation to Aphrodite, imploring the aid of the goddess in the poet's relation with a beloved girl.

triceps is the muscle that extends the arm and has three portions of attachment or "heads" (tri- + Latin *caput*, "head"). Despite the final "s," "triceps" is singular, not plural; there is no "tricep."

trichi-, tricho- are combining forms indicating a relation to hair and taken from the Greek *trikhos*, the genetive of *thrix*, "the hair, both of man and beast."

trichiasis is, literally, a hairy condition (*see* **trichi-, tricho-**), but in medicine it refers specifically to a condition of ingrown hairs about an orifice, such as ingrowing eyelashes that irritate the cornea.

trichina is a worm of the nematode genus *Trinchinella*, so called because its members give the appearance of little hairs.

trichinelliasis, trichinosis are designations of the disease consequent to infection by *Trichinella spiralis* (diminutive of tricho- Latin *spira*, "a coil"), a nematode ingested in raw or undercooked pork. Ambrose Bierce described trichinosis as "the pig's reply to proponents of porcophagy."

trichobezoar is a concretion of swallowed hair (*see* **bezoar**), typically found lodged in the stomachs of persons given to **trichotillomania**, a demented state in which the afflicted person habitually pulls out his or her own hair.

Trichomonas is a genus of pear-shaped protozoa characterized by hairlike flagella (tricho- + Greek *monas*, "a unit," as a unicellular organism).

Trichophyton is a genus of fungi that grow as branched, hairlike filaments (tricho- + Greek *phyton*, "plant").

Trichuris is a genus of intestinal nematodes, commonly called whipworms, so named because of their hairlike tails (tricho- + Greek *oura*, "tail").

tricuspid describes the valve between the right atrium and ventricle of the heart; it has three pointed leaflets (tri- + Latin *cuspis*, "pointed end, as of a spear"). A tricuspid tooth has three projections on its chewing surface.

trigeminal is taken from the Latin *trigeminus*, "threefold" (the plural *trigemini* means "triplets"). The trigeminal or fifth cranial nerve is so called because of its three divisions (mandibular, maxillary, and ophthalmic).

trigeminy is a disturbance wherein three heartbeats occur in rapid succession, often repetitively. Students with a smattering of Latin are sometimes confused by *trigeminus*. If *tri-* means "three" and *gemini* are "twins," doesn't *trigemini* mean "three twins"—and isn't that an oxymoron? Not really. The English "twins" means "two of a kind," but the Latin *geminare* means "to repeat, to replicate." Therefore, the Latin *gemini* are "twins" more in the sense of being replicas rather than their being only "two of a kind." To use the Latin-derived **bigeminy** specifies a like pair, but in English to say "a pair of twins" is redundant. But then, as Bergen and Cornelia Evans point out, aren't twins a living redundancy?

trigone is a term applied to various triangular areas in anatomy and is derived from the Greek *trigōnon*, a plane figure with three angles, i.e., a triangle. The trigone of the urinary bladder is a triangular portion of the mucosa at the base of that organ, where the three angles are marked by the two ureteral orifices on either side posteriorly and the midline urethral orifice anteriorly. The urogenital trigone or diaphragm is the layer of musculomembranous tissue extending between the ischiopubic rami and surrounding the urogenital ducts.

trimester is commonly used to refer to the equally divided early, middle, and late stages of pregnancy, but the term does not mean a division of time generally into three periods. "Trimester" means a period of 3 months and is derived from the Latin *tri-*, "three," + *mestris*, a variant of *menstruus*, "monthly" (the Vulgar Latin dropped the "n" before the "s"). There are 3 trimesters in the course of normal human gestation, but an elephant's gestation may occupy 6 or 7 trimesters. Similarly, the meaning of semester often is mistaken. This word is a combination of the

Latin *sex*, "six," + *mestris*. The "se-" has nothing to do with "semi-," though it is a coincidence that 6 months equal half a year. "Semester" also stretches a point in that the average academic semester does not last 6 months nowadays.

triploid (*see* -ploid)

trismus is a near borrowing of the Greek *trismos*, "a squeaking," the related Greek verb being *trizein*, "to squeak or croak." In medicine trismus is an inability to open the jaw because of intense muscular spasm. It can be due to a motor disturbance in the trigeminal verve and, as such, is a frequent symptom of tetanus, commonly known as **lockjaw**. The only sound utterable by a patient so afflicted is a squeak. **Laryngismus** shifted, long ago, from its classical meaning of "an act of shouting" to "spasm of the vocal cords," probably by mistaken identification with "trismus." Following this tortuous path, J. Marion Sims (1813-1883), a New York gynecologist, conceived **vaginismus** as a term for painful spasm of the vagina. On this subject the celebrated savant William Osler once contributed to the medical literature, writing under his pseudonym of Edgerton Yorrick Davis (*Med News.* 1884;45:637).

trisomy (*see* -ploid)

trituration is the reduction of larger solid particles to powder by means of rubbing, grinding, or milling. The term is taken from the Latin *tritus*, the past participle of *terere*, "to rub, crush, or grind," as of kernels of corn to make cornmeal or flour. There was a time when pharmacists made and mixed medicinal "powders," employing a shallow ceramic, glass, or metal dish called a **mortar** (a *mortarium* was a flat board or vessel used by Romans in mixing sand and lime with water to make mortar) and a club-shaped grinding utensil called a **pestle** (from *pistillum*, a diminutive verbal noun related to the Latin *pinsere*, "to pound"). Dentists still use a similar process to prepare an amalgam for filling cavities in teeth. In the early 19th century, when physiology was just emerging as a science, there was serious debate as to whether alimentary digestion was mechanical trituration or chemical dissolution; eventually it was established that trituration was a function of teeth but not of the stomach. A related term is **detritus**, particulate matter resulting from the disintegration of any substance, including bodily tissues.

trocar is a sharply pointed shaft used as an obturator in a cannula with which a body cavity can be pierced, thus permitting entry of the cannula. Typically, a trocar has a three-sided or tribeveled point. The name is an adaptation of the French *trocart*, which is derived from *trois*, "three," + *carre*, "side."

trochanter is an almost direct borrowing of the Greek word for "a runner" and is related to *trokhos*, "a wheel." The Greek *trokhanter* originally was used in anatomy as a name for the globular head of the femur, which turns in its socket like a wheel. Later, the usage of the term slipped down the neck of the femoral head and became applied to the lateral process (the greater trochanter) and the medial process (the lesser trochanter), to which the hip and thigh muscles are attached.

troche is a small, circular, medicinal **lozenge** intended to dissolve in whatever orifice it might be placed, thereby releasing its content. The name comes from the Greek *trokhiskos*, "a little wheel," the related Greek verb being *trekhein*, "to run." "Troche" is properly pronounced "troh-key," though occasionally one hears "trohsh," from a mistaken assumption it is a French word.

trochlea is the Latin word for a pulley block, a device by which heavy loads can be lifted. The related Greek words are *trokhilia* and *trokhalia*, in turn related to *trokhos*, "a wheel." The trochlea of the humerus is an articular cylinder that fits the semilunar notch in the proximal ulna to form the principal joint of the elbow. More like an actual pulley are certain structures through which tendons move so that the direction of pull by a muscle is changed. The best example is the fibrocartilaginous loop in the orbit through which the tendon of the superior oblique muscle passes before it is attached to the eyeball. By this arrangement, contraction of the muscle rotates the eye down and outward. The fourth cranial nerve, whose sole purpose is to supply this one small muscle, is named the trochlear nerve.

-trop- is a combining form that refers to a changing, especially of position or orientation, but also is used in the sense of stimulation, and is derived from the Greek *tropos*, "a turning." **Tropism** can be positive (turning toward) or negative (turning away from). Corticotropin is a hormone elaborated by the pituitary gland that is directed to (or turned toward) the adrenal cortex, wherein it stimulates hormonal activity. Similarly, a gonadotropin is directed to and has a stimulating effect on the gonads or organs of procreation. One must be careful to avoid confusion between "-trop-" (changing or stimulation) and "-troph-" (growth).

-troph- is a combining form that refers to growth and is taken from the Greek *trophē*, "food or nourishment." **Trophic** describes whatever regulates the growth or metabolism of a part, usually a nerve or hormone. **Atrophy** is a failure or reversal of growth, **hypotrophy** is diminished growth, and **hypertrophy** is an excessive growth. There is an important distinction between hypertrophy and hyperplasia. Both can result in enlargement of a part of an organ. When the enlargement is due to an increase in size but not in the number of component cells, the condition is known as "hypertrophy"; when the number but not necessarily the size of component cells increases, as by proliferation, the condition is known as "hyperplasia." Also, as noted under **-trop-**, a distinction between "-troph-" and "-trop-" must be made to avoid inadvertent and mistaken exchange. Incidentally, "trophy" as a memorial to victory or success comes not from the Greek *trophē* but rather is related to *tropē*, "a turning," as in the sense of an enemy being routed or turned back. Somewhere, sometime, there occurred a shift in pronunciation of "p" to an "f" sound.

trophic describes a nerve or hormone that regulates the metabolism or growth of a part.

trophoblast is the forerunner of the placenta or nourishing organ of the developing embryo (tropho- + Greek *blastos*, "germ or sprout").

trophozoite is a unicellular organism in its active, feeding stage, as contrasted to its dormant, encysted stage (tropho- + Greek *zōon*, "an animal").

trunk (*see* **torso**)

truss is a supporting device that includes a pad designed to hold in or prevent protu-

berance of a hernia. The term is an Anglicization of the French *trousse*, "a bundle or a pack." Incidentally, a "trousseau" is "a little bundle" of a bride's belongings that she takes along after her wedding.

Trypanosoma is a genus of protozoa among which certain species are pathogenic to animals and man. The name combines the Greek *trypanon*, "borer," + *sōma*, "body," indicative of the invasiveness of the infection. Most widely known of the diseases caused by this protozoa are African trypanosomiasis (sometimes called "sleeping sickness"), transmitted by the tsetse fly, and, in South America, Chagas' disease (named for Carlos Chagas [1879-1934], a Brazilian physician), transmitted by certain beetlelike bugs. Incidentally, "tsetse" as a name for the vector fly came into English through Afrikaans from *setswana*, the language spoken by the Tswana people who inhabit an area in western Africa.

trypsin is a proteolytic enzyme that was so named in 1874 by Willy Kühne (1837-1900), a German physiologist. The name was taken from the Greek *tripsis*, "a rubbing," because the substance was first obtained by rubbing or macerating the pancreas. Like pepsin, trypsin (while an enzyme) lacks the customary "-ase" ending. The explanation is that both were named before "-ase" became the conventional suffix denoting an enzyme.

tryptophan is an amino acid obtained by proteolytic enzymatic hydrolysis, is so called because with halogenation it produces a rather bright violet color (trypto-, indicating a relation to the enzyme trypsin, + Greek *phanos*, "bright").

tsetse (*see* ***Trypanosoma***)

tsutsugamushi disease is another name for scrub typhus. The term is a combination of the Japanese *tsutsuga*, "dangerous," + *mushi*, "bug," which is appropriate because the causative organism, an Oriental rickettsia, is transmitted by the bite of larval mites or chiggers. The disease has been known also as "inundation fever," the reason being that those who tend rice paddies are commonly exposed to the vector when the paddies overflow their banks. Several commentators have suggested that tsutsugamushi disease is "the coolie disease from Sumatra" that Sherlock

Holmes feigned in "The Adventure of the Dying Detective."

tube comes from the Latin *tuba*, "a trumpet," and is used in anatomy for various structures that might be fancied to bear some resemblance to a trumpet. The diminutive **tubule**, of course, refers to a little tubelike structure.

tubercle is taken from the Latin *tuberculum*, the diminutive of *tuber*, "a lump or bump." Various small anatomic bumps or excrescences are called tubercles.

tuberculosis is so called because its characteristic lesion is a tiny nodule (a tubercle) which, microscopically, is composed of epithelioid and giant cells. This is a granuloma resulting from infection by *Mycobacterium tuberculosis*. These lesions were first called "tubercles" in 1689 by Richard Morton (1637-1698), a London physician, in his classic treatise *Phthisiologia*. The disease, endemic for centuries, was otherwise known as **phthisis** (Greek for "wasting or decay") and, commonly, as "consumption," because persons so afflicted became wasted, as if they were being consumed by the disease.

tularemia is a disease resembling plague and is the result of infection by the bacterium *Pasteurella tularensis*, which is transmitted among rodents by insect bites. The infection is acquired by man from handling diseased animals. The name for the disease, coined in 1919 by Edward Francis (1872-1957), an American epidemiologist, combines Tulare, the name of a rural county in the central valley of California where the disease was first identified, and the Greek *haima*, "blood," to stress that the disease is bacteremic in animals.

tumor is a Latin word meaning "a swelling, bulging, or elevation" and, figuratively, "excitement, anger, or arrogance." The related Latin verb is *tumere*, "to swell up." In bygone days, "tumor" was used to designate a swelling of any cause (and can still be so used). Celsus included *tumor* as one of the cardinal features of inflammation (the others: *rubor* or redness, *calor* or heat, and *dolor* or pain). In the 19th century "tumor" tended to be restricted to chronic swellings or lumps and, later, further restricted to the masses caused by neoplasia. To many patients today "tumor" means cancer, an unfortunate connotation because many tumors are relatively benign.

tunica is the Latin word for "a skin, peel, husk, or other covering." To the Romans it also meant an ordinary sleeved garment (a tunic) worn by men and women. All sorts of coverings and coats in anatomy are called *tunica* (or, in the Latin plural, *tunicae*).

turbinate is taken from the Latin *turbo, turbinis*, "a whorl, an eddy, or a tornado." The related Latin verb is *turbare*, "to throw into confusion." The Latin *turbo* could also refer to a spiral shell, and probably it is in this sense that "turbinate" was given as a name for the curled shelves of bone protruding from the lateral walls of the nasal cavity.

turd is disdained by most standard dictionaries as vulgar slang. Like certain other four-letter words, its origin is in the murky past of Anglo-Saxon verbiage. The word has always meant a piece of dung, a fecal fragment. Regrettably, we have no acceptable, more elegant word that means exactly the same thing. We have "feces" and "excrement" as collective terms; we have the awkward "bowel movement" (which is rather ridiculous); we have the prissy "number 2." It seems odd that so many filthy words, previously scorned, have been embraced by the popular media, while a perfectly useful term like "turd" has been kept hidden, as it were, in the water closet.

tweezers (*see* **forceps**)

tympanum is the anatomic name for the cavity of the middle ear, demarcated laterally by the tympanic membrane or eardrum. The Latin *tympanum* and the Greek *tympanon* are words for "a drum," these being related to the Greek verb *typtein*, "to strike or to beat." The Greek *tympanias* referred to a form of dropsy wherein the swollen belly was taut as a drum.

tympany is the hollow, drumlike sound elicited at physical examination when a gas-containing cavity, such as the chest or distended abdomen, is sharply tapped. (*see* **tympanum**)

typhlitis is an old but still useful term for inflammation of the cecum. In times past, the term was sometimes used for what we now know as appendicitis. It is derived from the Greek *typhlos*, "blind," and thus refers to the cecum as a "blind" pouch, situated where the end of the small intestine is joined to the medial side of the proximal ascending colon. The Latin *caecum* also means "blind." (*see* **cecum**)

typhoid is a term concocted in 1829 by Pierre Charles Alexandre Louis (1787-1872), a celebrated French physician, as a name for a disease that resembled, but became recognized as distinct from, typhus. Louis simply tacked the suffix taken from the Greek *eidos*, "like," onto the stem of "typhus." Before the early 19th century, the two diseases were often confused. Later, it was found that typhoid fever could be further divided, and the term **paratyphoid** (Greek *para*, "beside") was coined.

typhus represents a widespread group of infectious diseases caused by rickettsial organisms. The condition was known to ancient physicians, though probably mixed up with other acute, febrile diseases. Typhus is featured by high, sustained fever, intense headaches, and often febrile delirium. The Greek *typhos* means "smoke or mist" but was also used in the metaphysical sense of "dullness or stupor."

tyrosine (*see* **amino acids**)

Ulcer comes through the French *ulcere* from the Latin *ulcus, ulceris,* "a sore or ulcer." The related Greek word is *helkos,* "a wound," and later, "an ulcer or abscess." If one remembers that when spelling certain Greek words, such as *helkos,* with Roman letters, the initial "he-" represents the Greek letter *eta* with an accent (circumflex) mark, then the Greek *helkos* begins to look a little more like the Latin *ulcus.*

ulna is the Latin word for "elbow." The related Greek *ōlenē* also means "elbow" (hence, **olecranon,** + Greek *kranion,* "skull," i.e., the "head" of the ulna), but more particularly the arm from the elbow to the wrist, what we call the forearm. Similarly derived is "ell," an archaic unit of linear measure. This was variously taken as the distance from the elbow, the shoulder, or the tip of the nose to the fingertips, so it is not surprising that an "ell" varied considerably from place to place and from time to time, and it is for good reason that the term became obsolete.

ultra- is a combining form directly borrowed from the Latin adverb and preposition meaning "beyond, farther."

ultrasonography is a means of producing an image by recording the echoes of acoustic frequencies that are above and beyond the range audible to the human ear (> 20,000 cycles per second). The term combines ultra- + Latin *sonus,* "sound," + Greek *graphein,* "to write." (*see* **echography**)

ultraviolet refers to that segment of the electromagnetic spectrum whose rays are of a wavelength above and beyond that for the violet of visible light (and below that for X-rays), whereas **infrared** rays, which convey heat, are of a wavelength just below that for visible red light. Incidentally, a mnemonic device for recalling the order of the visible light spectrum is a man's name: Roy G. Biv (red, orange, yellow, green, blue, indigo, violet).

Ulysses' syndrome is a term coined by Mercer Rang (*Can Med Assoc J.* 1976;106:122) in reference to a long and trying journey by a patient and his physician consequent to the discovery of a falsely positive finding on routine screening. Such a spurious finding can initiate a series of wearing, wearying diagnostic adventures and misadventures, with ultimate return, empty-handed, to the point of departure, as Ulysses returned to Ithaca after his harrowing 10-year odyssey.

umbilicus is the Latin word for the belly button (*see* **navel**). This is a diminutive of *umbo,* "the boss of a shield," i.e., the ornamental stud at the center of a warrior's shield. The allusion is evident, although the belly button in most people is concave rather than convex. In pathology an indentation or dimple, particularly in a elevated lesion, is called an **umbilication.**

umbo is the name given to the little knob-like projection at the center of the outer surface of the ear drum.

uncinate comes from the Latin *uncus,* "a hook," and describes any hooklike process or extension. Similarly, **unciform** (+ Latin *forma,* "shape") can refer to anything shaped like a hook, e.g., the unciform bone of the wrist, also called the **hamate** (Latin *hamus,* "a hook").

under the weather is a colloquial expression for a state of confining illness. A patient kept from his usual activities because of the flu might say, "I've been under the weather these past few days." The phrase has been attributed to seafarers being obliged, in the teeth of a gale, to seek shelter below deck, thus being, literally, "under the weather." The expression can also be a euphemism for incapacitating inebriation, as a sailor too drunk to gain the weather deck. A contrasting term, also of maritime origin, is **A-1,** meaning "wholly fit, in top condition." When conscription was in effect during World War II, a draftee found to be fully qualified for military service was labeled "1-A"; whoever was physically unfit was "4-F." In the 18th century Lloyd's of London, the marine insurance consortium, rated the seaworthiness of a given ship by assigning a letter-number sequence. The letter pertained to the condition of the hull and the numeral to that of the rigging and gear. "A-1" was the top rating.

undulant comes from the *undula*, the diminutive of the Latin *unda*, "a wave or billow." Undulant fever, more properly known as *brucellosis*, is so called because of the typical wavelike pattern of the patient's temperature chart. An appropriate slogan for those who engage in the sport of surfing is the Latin adage: *Unda fert nec regitur* ("You can ride the wave but not control it").

ungual is an adjectival form taken from the Latin *unguis*, "a fingernail or a toenail." A **subungual** infection occurs underneath a fingernail or toenail.

unguent (*see* **ointment**)

urachus is the fetal canal that connects the urinary bladder with an outpouching of the hindgut called the **allantois** (Greek *allas*, "sausage," + *eidos*, "like"). "Urachus" combines the Greek *ouron*, "urine," + *cheō*, "I pour." A modified urachus persists in the adult as the median umbilical ligament.

urano- is a combining form referring to whatever relates to the palate or roof of the mouth. The term is taken from the Greek *ouranos*, "the vault of heaven, the sky." In Greek mythology Uranus was the earliest supreme god, the personification of heaven. The Greeks used *ouranos* also as a word for any manmade vault or ceiling and for the roof of the mouth.

uranoplasty is a surgical reshaping of the palate (urano- + Greek *plassein*, "to mold").

uranoplegia is paralysis of the palate (urano- + Greek *plēgē*, "a stroke").

uranoschisis is a learned term for cleft palate (urano- + Greek *schisma*, "a fissure").

urea is taken from the French *urée*, a name for the essential salt of urine. The relation to the Greek *ouron*, "urine," is obvious.

uremia is the toxic condition marked by a retention in the blood of nitrogenous substances, notably urea, that normally are excreted with the urine (ur-, referring to urea + Greek *haima*, "blood").

ureter as a name for the conduit through which urine is led from the kidney is derived from the Greek *ourein*, "to make water." From the same source comes **urethra**. Ancient writers used the singular of the derived noun for the single urinary duct leading from the bladder to the exterior of the body, and the plural for the paired ducts leading to the bladder from the kidneys.

urethra (*see* **ureter**)

uric acid is so called because it was first found in urinary bladder stones.

urinalysis (*see* **analysis**)

urine is a direct borrowing of the French word that comes from the Latin *urina* and the Greek *ouron*, all meaning "urine" and all traceable to the postulated Indo-European root word *awer*, "wet, or to flow." In Latin there is a curious bifurcation in that whereas *urina* means "urine," the verb *urinare* means "to dive," and to the Romans a urinator was a diver. This is a good example of what Professor Alexander Gode (*JAMA.* 1967;199:145) called "deceptive cognates," i.e., etymologically identical words with riskily divergent meanings. Professor H. A. Skinner points out that Galen thought that urine was excreted directly from the vena cava and that the composition of urine was an indication of the nature of blood at any given time. Consequently, meticulous examination of the urine, or "uroscopy" as it was called, since ancient times has been a strong point in diagnosis. Every medieval physician worthy of the name carried a small flask in which to collect, then contemplate, his patient's urine. Almost every language has had sets of both vulgar and delicate words to describe common, natural acts. In Latin, *mingere* means "to urinate" and *micturire* means "to want to urinate." From the latter is taken the somewhat precious English verb **micturate** as a verb and **micturition**, the act of urinating. At the other end of the scale is **piss**, which serves as both noun and verb. This is actually an old word descended from the Middle English *pisse*, the Old French *pissier*, and the Vulgar Latin *pisiare*, all of these being obviously echoic of the sound of the act. To lessen the vulgarity, some people refer to the act and its product simply by the letter "**p**"(sometimes spelled out as "pee"). Of the billions of people who pass water every day, probably less than a million "urinate," and surely very few "micturate."

urso- is a combining form taken from the Latin *ursus*, "a bear." Ursodeoxycholic acid was originally found in the bile of bears and now, in synthetic form, is used medically in the dissolution therapy of gallstones, as well as in certain cases of cholestasis. (*see* **cheno**-)

urticaria comes from the Latin *urtica*, "a nettle," and by extension "a sting or itch." The nettle is an herb covered with fine hairs that, when touched, produce a stinging sensation and inflammatory reaction in the skin. *Urticaria* is the Latin term for the sting of a nettle. Today, the term applies to a focal, pruritic edema in the skin or mucous membranes signifying an acute allergic reaction to any sort of antigen.

uterus is the Latin word for the womb, but used by the Romans also for the belly or paunch of a man. Presumably, the term relates to the Latin *uter*, "a bag or bottle for wine or water" made from the hide of an animal.

uvea is a collective term for the iris, the ciliary body, and the choroid of the eye and is taken from the Latin *uva*, "a grape." If one plucks the stem from a grape, the hole can be imagined as the pupil and the grape as the eyeball. The term is a convenient one in that **uveitis** signifies an inflammation affecting all components of the uveal tract.

uvula is the Latin diminutive of *uva*, "grape," although classical anatomists never used that name for the little elongated appendage to the back of the soft palate, the shape of which is actually more like a little worm than a little grape. Not until the Middle Ages did Guy de Chauliac (1300-1368), a French surgeon, apply "uvula" to describe the appearance of the structure in an abnormally swollen state. Later, the term was preserved as a name for the appendage, swollen or not.

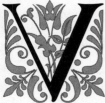**V**accine is taken from the Latin *vacca*, "a cow," and **vaccinia** is a viral disease of cattle, sometimes called **cowpox**. Edward Jenner (1749-1823), a country physician who practiced in Berkeley, Gloucestershire, England, took seriously the folk belief that dairymaids who contracted a mild reaction to cowpox were thereafter spared the risk of the dreaded smallpox. The idea of protecting against infectious disease by inoculating one person with pus taken from another person's lesion—a procedure known as "variolation"(*see* **variola**)—was not new with Jenner. Such attempts to prevent smallpox had been made for many years in the Orient, with varying degrees of success and disaster. In fact, the idea was introduced to England in 1717 by no less a personage than Lady Mary Wortley Montagu, wife of the British ambassador to Turkey. What Jenner contributed was his recognition of the cross-immunity between cowpox and smallpox and the proof, by experiment, that persons inoculated with cowpox showed no reaction when later deliberately inoculated with smallpox. This required of Jenner a good deal of perspicacity and courage. It was on 14 May 1796 that Jenner inoculated a young friend, 8-year-old James Phipps, with material taken from a pustule on the hand of Sarah Nelmes, an obliging local dairymaid. On 1 July and again several months later, Jenner demonstrated that material taken from an actual smallpox pustule elicited no reaction when inoculated into James Phipps. In 1797 Jenner submitted a paper describing his observation to the Royal Society. It was rejected with the admonition that Jenner "ought not risk his reputation by presenting to the learned body anything which appeared so much at variance with established knowledge, and withal so incredible." In 1798 Jenner privately published a pamphlet on the subject, bolstered by further evidence. Thereupon Jenner was engulfed by waves of adulation and condemnation, but he was serenely confident that he had conferred on mankind a boon. Originally, the term **vaccination** was limited to the inoculation of a preparation derived from cowpox. Later, it was extended to the injection of any microbial antigen for the purpose of inducing immunity to a corresponding disease.

vacuole is a diminutive taken from the Latin adjective *vacuus*, "empty," and hence is a term for any little empty space, particularly that apparent in the cytoplasm of cells.

vagina is the Latin word for "a scabbard or sheath," such as might be used to contain a *gladius*, "a sword." The Romans sometimes used *gladius* as another name for the penis and *vagina* (from the past participle of introire, "to go in, to enter") for the female genital introitus.

vaginismus (*see* **trismus**)

vagus as a name for the 10th cranial nerve is appropriate in that this nerve takes a long and meandering path from its origin in the midbrain to the far reaches of the peritoneal cavity. Thus, it was known as "the wanderer," and its name was appropriated from the Latin adjective *vagus*, meaning "wandering or inconstant." From the same source come vagabond, vagary, vagrant, and vague.

valetudinarian describes a person who, while not necessarily physically ill, is constantly preoccupied with his health and perturbed by his bodily functions. The term comes from the Latin *valetudo*, "a state of health," this being related to the Latin verb *valere*, "to be strong." A Roman *valetudinarium* was a sort of hospital.

valgus is the Latin word for "bowlegged" and has been adopted in medicine as an adjective meaning "bent outward." Its ending depends on the gender of the Latin term that is thereby modified, as in **coxa valga** (Latin *coxa*, "hipbone"), in which the thigh is bent outward; **genu valgum** (Latin *genu*, "knee"), which is an apparent contradiction because to most radiologists and orthopedists this means **knock-kneed**, i.e., the inner surfaces of the paired knees knock together; **hallux valgus** (Latin *hallux*, "the big toe"), a deformity wherein the big toe is bent so as to overlap the adjacent toes; and **talipes valgus** (Latin *talipes*, "clubfoot," from *talus*, "ankle," + *pes*, "foot"), in which the heel is turned sharply outward. Deformities that are the opposite of valgus, i.e., wherein the affected part is bent inward, are described by forms of the adjective *varus*, the Latin word for "knock-kneed." Again, there is a peculiar confusion in that **genu varum** is now customarily taken to be a **bowleg**. The sense depends on whether one looks at the direction in which the joint is deformed or the direction in which the affected limb is bent. All of this is the subject of an intriguing essay by C. Stuart Houston and Leonard E. Swischuk (*N Engl J Med.* 1980;307:471), who offer the sensible suggestion that, insofar as current usage is confused and confusing, the simple English words "bowlegged" and "knock-kneed" be used in preference to the Latin *genu valgum* and *genu varum*, and that **bunion** be used rather than *hallux valgus*. One would still have to distinguish an inwardly or outwardly bent clubfoot as talipes varus or talipes valgus, or simply say which way the heel is bent. Referring to the angle between the femoral head and shaft, **coxa vara** means a decrease in the angle, whereas **coxa valga** means an increase in the angle. In any case, prudence dictates the clear definition of any term used and the choice of the least ambiguous name available.

vallecula is the diminutive of the Latin *valles*, "a hollow or valley," and is used to describe various anatomic depressions or furrows. Used alone, the term usually applies to the cleft between the pair of longitudinal mucosal folds in the throat that extends on either side from the base of the tongue to the epiglottis.

valve is derived from the Latin *valvae*, used in the plural by the Romans for "a pair of folding or double doors." The valves of the heart and the veins function, in a way, as doors that open to permit traffic in one way but close to impede traffic in the opposite direction. The **valvulae conniventes** are circular folds in the mucosa of the small intestine. They are so named because they are small (hence the diminutive *valvulae*) and because they tend to come and go, as implied by conniventes (from the Latin *connivere*, "to wink or blink").

varicella (*see* **variola**)

varicose describes veins that are distended and tortuous, such as those that become prominent on the surface of the legs, or those that bulge into the lumen of the esophagus because they are burdened with blood that normally would course through the portal circulation but is blocked by disease in or near the liver. The term is a near borrowing of the Latin *varicosus*, which describes the condition of a *varix*, the name given by the Romans to an overly dilated vein. We still use **varix** and the Latin plural **varices** in the same way today. All these terms can be related to the Latin *varus*, "crooked." A **varicocele** (+ Greek *kēlē*, "a swelling") is an abnormal distention and tortuosity of the veins of the **pampiniform** (Latin *pampinus*, "a tendril of a vine," + *forma*, "shape") plexus associated with the spermatic cord and palpable within the scrotum.

variola is the Late Latin name for smallpox, having been adapted from the classical Latin *varius*, "spotted or variegated." "Variola" was used generally for a variety of mottled rashes as early as the 6th century, but was applied specifically to what later became commonly known as smallpox when that disease was fully described and differentiated from measles in the 10th century by Abu Bakr Muhammed Ibn Zalariya (850-932), the brilliant Persian physician better known as Rhazes. Before the spread of syphilis in Europe toward the end of the 15th century, variola was known simply as "the pox." Because syphilis was regarded as so formidable, it was called in French *la grosse véreole* (the great pox), and variola became *le petite vériole* (the small pox). Later, **chickenpox** was recognized as a much milder disease and given the name **varicella**, a diminutive of variola. (*see* **vaccine**)

varix, varices (*see* **varicose**)

vas is the Latin word for "a dish or vessel." The term was early applied in anatomy to tubular structures, such as blood vessels, that were identified as carrying fluids. A small blood vessel was called by the diminutive *vasculum*, and from this is derived our adjective **vascular**. Similarly, **vaso-** has come to be a combining form to denote a relationship to blood vessels. Vasomotor nerves are those that control the volume of flow through blood vessels by regulating the tone of their muscular walls. Larger blood vessels themselves must be nourished, and so they are served by fine vascular channels of their own. These are called **vasa vasorum**, a term using both the Latin plural noun and its possessive plural form. The **vas deferens** (or spermatic duct) is so called because it is a vessel that "carries away"(Latin *de-*, "away," + *ferre*, "to carry") the sperm-laden fluid from the male genital glands.

vector is the Latin word for "a bearer" and is related to the verb *vehere*, "to convey or transport." In medicine a vector is an intermediary "vehicle," usually an arthropod but sometimes another animate or inanimate object, that is capable of transferring an infectious agent from one host to another. The transfer can be from man to man or from animal to man or vice versa. Contagious diseases can, in some instances, be suppressed by identifying and then eradicating the vector.

vein clearly is derived from the Latin *vena*, but it is interesting to note that the Latin word has a number of meanings other than blood ves-

sel, as does its Greek counterpart *phlĕps*. Among these are a spring of water, a course of metal or ore in a mineral deposit, and a distinctive streak of color in a slab of marble. This is carried into English, where, by extension, a vein can also be a quality, manner, or style. Someone can speak "in a jocular vein" or can write "with a humorous vein coursing through otherwise turgid prose." It seems the use of "vein" as a name for an afferent blood vessel is almost incidental.

velum is the Latin word for "a sail, a curtain, or an awning." In anatomy the term is used for various veil-like coverings or membranes. The soft posterior portion of the palate was once called the *velum palati*.

venereal can be traced to the Sanskrit *was, van*, "to love, to honor, to desire," which gave rise to a string of more or less related Latin words, including *venus, veneris* "beauty, pleasure of love, sexual indulgence"; *venari*, "to hunt"; and *venenum*, "a love potion, sorcery, or poison"(hence **venom**). The ancients were wont to personify concepts and ideas, and so arose the mythologic Venus, goddess of beauty and love. Venus figures in all sorts of fascinating tales involving anthropomorphic deities and godlike humans. Alas, a price is paid for sexual indulgence. Part of the price is the risk of acquiring a *morbus venerus*, or venereal disease, such as syphilis, gonorrhea, or, more recently, herpes. The **mons veneris** ("the mount of Venus") is the pubis of a woman. (*see* **aphrodisiac**)

ventral is taken from the Latin *venter*, "the belly." As a term of anatomic reference, "ventral" refers to whatever is oriented toward the belly or toward the front of the body.

ventricle is a term adapted from the Latin *ventriculus*, the diminutive of *venter*, hence, "a little belly." In early anatomy *ventriculus* was the name given to the visceral stomach, but later *ventriculus* or "ventricle" was applied to the bulbous part of a muscle; for the pouch between the true and false vocal cords in the larynx; for the heavy-walled muscular chambers of the heart; and for the cavities in the brain that connect with the central canal of the spinal cord and contain cerebrospinal fluid. Incidentally, a ventriloquist (+ Latin *loqui*, "to speak") is "one who talks from his belly."

vermis is the Latin word for "a worm." The **vermis cerebelli** is the median portion of the cerebellum, which can be fancied in the shape of a worm. Even more wormlike is the **vermiform** (+ Latin *forma*, "shape") appendix (Latin for "addition or supplement"), which is stuck on the base of the cecum for no apparent reason in man but to serve as a seat for appendicitis. Out of familiarity, we seldom use the full name of this little organ; we call it simply the appendix. A **vermifuge** (+ Latin *fugare*, "to chase away") is a medicine that expels worms or similar vermin from the gut.

vernix is the Latin word for "varnish." The **vernix caseosa** is a cheesy or unctuous substance composed of sebum and desquamated epithelial cells that covers the skin of the fetus.

verruca is the Latin term for "a wart." A little boy holds out his finger and says, "Look, I have a wart!" The doctor observes the finger closely and pronounces, "Aha! You have a verruca vulgaris." Both are saying the same thing, but the doctor is identifying the excrescence as a common wart (Latin *vulgaris*, "the common or usual," from *vulgus*, "the masses or the common herd"). Occasionally, one encounters the Spanish spelling as **verruga**. Whatever is **verrucous** is wartlike. "Wart" comes from the Old English *wearte*, used as a term for excrescences of the skin as early as the 8th century.

version as used in obstetrics hews closely to its origin in the Latin verb *vertere*, "to turn." An **obstetrical version** is the maneuver whereby the polarity of the fetus is turned, in reference to the body of the mother, in order to facilitate delivery. Thus, a **cephalic version** brings the fetal head into the maternal birth canal. A **podalic** (Greek *pous*, "foot") **version** brings the fetal legs down into the maternal pelvis.

vertebra is the Latin word for "a joint or a bone of the spine," being taken from the Latin verb *vertere*, "to turn or to tilt." Altogether there are 33 **vertebrae** (the Latin feminine plural) making up the spinal column: 7 cervical (Latin *cervix*, "neck"); 12 thoracic (Greek *thōrax*, "chest") or dorsal (Latin *dorsum*, "back"); 5 lumbar (Latin *lumbus*, "loin"); 5 sacral (Latin *sacrum*, "holy vessel");

and 4 coccygeal (Greek *kokkyx*, "cuckoo bird") vertebrae. The sacral and coccygeal vertebrae are fused into two composite bones.

vertex is the Latin word for "a whirlpool, a whirlwind or tornado, the summit of a mountain, or the top of the head," all connected by the sense of spiraling and being related to the Latin *vertere*, "to turn." It is said the top of the head was called the vertex because it is there that the hairs of the scalp form a whorl.

vertigo is a hallucination of movement wherein one's surroundings or one's self seems to be whirling around (vert-, from Latin *vertere*, "to turn," + -igo, a condition). True vertigo, a rotary phenomenon usually signifying an inner ear disturbance, is not to be confused with simple, and much more common, lightheadedness or giddiness. Patients tend to use the term **dizzy** (from the Anglo-Saxon *dysig*, "foolish," related to the Teutonic form *dwaes*, "a god," hence the sense of a peculiar divine influence) for both vertigo and giddiness. Incidentally, **giddy** (from the Old English *gydig*, "mad") also originally meant "god-possessed."

verumontanum is an alternative term for the seminal colliculus (a diminutive of the Latin *collis*, "a hill," hence "a little mound"), the prominent portion of the urethral crest where join the orifices of the ejaculatory ducts and the sac of the prostate gland. *Verumontanum* is Latin for "the crest or top of a hill or mountain."

vesicle is taken from the Latin *vesiculum*, the diminutive of *vesica*, "a bladder or bag." A vesicle in anatomy can be any one of a number of small pouches in various organs, whereas in dermatology a vesicle is a small blister. The anatomic adjective **vesical**, a different word even though pronounced the same, is derived directly from *vesica* and does not denote the diminutive but simply describes whatever pertains to the urinary bladder.

vestibule is the Latin term for an entrance or a forecourt, like an enclosed porch. In anatomy a vestibule is a space or cavity at the entrance of a canal or other sort of channel or vessel. The vestibule of the ear is the oval cavity in the middle of the bony labyrinth.

vestige denotes the nonfunctioning remnant of a structure which, in an antecedent of the species or in a previous stage of individual development, may have had a defined function that no longer pertains. For example, the navel is a vestige of the former entrance of the umbilical cord, vital to the fetus but of no use to the adult. The term is derived from the Latin *vestigium*, "a footprint," as a trace of something that has gone before. The wings of an ostrich are vestigial. But as Ambrose Bierce in his *Devil's Dictionary* observed of the ostrich, "The absence of a good working pair of wings is no defect for, as has been ingeniously pointed out, the ostrich does not fly." **Investigation** is a pursuit essential to medical progress. The word relates to the Latin verb *investigare*, "to track or to search after," this, of course, being related to *vestigium* "a footprint." Thus, an investigator is one who looks for traces or footprints in quest of whatever is sought. An investigator also seeks to pick up a **clue** as a guide to solving a problem. (*see* **labyrinth**)

veterinary refers to whatever pertains to domestic animals, including veterinary medicine, which treats of their diseases. The Latin adjective *veterinus* refers to carrying burdens; the feminine and neuter plural *veterinae* and *veterina* refer to beasts old enough to bear burdens. The root Latin word is *vetus, veteris*, "old." The relation to "veteran" is evident.

viable is borrowed from the French and is related to the French *vie*, "life," and thus means "capable of living." A viable fetus is one that has matured to a stage of development at which it is capable of life independent of the uterus.

Vibrio is a genus of slightly curved, actively motile, gram-negative bacteria. The name comes from the Latin *vibrare*, "to quiver." Among the best known species is *Vibrio comma*, so called because it is shaped like the punctuation mark (,). Infection by this organism is the cause of Asiatic cholera, a devastating disease characterized by profuse, often lethal diarrhea.

vibrissa (*see* **hair**)

vicarious is sometimes used in medicine to describe that which acts in place of another or occurs at an unaccustomed site. For example, **vicarious menstruation** is bleeding in a woman from an extragenital source coincident with the regular menstrual cycle, presumably because of generally increased capillary permeability. The Latin *vicarius* means "a substitute." An ecclesiastical vicar is one who serves in Christ's stead.

vigor (*see* **vital**)

villus is the Latin word for "shaggy hair or fleece"(*see* **hair**). The mucosal surface of the small intestine, when looked at with a magnifying glass, appears to be made up of minute, hairlike projections resembling the nap of a rug. These are called the intestinal villi (from the Latin masculine plural). The epithelial cells covering the mucosa, when viewed by electron microscopy, are seen to bear, on their luminal surfaces, even more minute projections of their own cell membranes. These are called **microvilli** (Greek *mikros*, "small"). The busy absorptive surface of the small intestine is thus progressively increased by its corrugated folds, by its villi, and finally by microvilli. Someone has estimated, taking all these devices into account, that the actual surface area of the human small intestine, approximates that of a basketball court.

vim (*see* **vital**)

virus is a Latin word meaning "slime," particularly that which is foul or poisonous. In 16th century English, "virus" was a synonym for "venom." Later, it came to refer to the noxious or infectious essence of pus. After bacteria were discovered in pus and identified as pathogenic microorganisms, it became apparent that even smaller transmitters of disease exist, because certain types of pus could be passed through exceedingly fine filters and still cause infection. Hence, it was postulated that there exist "filterable viruses"(they never were, are, or should be called by the quasi-Latin "viri"). Only much later, with the advent of electron microscopy, were certain viruses morphologically defined. Viruses have yet to be classified as systematically as bacteria and other pathogenic organisms, but many, when discovered, have been named according to their configuration, their place of origin, or their predilection, sometimes as acronyms. A few examples are given:

adenovirus originally "adenoid degenerative virus" or "adenoid-pharyngeal-conjunctival virus"

arborvirus *ar*thropod-*bor*ne virus

arenavirus a sandlike appearance (from Latin *arena,* "sand")

Brunhilde virus presumably from the name of a patient

bunyavirus from the Bunyamwera region of Uganda where this form of arbovirus causes a mild febrile illness

coronavirus from the Latin *corona,* "crown"; its outer surface is spiked like a crown

Coxsackie virus from the name of a town along the Hudson River in New York, south of Albany, where the virus was first recognized

cytomegalic virus from the Greek *kytos,* "cell," + *mega-,* "huge"; so called because cells infected by this virus become notably swollen

flavivirus of the type that causes yellow fever, from the Latin *flavus,* "yellow"

hantavirus a family of viruses named originally for the Hantaan River in South Korea where the prototype virus was discovered and linked to an outbreak of acute hemorrhagic fever among U.S. troops deployed there. A more recent notoriety relates to an occurrence of a potentially lethal pulmonary syndrome in the southwest United States (*N Engl J Med.* 1994;330:949,1004)

HIV human immunodeficiency virus, to which AIDS has been attributed

Lansing virus a prototype of poliovirus-2, first isolated in Lansing, Michigan

louping ill virus causes "louping ill" or "the trembles" in sheep and is transmissible to man

masked virus ordinarily noninfectious and can be demonstrated by indirect methods that activate (or "demask") it, such as by a blind passage through an experimental animal

Newcastle virus causes a viral disease in birds that is transmissible to man; first demonstrated in Newcastle, England

Norwalk virus first recognized as the cause of an outbreak of illness among schoolchildren in Norwalk, Ohio

oncovirus any virus known or purported to instigate neoplasia; from the Greek *onkos,* "a mass or tumor"

orbivirus from the Latin *orbis,* "a circle"; its inner shell is ring-shaped

orphan viruses so named because of being, when discovered, bereft of associated diseases; some of these are best known by acronyms, e.g., **ECHO** (enteric, *c*ytopathogenic, *h*uman, *o*rphan) **virus**; an echovirus can also be an orphan virus in the sense of being a signal of a nonvisible disease; also **reovirus** (*r*espiratory and *e*nteric *o*rphan virus)

papovavirus papilloma-polyoma-vacuolating-agent

parvovirus a very small virus, from the Latin *parvus,* "small"

picornavirus often pronounced "pike-orno-virus" but probably should be "peek-oh-RNA-virus"; characterized by a very small ribonucleic acid molecule, from the Spanish *pico,* "a small quantity"

retrovirus a form that replicates by means of reverse transcriptase, i.e., from RNA-to-DNA, rather than the usual DNA-RNA sequence

rhabdovirus rod-shaped, from the Greek rhabdos, "rod"

rhinovirus an agent typically causing nasal infections, from the Greek *rhis, rhinos,* "the nose"

rotovirus shaped like a wheel, from the Latin *rota,* "a potter's or chariot wheel"

Rous sarcoma virus named for Francis Peyton Rous (1879-1970), an American pathologist who, when he found he could transmit tumors of chickens by passage of a filterable agent, demonstrated the prototype of postulated oncogenic viruses

slow virus a viral agent that causes disease only after an unusually long incubation period, as in **scrapie** of sheep and **kuru** of man

togavirus a coated virus, from the Latin *toga,* "a cloak"

viscera (*see* **viscus**)

viscid describes a glutinous or sticky substance, and **viscous** describes a fluid that exhibits a high resistance to flow. Both adjectives are applied to certain body fluids and exudates, and both are taken from the Latin *viscum,* the name used by the Romans for the evergreen shrub mistletoe and for "birdlime." Birdlime is a sticky substance obtained from the waxy white berries of the mistletoe, then smeared on the twigs of a tree in order to ensnare small birds.

viscus is the Latin word for "an organ of the body," specifically an internal organ contained within the chest or abdomen, particularly the latter; the Latin plural is **viscera.** The noun "viscus" is not to be confused with the adjective "viscous," although the two words are pronounced the same and are etymologically related to the Latin *vis-cum* (*see* **viscid**). Presumably, internal organs were so named because when handled in their fresh state they are impressively sticky.

vital is an almost direct borrowing of the Latin *vitalis*, the adjectival form of vita, "life," related to the Latin verb *vivere*, "to live, to be alive." In biology and medicine **in vivo** refers to an observation or occurrence within a living organism or tissue. **In vitro** (Latin *vitrum*, "glass"; the neuter plural *vitrea* means glassware) refers to an observation of occurrence outside a living organism, i.e., in a glass receptacle, such as a test tube. Conception in the usual and natural manner is said to occur *in vivo*; the artificial process of uniting a sperm and an ovum in a **petri** dish (a shallow glass receptacle named for Julius Richard Petri [1852-1921], a German bacteriologist) is said to occur *in vitro*. Vital capacity is the maximum volume of gas that can be expelled from the lungs after a maximal inspiration. In only a limited sense is this a measure of one's capacity for life. In vital staining a dye is applied that is compatible with the life of the tissue or cell being examined, thus permitting the study of living cells. One often hears mention of the triad "Vim, vigor, and vitality." **Vim** is the accusative of the Latin *vis*, "force." **Vigor** is taken from the Latin *vigere*, "to thrive."

vitamin is a term coined by the Polish-born biochemist Casimir Funk (1884-1967) in 1911, while he was working in England. He had isolated a substance he believed to prevent neuritis in chickens raised on an otherwise deficient diet. Funk spelled the word "vitamine" because the substance he isolated had the chemical characteristics of an amine and because he believed it exerted a protective effect necessary to life. A more general term had been formerly used for such postulated substances: "vital accessory factors." It turned out that the substance found by Funk was an amine of nicotinic acid, the antipellagra factor, rather than the anti-beriberi factor as first supposed. In 1920 J. C. Drummond (1891-1952) suggested dropping the "e" because it was then known that these factors are not necessarily amines. As more vitamins were discovered, and before they were chemically characterized, they were assigned letter-names in alphabetical sequence: A, B, C, D, and so on. An exception is vitamin K, the blood-clotting factor, given its initial, for *Koagulation*, in 1935 by its discoverer, Henrik Dam, a Danish investigator.

vitelline is taken from the Latin *vitellus*, the diminutive of *vitulus*, "a yearling, especially a calf," hence literally "a little calf" but also used by the Romans as a word for the yolk of an egg. The **vitelline membrane** envelops the yolk, and the **vitelline duct** is the yolk sac of an embryo.

vitiligo (*see* **lentigo**)

vitreous means "glasslike or hyaline" and is taken from the Latin *vitrum*, "glass." "Vitreous" is an adjective, but in anatomy and medicine it is applied almost exclusively to that body of transparent substance that fills the lumen of the eyeball between the lens and the retina, thereby becoming, when used alone, a noun.

vivisection is the performance of experimental surgical procedures on living animals, especially in the pursuit of biomedical research (vivi-, from the Latin *vivere*, "to be alive," + *secare*, "to cut").

volar is taken from the Latin *vola*, "the palm of the hand or the sole of the foot." In anatomy "volar" describes whatever is related to the palm of the hand, such as the volar surface or the volar artery. The Romans actually used *palma* to refer to the outstretched palm of the hand. The relation of *vola* as a term for the palm might be to the Latin *volens*, "willing," from *volo*, "I wish," perhaps in the sense of the open hand as a gesture of willingness or supplication. It has been suggested, too, that *vola* may be related, by transliteration, to the Greek *bolē*, "a throw."

volatile is a near borrowing of the Latin *volatilis*, "flying or fleeting." Whatever is volatile tends to evaporate quickly and seems to "fly away."

volvulus is the Latin word for "rolled up or twisted" and is related to the Latin verb *volvere*, "to roll or to turn about." In medicine a volvulus is a twisted obstruction in a seg-ment of the gut that is supported by a mesentery (rather than being firmly attached by a peritoneal membrane) and hence liable to twisting on its longitudinal axis. Thus, the stomach, the mesenteric small intestine, the cecum, and the sigmoid segment of the colon are all subject to volvulus. The risk is not so much in the twisting alone but more in the consequent constriction of mesenteric blood vessels, which can lead to infarction.

vomer is the Latin word for "a plowshare," related to the verb *vomere* (*see* **vomit**), the allusion being to the soil thrown up by use of this implement. The bone in the nasal septum was given the name "vomer" because of its fancied resemblance to a plowshare.

vomit comes from the Latin *vomere*, "to throw up from the stomach," which is related to the Greek *emein*, meaning the same. (*see* **emesis**)

vulgaris is the Latin word for "common, gen-eral, or usual," and has been incorporated into several medical terms to mean "of the ordinary type" or "common in the general population." **Acne vulgaris** is so ordinary as to be almost a rite of passage for young-sters. **Lupus vulgaris** is a form of tubercu-lous dermatitis, once common, now rare.

vulva is a direct borrowing of the Latin word for "a wrapper." It can also be spelled *volva*, which would seem to indicate its origin in the Latin verb *volvere*, "to roll or turn about." To the Romans *vulva* also was a word for the womb (a sort of wrapper), par-ticularly that of the sow; the term was later applied to the female genital tract and became restricted to the labia majora, its current designation. Another version has "vulva" related to the Latin *valvae*, "folding or double doors." The sense seems apt but, beyond that, evidence is lacking.

Waist refers to that part of the body between the lowest ribs and the hips, usually at the smallest circumference, also known as the midriff (Old English *hrif*, "belly"). "Waist" can be traced to the Indo-European *aweg*, "to increase," which became the Anglo-Saxon *weaxin*, "to grow." This, of course, accounts for "wax" in the phrase "wax and wane." In Middle English, *wast* was "the growth of a man," the part of the body where size and strength were evident. The sense is similar to that of "well girded" or "in fine fettle." Nowadays, most people strive for a slim waist, but a thin middle was not always admired.

warfarin is the generic name for a major anti-coagulant agent and currently the most widely used drug for the prevention of blood clotting. Sweet clover was planted in the Dakota plains and Canada in the late 19th century because it flourished in poor soil and substituted for corn as fodder. In 1924 appeared the first report of a hemorrhagic disorder in cattle resulting from ingestion of spoiled, sweet clover silage. The cause was identified as a toxic reduction in plasma pro-thrombin, and the agent responsible was identified as coumarin, one of the potent anticoagulant principles of which is bishy-droxycoumarin (**dicumarol**). An effective synthetic form of the substance evolved from work at the University of Wisconsin. A patent for this new agent was granted to the Wisconsin Alumni Research Foundation. It was called racemic "warfarin," a name incorporating an acronym of the patent holder, together with the suffix "-arin," denoting a relation to coumarin. Originally, warfarin was used as a rodenticide. Later, an unsuccessful suicide attempt with this rat poison led to clinical trials of the agent as an anticoagulant medication. **Coumarin** is taken from *cumara*, the Arawak Indian name for the tonka bean tree, originally a well known source of the substance.

wean can be traced to the Anglo-Saxon *wenian*, "to accustom." The true meaning of "wean" is to accustom a child to food other than its mother's milk. But a secondary and frequent use of the word is in a seemingly contradic-tory sense of weaning *away* from the breast, i.e., to deprive or disaccustom, rather than weaning *to* solid food.

Western blot test is the name given to the cur-rently most specific assay for infection by the AIDS virus. An **ELISA** (enzyme-linked *immunoabsorbent assay*) test is a fairly sen-sitive screening method used to detect anti-bodies to the AIDS virus, but this test lacks specificity; therefore, the need for a comple-mentary means of confirming the validity of a "positive" ELISA for AIDS. The Western blot test fills this need. The technique evolved from a procedure described (*J Mol Biol.* 1975;98:503) by E. M. Southern, an investi-gator from the department of zoology at the University of Edinburgh (though much of the work was done while Dr. Southern was on leave at the University of Zürich). He described a method of transferring fragments of DNA from agarose gels to cellulose nitrate filters, the fragments then being hybridized to active RNA and detectable by radioautog-raphy. This procedure became known as the "Southern blot test." A subsequent, similar assay for RNA was called the "Northern blot test," as a play on Southern's surname. Later, the "Western blot test" was so designated as a further whimsical extension. There is yet no "Eastern blot test," but Dr. M. E. Williams of the University of Virginia informs me that there has evolved a "Southwestern blot test" by which DNA-protein binding is analyzed.

whiplash is a highly descriptive word that con-veys a clear meaning, an abrupt wrenching of the neck resulting in a cervical sprain, though few persons who use the word have ever held a whip in their hands or felt the sting of a lash. "Whiplash" is a vivid picture-word. The French refer to a sharp wrenching of the neck as a *coup de lapin*, literally a **rabbit punch**. To be prepared as food or pelts, rabbits customarily were killed by being held by their hind legs and struck sharply at the nape of the neck by the edge of the hand.

whitlow is a suppurative inflammation or abscess at the tip of a finger or toe, also called a felon. According to the Reverend Skeat, "whitlow" is a corruption of "whickflaw," wherein "whick" is a north England pronunciation of quick, the sensitive part of the finger around and under the nail. "Quick" at one time meant living or lively. The **quick** of the nailbed and of the dermis generally is so called because of its keen sensitivity (hence the expression, "He hurt me to the quick.") "Flaw" was, and is, a defect, more specifically a crack, a breach, or a sore. **Felon** has two meanings: one in law and one in medicine. Both can possibly be traced to the Latin *fel*, "bile or gall" and, figuratively, "bitterness or animosity." One who is full of fel is likely to be a wicked person. The Old French *felon* was "a traitor." In law a felony is an offense greater than a misdemeanor and punishable by a loss of citizens' rights and imprisonment. In medicine a felon was first any inflamed sore (perhaps as bitterness coming to a head), then was restricted to a sore and swollen finger. The classical designation is **paronychia**, from the Greek *para-*, "beside," + *onyx*, "nail."

whopper-jawed is a colloquial expression for anything asymmetric or out of line. Originally the term referred to a condition, also known as "lumpy jaw" in cattle, that sometimes produced a grotesque swelling on one side of the mandible. Lumpy jaw is the result of inflammation consequent to infection by actinomyces. "Whopper-jawed" is a change (some call it a mistake) in the spelling of "wapper-jawed." Wapper (or whopper) is of uncertain origin. Possibly the relation is to wap (or to whop), "to throw or to beat violently." A violent blow to the jaw is well known to induce swelling.

wryneck (*see* **torticollis**)

X **anth-** is a combining form taken from the Greek *xanthos*, "yellow."

xanthelasma is a flat, plaquelike xanthoma (*see* **xanthine**), typically appearing in or near the eyelid (xanth- + Greek *elasma*, "a plate").

xanthine is a white, amorphous base, 2,6-dioxypurine, and it is found in most body tissues; its nitrate compound is yellow, hence its name.

xanthinuria is a rare genetic disorder in which xanthine oxidase is deficient; consequently xanthines, rather than uric acid, are excreted in the urine (xanthin- + Greek *ouron*, "urine") as the end products of purine metabolism.

xanthoma is a yellow, circumscribed nodule (xantho- + Greek *-ōma*, "a swelling") in the skin or mucous membrane that is composed of lipid-laden foamy histiocytes.

xeno- is a combining form taken from the Greek *xenos*, "strange or foreign."

xenobiotic denotes a chemical agent that may be used therapeutically but one not normally found in biologic systems, i.e., "foreign to the organism."

xenodiagnosis involves a procedure whereby a previously uninfected, laboratory-bred animal host is exposed, usually by inoculation, to presumably infectious material taken from a patient; if the animal develops lesions compatible with the disease of the donor, then it is inferred that the substance to which the animal was exposed carried the causative agent. Years ago it was by intraperitoneal injection of rabbits with a preparation of sputum from a consumptive patient that a diagnosis of tuberculosis was established.

xenograft is a transplantation of tissues between different species.

xenorexia is a perversion of appetite leading to repeated swallowing of foreign objects not ordinarily ingested.

xero- is a combining form taken from the Greek *xeros*, "dry or parched."

xeroderma is a condition marked by dry, rough, scaly skin (xero- + Greek *derma*, "skin").

xerophthalmia is a dryness of the conjunctiva which, in more advanced stages, also affects the cornea (xero- + Greek *ophthalmos*, "eye").

xerostomia is excessive dryness of the mouth (xero- + Greek *stoma*, "mouth") due to a lack of saliva from any cause. Dryness in the eyes and mouth is a principal feature of the **sicca** (Latin *siccus*, "dry or thirsty") complex, an early manifestation of Sjögren's syndrome, an immunopathic disorder marked, in part, by degeneration in the lacrimal and salivary glands.

xiphoid is one of the names for the pointed cartilage attached to the lower end of the breastbone or sternum. The name combines the Greek *xiphos*, "a straight sword," + *eidos*, "like." By the same allusion to its shape, the structure also is called the **ensiform** cartilage (Latin *ensis*, "sword," + *forma*, "shape").

X-rays were so named by their discoverer, Wilhelm Konrad Röntgen (1845-1923), a German physicist, who first observed their remarkable property of penetrating soft tissues on 8 November 1895, at Würzburg. Röntgen called them *X-Strahlen*, naturally using the German word for rays. Röntgen's use of "X" was appropriate because the nature of the rays and the phenomenon they produced was then unknown. How "x" came to be a symbol of an unknown quality or quantity is itself unknown or uncertain. According to Professor Alexander Gode (*JAMA.* 1965;191:648), it may have begun with the word used by early Arabic mathematicians, *shei*, "a thing," which came to be spelled with an initial "x" by the Spaniards. Descartes, the 17th-century French philosopher and mathematician, seems to have established the systematic use of "x," "y," and "z" as symbols for unknown quantities or qualities.

xyl- is a combining form taken from the Greek *xylon*, "wood."

xylene is a volatile hydrocarbon, also called **xylol** (xyl- + Latin *oleum*, "oil"), originally obtained from wood alcohol. It is used in microscopy as a solvent and a clarifier.

xylol (*see* **xylene**)

xylose is a pentose monosaccharide and is sometimes called "wood sugar" (xyl- + -ose, signifying a sugar) because it can be obtained from certain species of woody plants. The urinary excretion of ingested D-xylose is used as a test of intestinal absorption.

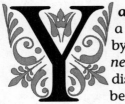**aws** is one name for a tropical infection by a spirochete, *Treponema pertenue*. The disease is marked by berrylike excrescences, sometimes pustular and ulcerated, in the skin of the face, hands, feet, and genital area. The disease is thought to have originated in Africa, and *yaw* may have been an African word for "berry." Or, the term may have come, through Spanish, from the Carib word *yaya*, "a sore." Another name for the disease is **frambesia tropica**, this being taken from the French *framboise*, "raspberry."

yellow fever is an acute, systemic, infectious disease occurring chiefly in tropical America and Africa, so named because it is characterized, in severe cases, by intense jaundice and high fever in addition to hemorrhagic lesions in the skin and mucous membranes and tubular necrosis in the kidneys. At one time the disease was a scourge of port cities in the United States during the summer months and caused thousands of deaths in New Orleans, Philadelphia, and New York. A common name for the disease was **yellow jack** (the "jack" being a colloquial substitute for "fellow," as in "lumberjack" or "jack-of-all-trades"). Yellow fever in Cuba claimed more victims by far than did bullets in the Spanish-American War of 1898. Control of the disease was made possible by the valiant investigation of Walter Reed (1851-1902), an American army doctor, who proved that the vector was the mosquito *Aedes aegypti*. In so doing Reed substantiated the hypothesis advanced by Carlos Finlay (1833-1915), a Cuban physician, whose prior evidence Reed graciously acknowledged. Only much later was the causative agent found and named a **flavivirus** (Latin *flavus*, "yellow").

Yersinia (*see* **plague**)

yolk as the name for the nutritive substance available to an embryo is derived from the Old English *geolca*, from *geolu*, "yellow." The most familiar yolk is that of a hen's egg, which is, indeed, yellow. In Middle English the word became *yolke*, and from that it was a short step to "yolk."

Zeiosis is an appearance of bubbling or blebbing at the periphery of certain cells cultured in artificial media, suggesting a process of boiling in slow motion. The term is taken from the Greek *zeiein*, "to boil or seethe."

zest is hearty or spirited enjoyment, something we all seek for ourselves and admire in others. The word, originally French, was used as a name for the thick coat or peel of a citrus fruit, and a piece of zest was added to a beverage to impart a piquant flavor. Much talked of these days is "quality of life." Mere survival is insufficient; we all strive for survival with a little zest.

zona is Latin for "a belt or sash" and a lead-in for various terms in anatomy. An example is zona **pellucida** (from the Latin *perlucidus*, "thoroughly clear"), the area of translucency surrounding an oöcyte. There are three *zonae* or zones that make up the cortex of a suprarenal gland: the thin, outer zona **glomerulosa** (from the Latin word meaning "a little ball"); the thick, middle zona **fasciculata** (from a diminutive of the Latin *fascis*, "a bundle"); and the inner zona **reticularis** (from a diminutive of the Latin *rete*, "network").

zoology is the science of animals, combining the Greek *zōon*, "a living animal," + *logos*, "study or treatise." Everyone knows this, but the discerning speaker also remembers that the root contains, in sequence, both an omega and an omicron, which in Greek are two distinct letters. Therefore, "zoölogy" is properly pronounced "zoe-ah-logee," not "zoo-ah-logee." There was a time when the word was written "zoölogy," the diacritic mark (¨) over the second "o" being a reminder of the distinction. This is no longer done; we are supposed to remember without being told. Proper pronunciation is especially important when dealing with a word such as **zoönosis**, which means a disease of animals transmissable to man.

zwitterion (*see* **rifampin**)

zygomatic describes the quadrilateral bone of the skull that forms the bony prominence of the cheek and the lateral wall of the orbit. The term also describes the bony arch by which a barlike projection of the temporal bone is joined by a fixed suture to the zygomatic bone. The anatomic adjective is taken from the Greek *zygon*, "a yoke or crossbar by which two draft animals can be hitched to a plow or wagon."

zygote is the cell resulting from fusion (or "yoking together"; *see* **zygomatic**) of two gametes, i.e., the fertilized ovum. An odd-looking and odd-sounding word is **syzygy** (Greek *sy[n]*, "together," + *zygon*), used to denote conjunction, as of heavenly bodies when they are aligned in space, or in biology to denote a fusion of microorganisms.

zym- is a combining form taken from the Greek *zymē*, "a leavening agent or a ferment."

zymase (zym- + -ase, denoting an enzyme) was detected in 1897 by Eduard Buchner (1860-1917), a German biochemist, as the active substance in yeast that could produce fermentation in the absence of living yeast cells. For this achievement, Buchner was awarded the Nobel Prize for chemistry in 1907. Buchner died in 1917 of a wound sustained in World War I. Buchner's discovery was preceded almost 40 years by the hypothesis that fermentation could be induced by an inanimate substance, a notion that Louis Pasteur thought preposterous. The hypothesis was advanced in 1858 by Moritz Traube (1826-1894), a Prussian botanist, who went so far as to coin a word for the supposed substance contained in yeast: **enzyme** (Greek *en*, "within," + *zymē*). It was about the time of Buchner's work that Rudolf Heidenhain (1834-1897), a physiologist at Breslau, observed that a carbohydrate-splitting enzyme was derived from a product of pancreatic acinar cells. He called this potentially enzymatic material **zymogen** (+ Greek *gennaō*, "I produce") because it is a precursor of the active principle. Only recently have **zymodemes** (+ Greek *demos*, "population") been proposed as a means of classifying microorganisms according to their isoenzyme patterns by electrophoresis (*N Engl J Med.* 1986;315:353).

zyzzyva is not exactly a medical term—rather it is the name of a tropical American weevil destructive of plants, not known to be otherwise harmful to man—but what better word with which to end a lexicon?

ABOUT THE AUTHOR

William S. Haubrich, MD, FACP, is Clinical Professor of Medicine at the University of California, San Diego, and Senior Consultant Emeritus at the Scripps Clinic & Research Foundation. Dr. Haubrich is the author or coauthor of more than 115 original or review articles in major medical journals. He has contributed more than 65 chapters to various textbooks, including the four-volume 5th Edition of *Bockus Gastroenterology*, of which he is coeditor. Dr. Haubrich served as a consultant in the life sciences for *The American Heritage Dictionary of the English Language*, 3rd Edition.